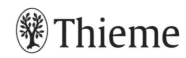

Pediatric Imaging Essentials

Radiography, Ultrasound, CT,
and MRI in Neonates and Children

Michael Riccabona, MD
Professor
Department of Radiology
Division of Pediatric Radiology
Graz University Hospital
Graz, Austria

With contributions by

Ingmar Gassner, Gabriele Hahn, Wolfgang Hirsch,
Marcus Hoermann, Thekla von Kalle, Kathrin Maurer,
Heimo Nemec, Gerald Paertan, Brigitte Povysil,
Ianina Scheer, Jens-Peter Schenk, Gisela Schweigmann,
Maria Sinzig, Erich Sorantin, Gundula Staatz,
Peter Waibel, Doris Zebedin

633 illustrations

Thieme
Stuttgart · New York

Library of Congress Cataloging-in-Publication Data

Trainer Kinderradiologie. English.
  Pediatric imaging essentials : radiography, ultrasound, CT, and MRI in neonates and children / [edited by] Michael Riccabona ; with contributions by Ingmar Gassner, Gabriele Hahn, Wolfgang Hirsch, Marcus Hoermann, Thekla von Kalle, Kathrin Maurer, Heimo Nemer, Gerald Paertan, Brigitte Povysil, Ianina Scheer, Jens-Peter Schenk, Gisela Schweigmann, Maria Sinzig, Erich Sorantin, Gundula Staatz, Peter Waibel, Doris Zebedin.
     p. ; cm.
  "This book is an authorized translation of the German edition entitled Trainer Kinderradiologie published and copyrighted 2010 by Georg Thieme Verlag, Stuttgart."
    Includes bibliographical references and index.
    ISBN 978-3-13-166191-3 (paperback) –
    ISBN 978-3-13-166211-8 (e-ISBN)
    I. Riccabona, M. (Michael), editor of compilation. II. Title.
    [DNLM: 1. Diagnostic Imaging–methods. 2. Adolescent. 3. Child. 4. Infant. WN 240]
    RJ51.D5
    618.92'00754–dc23   2013030053

This book is an authorized translation of the German edition published and copyrighted 2010 by Georg Thieme Verlag, Stuttgart. Title of the German edition: Trainer Kinderradiologie. Röntgen, Ultraschall, CT und MRT im Neugeborenen- und Kindesalter

Translator: Terry C. Telger, Fort Worth, TX, USA

Illustrator: Andrea Schnitzler, Innsbruck, Austria

MIX
Paper from responsible sources
FSC
www.fsc.org   FSC® C012521

© 2014 Georg Thieme Verlag KG,
Rüdigerstrasse 14, 70469 Stuttgart, Germany
http://www.thieme.de
Thieme Medical Publishers, Inc., 333 Seventh Avenue,
New York, NY 10001, USA
http://www.thieme.com

Cover design: Thieme Publishing Group
Cover graphics: Martina Berge, Erbach, Germany
Typesetting by Ziegler und Müller, Kirchentellinsfurt, Germany
Printed in China by Asia Pacific Offset

ISBN 978-3-13-166191-3

Also available as e-book:
eISBN 978-3-13-166211-8

Contributors

Ingmar Gassner, MD
Medical University of Innsbruck
Department of Radiology
Division of Pediatric Radiology
Innsbruck, Austria

Gabriele Hahn, MD
Department of Diagnostic Radiology
Carl Gustav Carus University Hospital
Dresden University of Technology
Dresden, Germany

Franz Wolfgang Hirsch, MD
Professor
Department of Pediatric Radiology
University of Leipzig
Leipzig, Germany

Marcus Hoermann, MD
Professor
City Diagnostic Center Bellaria
Vienna, Austria

Thekla von Kalle, MD
Department of Radiology of Olga Hospital
Stuttgart Medical Center
Stuttgart, Germany

Kathrin Maurer, MD
Medical University of Innsbruck
Department of Radiology
Pediatric Radiology
Innsbruck, Austria

Heimo Nemec, MD
Department of Radiology and Pediatric Radiology
Salzburg Regional Hospital
University Hospital Paracelsius
Private Medical University
Salzburg, Austria

Gerald Paertan, MD
Department of Radiology
Donauspital, Social Medical Center East
Vienna, Austria

Brigitte Povysil, MD
Department of Diagnostic Radiology
Linz Regional Women's and Children's Hospital
Linz, Austria

Michael Riccabona, MD
Professor
Department of Radiology
Clinical Division of Pediatric Radiology
Graz University Hospital
Graz, Austria

Ianina Scheer, MD
Zurich Children's Hospital
University Children's Hospital
Zurich, Switzerland

Jens-Peter Schenk, MD
Heidelberg University Medical Center
Division of Pediatric Radiology
Angelika Lautenschläger Hospital
Heidelberg, Germany

Gisela Schweigmann, MD
Medical University of Innsbruck
Department of Radiology
Division of Pediatric Radiology
Innsbruck, Austria

Maria Sinzig, MD
Klagenfurt Regional Hospital
Department of Diagnostic
and Interventional Radiology
Division of Pediatric Radiology
Klagenfurt, Austria

Erich Sorantin, MD
Professor
Department of Radiology
Clinical Division of Pediatric Radiology
Graz University Hospital
Graz, Austria

Gundula Staatz, MD
Professor
Instructor, Division of Pediatric Radiology
Department of Diagnostic
and Interventional Radiology
Mainz University Hospital
Mainz, Germany

Peter Waibel, MD
East Swiss Children's Hospital
Department of Radiology
St. Gallen, Switzerland

Doris Zebedin, MD
Department of Radiology
Clinical Division of Pediatric Radiology
Graz University Hospital
Graz, Austria

Preface

The role and importance of diagnostic imaging are changing. While more and more imaging studies are being requested—with a constantly growing workload of individual examinations—some radiology (sub)specialties are facing increasing staff shortages, making state-of-the-art services for all, particularly pediatric patients, difficult in some localities and countries. This development raises concern, especially as diagnostic imaging studies are becoming a central hub for prevention, (pre)clinical diagnosis, treatment planning and monitoring, and follow-up in a more individualized approach to medicine, which is the way of the future. With this new role of diagnostic imaging, comprehensive knowledge and expert skills in all imaging modalities are becoming an essential requirement for all (pediatric) radiologists. In addition, there is a growing desire within other specialties to implement imaging procedures. This threat to radiology can probably be met most effectively by giving focused attention to all aspects necessary for a particular subspecialty and by interdisciplinary cooperation, which ensures that all clinically relevant aspects are addressed with optimal professional skill in order to avoid any bias that might be engendered by being too closely involved, clinically. This approach can best be achieved by a profoundly educated radiologist performing the studies—in pediatric radiology this means, in particular, that the high radiation sensitivity of children needs to be specifically addressed.

Soon, in response to growing economic pressures, only a few centers will be able to provide tertiary care for children. These centers must also be able to guarantee training and continuing education in the subspecialty of pediatric radiology. Because many children are seen in office settings and primary care facilities, a sound basic knowledge and good working skills in pediatric imaging have become an essential part of specialty training in radiology. Equipment and resource-sharing with "adult radiology" continue to be important, which requires substantive knowledge in adapting protocols and equipment to ensure consistent, high-quality results for pediatric patients. It is obvious in this context that while pediatric radiology is functionally a branch of pediatrics, the laws regulating the occupational and training aspects of pediatric radiology make it more closely allied to the field of radiology in general. Although children are less socially powerful than other groups, they are the future of our society, and we must strive to provide universally accessible imaging tools and protocols available "24/7" throughout the year that are appropriate to their needs, just as we would for any other segment of society.

Imaging procedures should always have a valid indication and sound rationale that justifies every single investigation, especially in children. Actions in pediatric radiology should have an impact on diagnostic confidence, patient management, long-term outcome, and on public health whenever possible. The nature and application of all imaging modalities, the various imaging algorithms, and the interpretation of findings must conform to the special requirements of children, notably their greater radiation risk.

This textbook seeks to address these needs by summarizing essential knowledge in the subspecialty of pediatric radiology, conveying this information as clearly and concisely as possible, thus also helping students prepare for certification exams. Essential points are reinforced by ending each chapter with concise case reports that illustrate typical clinical questions and findings in children. These brief reports are also meant to highlight relevant aspects of good practice in pediatric radiology, such as the different roles of specific imaging modalities (especially ultrasound) compared to adult radiology, the special importance of radiation protection (especially in modality selection and dose adaptation, as when defining CT protocols), and a familiarity with child-specific diseases and clinical questions.

As imaging algorithms and indications for certain studies vary with differing health care systems (more or less inpatient care, different billing systems, other medico-legal requirements, etc.), none of such aspects are included or recommended here. By the very nature of the book and its authors, the treatment of some aspects may reflect the habitual use of practitioners in Austria, Germany, and Switzerland. However, great efforts have been made toward the goals of relevance and applicability across continents, in particular to North America, and to cater to the respective and specific needs of pediatric radiology in all countries. Still, for many reasons, not all aspects of imaging could be addressed.

But it is important to remember that diagnostic imaging should always primarily serve the patient/child, and should be performed at lowest possible invasiveness and (radiation) burden. Even though certain medicolegal and financial requirements must be kept in mind, diagnostic imaging should not primarily address (legal) needs and (financial) interests of lawyers or hospital administrations.

And though imaging should be performed cost effectively, financial success can never be accepted as the primary goal of any pediatric radiology activity. These beliefs are becoming more and more important; and some countries and institutions might well benefit from reconsidering and redefining their use of imaging, potentially also resulting in a significant reduction of imaging studies, which would not only better serve the patient, but also may contribute to relieve economic burden on health care systems.

I hope that my readers will enjoy this exposition of pediatric imaging. In addition I want to express my sincere thanks to all those who made this book possible, especially the staff at Thieme Medical Publishers, my dedicated coauthors, and everyone who helped out in any way. I am grateful for valuable suggestions from colleagues and technologists, and I extend special thanks to our young, motivating patients, and to my partner Barbara for her patience and support.

Michael Riccabona, MD

List of Abbreviations

AAo	Ascending aorta		BA	Biliary atresia
ABC	Aneurysmal bone cyst		BBB	Blood–brain barrier
AC	Anterior commissure		BV	Brachiocephalic vein
ACA	Anterior cerebral artery		b.w.	Body weight
aCDS	Amplitude-encoded color Doppler sonography, power Doppler		C4	Fourth cervical vertebra (etc.)
aCDU	Amplitude-encoded color Doppler ultrasound, power Doppler		CA	Carotid artery
			CAH	Congenital adrenal hyperplasia
ACR	American College of Radiology		CCAM	Congenital cystic adenomatoid malformation
ACF	Anterior cranial fossa			
ADC	Apparent diffusion coefficient		CCT	Craniocerebral trauma
ADEM	Acute disseminated encephalomyelitis		CDS	Color Doppler sonography, color duplex sonography
ADPKD	Autosomal dominant polycystic kidney disease		CCT	Craniocerebral trauma
			CDU	Color Doppler ultrasound
AEC	Automatic exposure control		ce-CT	Contrast-enhanced computed tomography
AFAP	Attenuated classic familial adenomatous polyposis		ce-MRA	Contrast-enhanced magnetic resonance angiography
AGS	Adrenogenital syndrome			
ALARA	As low as reasonably achievable		ce-MRI	Contrast-enhanced magnetic resonance imaging
ALD	Adrenoleukodystrophy			
ALL	Acute lymphoblastic leukemia		ce-US	Contrast-enhanced ultrasonography
AMA	American Medical Association			
AML	Angiomyolipoma; acute myeloid leukemia		ce-VUS	Contrast-enhanced voiding urosonography
ANA	Antinuclear antibodies		CF	Cystic fibrosis
APUD	Amine precursor uptake and decarboxylation		CFTR	Cystic fibrosis transmembrane conductance regulator
ARF	Acute renal failure		cGFR	Calculated glomerular filtration rate
ARPKD	Autosomal recessive polycystic kidney disease		CH I	Chiari malformation type I
AP	Anteroposterior; Annular pancreas		CH II	Chiari malformation type II
			CM	Contrast medium
APN	Acute pyelonephritis		CMV	Cytomegalovirus
ARF	Acute renal failure		CNS	Central nervous system
AS	Aortic stenosis		CoA	Coarctation of the aorta
ASD	Atrial septal defect		CPAM	Congenital pulmonary airway malformation
AVC	Atrioventricular canal			
AVF	Arteriovenous fistula		CPAP	Continuous positive airway pressure
AVM	Arteriovenous malformation			
			CPDN	Cystic partially differentiated nephroblastoma

CPR	Cardiopulmonary resuscitation		ESPR	European Society for Paediatric Radiology
CRMO	Chronic recurrent multifocal osteomyelitis		ESUR	European Society of Urogenital Radiology
cRNP	Congenital reflux nephropathy		EU	European Union
CRP	C-reactive protein			
CSF	Cerebrospinal fluid		FAST	Focused abdominal sonography for trauma
CT	Computed tomography		FAP	Familial adenomatous polyposis
CTA	CT angiography		FB	Foreign body
CTDI	CT dose index		FDG	Fluorodeoxyglucose
Cu	Copper (thickness)		FFE	Fast field echo
CVC	Central venous catheter		FISP	Fast imaging with steady-state precession
DA	Ductus arteriosus		FL	Fluoroscopy
DAP	Dose–area product		FLAIR	Fluid-attenuated inversion recovery
DASV	Dural AV shunt with aneurysmal vein of Galen dilatation		FNH	Focal nodular hypoplasia
DCIS	Ductal carcinoma in situ		FOV	Field of view
DD	Differential diagnosis		fs	Fat saturation
DDH	Developmental dysplasia of hip			
DDREF	Dose and dose rate effectiveness factor		Gd	Gadolinium
DDS	Duplex Doppler sonography		Gd-DTPA	Gadolinium diethylenetriamine penta-acetic acid
DGMP	German Society of Medical Physics		GE	Gastroenteritis
DHC	Common bile duct (ductus hepatocholedochus)		GER	Gastroesophageal reflux
DLP	Dose–length product		GERD	Gastroestophageal reflux disease
DMSA	Dimercaptosuccinic acid		GFR	Glomerular filtration rate
DORV	Double-outlet right ventricle		GI	Gastrointestinal
DQE	Detective quantum efficiency		GIST	Gastrointestinal stromal tumor
DR	Digital direct radiography		GLD	Globoid cell leukodystrophy
dRTA	Distal renal tubular acidosis		GMH	Germinal matrix hemorrhage
DSA	Digital subtraction angiography		GPOH	Society for Pediatric Oncology and Hematology
d-TGA	Complete transposition of the great arteries		GRE	Gradient echo
DTPA	Diethylene triamine penta-acetic acid		Gy	Gray
DVA	Developmental venous anomaly			
DWM	Dandy–Walker malformation		HASTE	Half-Fourier acquisition single-shot turbo spin echo
EA	Esophageal atresia		HCC	Hepatocellular carcinoma
ECG	Electrocardiography		HI	Harmonic imaging
ECMO	Extracorporeal membrane oxygenation		HIE	Hypoxic–ischemic encephalopathy
EDH	Epidural hematoma		HLA	Human leukocyte antigen
EMG	Electromyography; exomphalos–macroglossia–gigantism		HN	Hydronephrosis
			HPE	Holoprosencephaly
ER	Emergency room		HPS	Hypertrophic pyloric stenosis
ERCP	Endoscopic retrograde cholangiopancreaticography		HRCT	High-resolution computed tomography
			HU	Hounsfield units
			HUS	Hemolytic uremic syndrome

ICH	Intracerebral hemorrhage		MLD	Metachromatic leukodystrophy
ICRP	International Commission on Radiological Protection		MM	Megacisterna magna
			MMC	Myelomeningocele
ICU	Intensive care unit		MOPD	Microcephalic osteodysplastic primordial dwarfism
I.I.	Image intensifier			
INRG	International Neuroblastoma Risk Group		MR	Magnetic resonance
			MRA	Magnetic resonance angiography
INSS	International Neuroblastoma Staging System		MRCP	Magnetic resonance cholangio-pancreatography
IRDS	Idiopathic respiratory distress syndrome		MRI	Magnetic resonance imaging
			MRU	Magnetic resonance urography
IV	Intravenous		MRV	Magnetic resonance venography
IVC	Inferior vena cava		MS	Multiple sclerosis
IVH	Intraventricular hemorrhage		MSCT	Multislice computed tomography
IVP	Intravenous pyelography		MSK	Medullary sponge kidney
			mSv	Millisievert
JIA	Juvenile idiopathic arthritis		MU	Megaureter
JPI	Juvenile polyposis of infancy			
KERMA	Kinetic energy released to matter		NC	Nephrocalcinosis
KUB	Kidney–ureter–bladder radiograph		NEC	Necrotizing enterocolitis
			NF	Neurofibromatosis
			NHL	Non-Hodgkin lymphoma
LA	Left aortic arch		NICH	Non-involuting congenital hemangioma
LC	Left common carotid artery			
LCH	Langerhans cell histiocytosis		NPO	Nonprofit organization
LDA	Left descending aorta		NSAIDs	Nonsteroidal anti-inflammatory drugs
LDL	Left ductal ligament			
LE	Lupus erythematosus		NSF	Nephrogenic systemic fibrosis
LIH	Last image hold			
LIS	Lissencephaly		OSD	Open spinal dysraphism
LL	Lower lobe			
LLD	Left lateral decubitus		PA	Posteroanterior; pulmonary artery; pulmonary atresia
LP	Lumbar puncture; Left pulmonary artery		PAPVR	Partial anomalous pulmonary venous return
l-TGA	Corrected transposition of the great arteries		PC	Posterior commissure
LV	Lateral ventricle		PCA	Posterior cerebral artery
LS	Left subclavian artery		PCF	Posterior cranial fossa
			PCN	Percutaneous nephrostomy
mA	Milliampere, milliamperage		PCS	Pelvicalyceal system, pyelocaliceal system
MAG3	Mercaptoacetyltriglycine			
mAs	Milliampere seconds		PD	Pancreatic duct; proton density (MRI)
MCA	Middle cerebral artery			
MCD	Multicystic dysplasia		PDA	Patent ductus arteriosus
MCU	Micturating cystourethrogram		PEEP	Positive end-expiratory pressure
MD	Meckel diverticulum		PEG	Percutaneous endoscopic gastro-stomy
MI	Mechanical index			
MIBG	Metaiodobenzylguanidine		PET	Positron emission tomography
MIP	Maximum intensity projection		PFFD	Proximal femoral focal deficiency
mL	Milliliter		PFO	Persistent foramen ovale

PID	Pelvic inflammatory disease
PIE	Pulmonary interstitial emphysema
PKAN	Pantothenate kinase-associated degeneration
PMD	Pelizäeus-Merzbacher disease
PML	Progressive multifocal leukoence-phalitis
PNET	Primitive neuroectodermal tumor
PNP	Polyneuropathy
PNS	Peripheral nerve stimulation
POM	Primary obstructive megaureter
PPB	Pleuropulmonary blastoma
PRF	Pulse repetition frequency
PROPELLER	Periodically rotated overlapping parallel lines with enhanced reconstruction
PS	Pulmonic stenosis
PT	Pulmonary trunk
PTLD	Post-transplant lymphoprolifera-tive disease
PUV	Posterior urethral valve
PVEs	Periventricular echoes
PVH	Periventricular hemorrhage
PVL	Periventricular leukomalacia
PW-DDS	Pulsed-wave duplex Doppler sonography
RC	Right common carotid artery
RA	Right aortic arch
RAS	Renal artery stenosis
RDA	Right descending aorta
RDS	Respiratory distress syndrome
RES	Reticuloendothelial system
RF	Radiofrequency
RI	Resistive index
RICH	Rapidly involuting congenital hemangioma
RMS	Rhabdomyosarcoma
RNC	Radionuclide cystography
ROI	Region of interest
ROM	Range of motion
RP	Right pulmonary artery
RS	Right subclavian artery
RSV	Respiratory syncytial virus
RTx	Renal transplant
RV	Right ventricle, right ventricular

SAH	Subarachnoid hemorrhage
SAR	Specific absorption rate
SCIWORA	Spinal cervical injury without radiographic abnormality
SD	Standard deviation
SDH	Subdural hematoma
SE	Spin-echo
SEB	Subependymal bleeding
SIOP	International Society of Pediatric Oncology
SMA	Superior mesenteric artery
SMV	Superior mesenteric vein
SNR	Signal-to-noise ratio
SPECT	Single-photon-emission computed tomography
SPIR	Spectral presaturation with inver-sion recovery
SPR	Society of Pediatric Radiology
SSFP	Steady-state free precession
STIR	Short-tau inversion recovery
SV	Single ventricle
SVC	Superior vena cava
TA	Tricuspid atresia
TAC	Truncus arteriosus communis
TAPVD	Total anomalous pulmonary venous drainage
TAPVR	Total anomalous pulmonary venous return
TAR	Thrombocytopenia with absent radius
Tb	Tuberculosis
TCI	Transcranial imaging
TEF	Tracheo-esophageal fistula
TGC	Time gain compensation
TI	Thermal index
TIRM	Turbo inversion recovery magnitude
TOF	Tetralogy of Fallot
TORCH	Range of possible congenital infections: toxoplasmosis, rubella, cytomegalovirus, herpes simplex virus, HIV, syphilis
TR	Repetition time
TRH	Thyrotropin-releasing hormone
TrueFISP	True fast imaging with steady-state precession
TS	Tuberous sclerosis
TSE	Turbo spin-echo
TSH	Thyroid stimulating hormone

UGI	Upper gastrointestinal series	VGAM	Vein of Galen aneurysmal malformation
UPJ	Ureteropelvic junction	VGM	Vein of Galen malformation
UPJS	Ureteropelvic junction stenosis	VIBE	Volumetric interpolated
US	Ultrasound, sonography		breath-hold examination
UTI	Urinary tract infection	VIP	Vasoactive intestinal peptide
UVH	Univentricular heart	VSD	Ventricular septal defect
		VUR	Vesicoureteral reflux
VACTERL	Vertebral anomalies, cardiac malformation, tracheo-esophageal fistula, esophageal atresia, renal dysplasia and limb anomalies	WAGR	Wilms tumor, aniridia, genitourinary abnormalities
VATER	See VACTERL	WHO	World Health Organization
VENC	Velocity encoded (imaging)	WBS	Wiedemann–Beckwith syndrome
VCUG	Voiding cystourethrography		
VGA	Vein of Galen aneurysm	XPN	Xanthogranulomatous
VGAD	Vein of Galen aneurysmal dilatation		pyelonephritis

Contents

1 Special Imaging Issues in Children

1.1 General Introduction, Basic Considerations

Michael Riccabona

Children are not small adults. They have different body proportions, different heart and respiratory rates, different proportions of fat and connective tissue, and, to a degree, different tissue structure (e.g., nonossified skeletal structures, open cranial sutures, physiologic remnants of the fetal circulation, immature organs). Some organs occupy different relative positions and are less protected than in adults. Children are different in their movements, biomechanical loads, and even in their diseases (childhood illnesses, congenital anomalies, immaturity, dysfunction without frank organ damage, etc.).

Pediatric radiology covers a very broad area. In addition to less common but significant diseases that typically affect adults (e.g., stroke, diabetes), it includes numerous disorders and needs that are characteristic of children and newborns. As a result, imaging devices must be able to cover a very broad spectrum (from preterm infants weighing 400 g to obese adolescents weighing up to 150 kg), placing rigorous demands on equipment flexibility and adaptability. Radiologists who deal with children must address adult-type disorders as well as the specific clinical questions that arise in pediatrics. At the very least, they must be able to recognize these conditions, including various congenital syndromes or malformations and genetically determined (metabolic) diseases, and refer patients to a specialist as needed. They should also know how radiographic and sonographic organ morphologies differ from adult patterns, especially in small children, so that they can correctly interpret various phenomena. Examples are the difficulty of performing urinary contrast examinations in newborns due to immature renal function, immature lung structure causing a higher risk of atelectasis even with mild respiratory disease, and the paucity of fat, making it more difficult to distinguish intestinal structures on computed tomography (CT) scans of the pediatric abdomen.

Finally, everyone must recognize that the radiation risk to children is much higher than it is to adults, due not only to the higher rate of cell division but also to the longer life expectancy of children, allowing ample time for the manifestation of radiation-induced tumors. As a result, radiation-producing tests should be avoided in children whenever possible, and necessary tests should deliver the lowest possible dose in accordance with the ALARA principle ("**A**s **L**ow **A**s **R**easonably **A**chievable").

Ultrasound (US) imaging is of special importance in the pediatric age group owing to its high safety and efficacy. Less fat and smaller dimensions permit the use of high-resolution transducers. Cartilaginous structures that have not yet ossified can be clearly visualized with US, and structures underlying them can be evaluated. As a result, many investigations—especially in the neonatal neurocranium and thoraco-abdominal region—can be adequately accomplished without the use of X-rays. This allows formulation of several useful rules for pediatric imaging:

- US is generally preferred and has a wide range of applications in children.
- Given the risks, many clinical questions that were formerly addressed radiographically can be resolved today with US, such as hypertrophic pyloric stenosis (HPS), ileocecal intussusception and its reduction, the assessment of gastroesophageal reflux (GER) or vesicoureteral reflux (VUR), neonatal cerebral hemorrhage, genital anomalies, and abnormalities of the neonatal spinal cord.

- CT should be used with caution and in highly selected cases.
- Small children may need sedation for CT and magnetic resonance imaging (MRI).
- Fluoroscopy (FL) should be avoided whenever possible, and when necessary should be optimized to ensure minimal radiation exposure.

All of this is conveyed here in brief "checklist" format, resulting in a concise textbook that makes for fast and easy reference. The contents are reduced to a level of basic knowledge and general information ("What every radiologist should know"). A complete exploration of pediatric imaging is beyond the scope of this text, and readers are referred to the technical literature for more detailed accounts. Our intent is to convey a basic spectrum of knowledge that is essential for all imaging specialties, which will provide a fundamental understanding of child-specific imaging requirements. This book aims to support and promote the availability of correct and skillful pediatric imaging (including dedicated pediatric US) 24 hours a day throughout the entire year, as children also deserve the prudent and specific care that is generally considered state-of-the-art and natural for the various other (adult) specialties.

Bibliography

1 Babyn PS. Teaching Atlas of Pediatric Imaging. Stuttgart, New York: Thieme; 2006
2 Blickmann JG. Pediatric Radiology—the Requisites. St. Louis, Philadelphia: Mosby; 1994
3 Carty H, Brunelle F, Stringer DA, Kao SCS. Imaging Children, vols 1, 2. 2nd ed. New York: Elsevier; 2005
4 Riccabona M. Trainer Kinderradiologie. Stuttgart, New York: Thieme; 2010
5 Riccabona M. Pediatric Ultrasound, Requisites and Applications. Heidelberg: Springer; 2014
6 Schuster W. Kinderradiologie, vols 1, 2. Berlin, Heidelberg: Springer; 1990
7 Siegel MJ, Coley BD. The Core Curriculum: Pediatric Imaging. Philadelphia: Lippincott Williams & Wilkins; 2006
8 Siegel MJ. Pediatric Sonography, 4th ed. Philadelphia: Lippincott Williams & Wilkins; 2010
9 Slovis Th L. Caffey's Pediatric Diagnostic Imaging, vols 1, 2. 11th ed. Philadelphia: Mosby; 2008
10 Troeger J, Seidensticker P. Paediatric Imaging Manual. Heidelberg: Springer; 2008

1.2 Importance of Radiation Protection in Children

Gerald Paertan

Introduction

Impressive development of diagnostic imaging (especially CT, MRI) → increasing expectations among referring physicians and patients.

- Fear of litigation → medical examinations, which are often ordered even with pretest probabilities close to zero

However, diagnostic imaging may have side effects:

- Direct and indirect consequences of false-negative and false-positive findings
- X-ray modalities (radiography, fluoroscopy, and especially CT) → potentially harmful ionizing radiation

When we provide patients with **optimal instead of maximal** diagnosis and treatment, we are obliged to know and consider the risks and benefits of our actions and explain them to patients and families in understandable terms.

ALARA principle of radiation safety: keep the radiation dose from an examination as low as reasonably achievable (also considering social and economic factors).

However, using an image dose that is too low—resulting in image quality too poor for a specific diagnostic task and rendering the examination with its radiation exposure useless—is equally detrimental to patients. Also, withholding justified imaging may yield fatal consequences for both patients and doctors.

- It is the **patient** (not physicians or parents) who should benefit from a radiologic examination.
- Benefits outweigh risks only with well-indicated examinations.

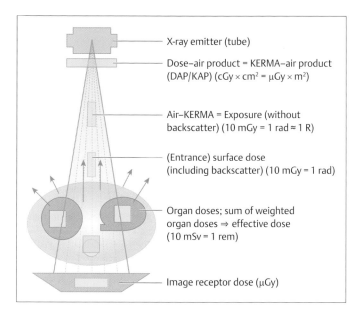

X-ray emitter (tube)

Dose–air product = KERMA–air product
(DAP/KAP) $(cGy \times cm^2 = \mu Gy \times m^2)$

Air–KERMA = Exposure (without
backscatter) (10 mGy = 1 rad ≈ 1 R)

(Entrance) surface dose
(including backscatter) (10 mGy = 1 rad)

Organ doses; sum of weighted
organ doses ⇒ effective dose
(10 mSv = 1 rem)

Image receptor dose (μGy)

Fig. 1.1 Diagrammatic representation of dose quantities. Blue boxes indicate sites of dose measurement/estimation (physical or mathematical).

Dosimetry Terms

Assessment of effects of ionizing radiation is not trivial; therefore, predominantly indirect methods are used. Different units, quantities and their derivations depend on place, method, and purpose of measurement **(Fig. 1.1)**.

"Physical" Quantities: Absorbed Dose, Kinetic Energy Released to Matter

- Energy deposited by secondary electrons (absorbed dose) or transferred from photons to electrons in matter—in this case, body tissue (Kinetic Energy Released to Matter—KERMA). At beam energies used for diagnostic imaging (< 1 MeV), both quantities are numerically the same.
- SI (Système International d'unités) unit = **1 J/kg**, expressed as **gray (Gy)**: in dose range of diagnostic radiography, fractional amounts such as cGy, mGy, or µGy are used.
- Measurement in X-ray beam with ionization chamber or thermoluminescent dosimeter, with the following operational quantities:

- **Entrance surface dose** (ESD, expressed in Gy, measured at body surface and thus taking into account additional backscattered dose proportion).
- **Dose–area product** (DAP, expressed as Gy times unit surface area, e.g., $cGy \times cm^2 = \mu Gy \times m^2$ and measured by ionization chamber at the beam exit of X-ray tube).
  (For Dose Length Product [DLP] and CT Dose Index [CTDI], see Sect. 1.5)
- **Image receptor dose** (usually stated in µGy); important for radiation protection and quality assurance; limited correlation with patient dose.
- Roughly comparable reference value in nuclear medicine: **administered activity** (dose unit: megabecquerel, MBq).
- These quantities give information about quality of examination with emphasis on dose emitted by X-ray device; useful for quality assurance.
- **Note:** before 1980, international unit of absorbed dose was the **rad** (1 rad = 10 mGy); furthermore, for roentgen and gamma radiation the obsolete quantity of **exposure** still exists. Units are **Coulomb** (C) per kg or **Roentgen** (R). Very roughly, 1 R = 1 rad (both still partially used in publications especially from United States).

"Radiation Risk" Quantities: Equivalent, Organ, and Effective Dose

- Quantification of radiation dose within body tissue to estimate biological effects and radiation risk. Only indirectly possible.
- **Equivalent dose:** SI unit—as in absorbed dose (above)—is 1 J/kg multiplied by the biological effectivity factor of type of radiation. Unit = **Sievert (Sv)**. For X-ray and gamma radiation biological effectivity factor = 1, and 1 Sv is equivalent to 1 Gy.
- **Organ dose:** For more accurate estimation of effects of radiation exposure, doses (expressed as **Sv**) absorbed by specific tissue or body organs with different radiosensitivities are determined. May only be estimated indirectly either by simulation of examination, placing dosimeters in anthropomorphic phantoms, or by calculating organ doses based on virtual mathematical body models.
- **Effective dose (E):** working term, tries to make different distribution of organ doses comparable between different X-ray examinations and reduce to common denominator for assessment of radiation risk = **sum of weighted organ doses** absorbed in given exposure, expressed as **Sv**.
- **Weighting factors** recently modified by International Commission on Radiological Protection (ICRP) in accordance with new epidemiologic findings: radiation risk of gonad exposure lower than previously assumed, radiation risk to breast tissue higher.[1]
- Reasonably accurate calculation of effective and organ doses: **dose calculation software** such as CT-Expo[2] and PCXMC.[3]
- Simpler but less accurate: calculate effective dose, multiply energy dose (e.g., DAP) by published examination-specific **conversion factors** (mSv per energy dose unit, e.g., mSv/cGy × cm²)—should be adapted for children.
- Radiation **risk** may be estimated by multiplying organ and/or effective dose with age and sex-specific risk factors (see following).

Radiation Risk

Deterministic Radiation Effects ("Tissue Reactions")

Generally, diagnostic exposures remain below the threshold for deterministic effects, but with possible exceptions:

- Skin reaction in patients of interventional radiology/cardiology procedures with protracted fluoroscopy time/without proper radiation protection precautions.
- Skin reactions in interventionalists, exposing hands repeatedly to primary X-ray beam.
- Repeated exposure of eye lens, e.g., patients with cranial CT without gantry tilt, or interventionalists with high occupational exposure of eye lens from scattered radiation.

Stochastic Radiation Effects

Cancer induction and (much less important) genetic effects.

Broad scientific consensus on the following assumptions (though evolution of knowledge on complex relationships between radiation-induced cell damage, repair processes, and carcinogenesis are still far from complete):

- Stochastic radiation effects subject to **linear dose–response relationship with no absolutely safe lower threshold** (LNT—linear no-threshold hypothesis).
- Risk of cancer induction **significantly higher in children than in adults** (**Fig. 1.2**), with about 10%/Sv for lethal cancer in males and almost 50%/Sv for nonlethal cancer in females if exposed in early childhood.[4]
- Radiation risk from **prenatal** exposure approximately equals that of small children, with additional 6%/Sv for developing cancer already in childhood (Oxford Survey of Childhood Cancers[5]); trend confirmed in results of recent study.[6]
- Latency period for leukemia, average 7 years, for solid carcinomas 20 years, with risk lasting about 10 years for the former and 20 to 40 years for the latter after exposure.
- Risk of single radiation doses **cumulates additively**.
- Children have different body proportions with more radiosensitive hematopoietic marrow in cranial and long bones.

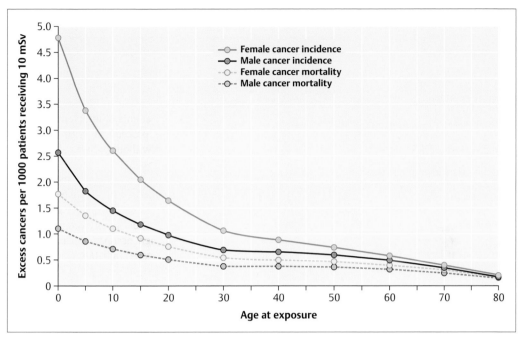

Fig. 1.2   Additional lifetime risk for developing cancer. (From Sodickson A, Baeyens PF, Andriole KP, et al. Recurrent CT, cumulative radiation exposure, and associated radiation-induced cancer risks from CT of adults. Radiology 2009; 251: 175–181, with permission.)

- **Genetic effects:** In ICRP publication, 103 weighting factors reduced in relation to other effects; about 10% of cancer risk, i.e., 0.3–0.5%/Sv in first generation and 0.5–0.9% in second generation, or 0.4–0.6% of natural hereditary disease rate.
- **Genomic instability:** Increased chromosome abnormalities in daughter cells of irradiated cells, which last for generations.
- **"Bystander" effect:** Transfer of destructive processes from irradiated to nonirradiated cells.
- Some effects occur spontaneously or result from other types of exposure (e.g., chemical).

Estimation of Individual Radiation Risk

Difficult to make individual risk assessments for particular patients and examinations owing to complexity of matter and assumptions rather than proof for doses < 50 mSv.

Even in small children, radiation risk is generally only small addition to natural incidence of around 25% during whole life. Considering, e.g., effective dose of 10 mSv from an abdominal CT, this addition may be estimated to be roughly 1 : 1000 from this exposure in early childhood. Typical sex-averaged effective doses from some radiologic examinations

for 5-year-old child given in **Table 1.1**. Dose for younger children and/or females slightly higher, for older children and/or males slightly lower compared with 5-year age group.

Note: concept of "effective dose" as defined by ICRP is somewhat controversial[8] and risk assessment should rather be done for populations and not for individuals.

> **Why is radiation protection even more important in children than in adults?**
> Because children:
> - have significantly higher risk of carcinogenesis per radiation dose
> - have longer life expectancy to develop cancer
> - have more time to experience cumulative effects from many radiographic examinations
> - receive more radiosensitive tissue exposure in certain examinations than adults due to body proportions and tissue distribution
> - receive higher organ radiation doses than adults from identical exposure settings
> - require more meticulous imaging technique due to small size and limited ability to cooperate, with higher relative dose needed to achieve diagnostically reliable imaging (less tissue, less fat)

Table 1.1   Typical effective doses for a 5-year-old child. Compare with annual natural background radiation of approx. 3 mSv

Imaging procedure	Effective dose (mSv)	Equivalent no. of CXRs
Ankle (3 view)	0.0015	0.07
Chest (PA + lateral)	0.02	1
Abdomen (2 view)	0.05	2.5
Tc-99m radionuclide cystogram	0.18	9
Tc-99m radionuclide bone scan	6.2	310
FDG PET scan	15.3	765
MCU/VCUG	0.1–1	5–50
Head CT	2–4	100–200
Chest CT	3–8	150–400
Abdomen CT	5–15	250–750

Abbreviations: CXR, chest radiograph; Tc-99m, technetium 99 m; FDG PET, fluorodeoxyglucose positron emission tomography; MCU, micturating cystourethrogram; VCUG, voiding cystourethrography.

Risks of Prenatal Radiation Exposure and Principles of Action

- Stochastic radiation effects on embryo or fetus assumed to be similar as for small children.
- Important radiation effects on cell maturation and migration of deterministic nature and as such do not occur below threshold dose of 100–300 mSv → induction of anomalies including CNS maturation disorders with severe mental retardation (**Table 1.2**).
- Normally, single diagnostic X-ray examination does not deliver dose necessary for deterministic radiation effects in unborn child (expressed by uterine organ dose):
  - Peripheral skeleton, chest (latter in CT as well): ≤ 1 mSv ("trivial threshold")
  - Abdominal radiographs: 0.5–10 mSv per image
  - Fluoroscopy (FL) examinations at 10 to maximum 40 mSv/min
  - Abdominal/pelvic CT: 15–35 mSv
- All women of reproductive age have to be asked whether they are or could be pregnant before undergoing X-ray examination.[11] Response should be documented. Reproductive age begins at 12 years—thus includes many patients in pediatric radiology (be tactful!). In most countries, jurisdiction allows for questioning by nonphysician staff members.
- Pregnancy is not an absolute contraindication to X-rays but does require rigorous risk–benefit analysis. If analysis does not support postponement or changing to MRI or US, dose optimization and radiation protection (shielding of nonexposed regions) is imperative. Document all dose-relevant imaging parameters in detail.
- Examinations with prospective uterine dose below 1 mSv (i.e., dose limit for general public) considered harmless.
- All other X-ray examinations: In slightest doubt (unstable cycle, communication problems, question as to legal adulthood), perform pregnancy testing (less sensitive during first weeks).
- In life-threatening situations (e.g., CT for multiple injuries), wellbeing of (potential) mother precedes. Do not delay imaging by testing for pregnancy.
- Pregnancy requires greater caution, not only with ionizing radiation but also in MRI and all types of contrast studies.

Table 1.2 Biological effects of prenatal radiation exposure (modified from DGMP 2002[9])

Effect	Time after conception	Lower threshold dose (mSv uterine dose)	Risk coefficient (per mSv uterine dose)
Death during preimplantation stage	Up to 10 days	100	0.1% (above threshold)
Malformations	10 days to 8th week	100	0.05% (above threshold)
Severe mental retardation	Weeks 8 to 15	300	0.04% (above threshold)
	Weeks 16 to 25	300	0.01% (above threshold)
IQ reduction	Weeks 8 to 15	Questionable[10]	0.03 IQ points
	Weeks 16 to 25	Questionable[10]	0.01 IQ points
Carcinogenesis	Whole pregnancy	0 (stochastic radiation effect)	0.006%
Inheritable defects	Whole pregnancy	0 (stochastic radiation effect)	0.0003% male, 0.0001% female

Abbreviation: IQ, intelligence quotient.

Accidental Prenatal Radiation Exposure[8,9,11]

If a woman exposed to radiation is later found to be pregnant at time of exposure:

- Determine exact time interval from conception to radiation exposure.
- Estimate approximate uterine dose (e.g., from tables in literature[7,12]). If fetus outside beam or presumptive uterine dose < 10–20 mSv, no further action needed.
- Uterine dose > 20 mSv → precise dose calculation by medical physicist.
- Dose 100–200 mSv or higher → option of pregnancy termination may be discussed with patient (100 mSv = threshold dose for embryonic death or malformations, 200 mSv = doubling dose for malformations). Generally these doses occur only in interventional radiology procedures in pelvic region (e.g., embolization of myomas) or prolonged FL examinations in obese women.
- In dose range of *diagnostic* imaging, risk of invasive prenatal diagnosis (amniocentesis) usually exceeds radiation risk.
- Even at several hundred millisievert, no definite indication for pregnancy termination → more likely that baby normal than handicapped.

- May screen parents for syndromes with increased radiosensitivity (e.g., ataxia telangiectasia, Fanconi anemia, retinoblastoma).
- **Nuclear medicine:** standard nuclear medicine tests usually deliver uterine dose < 10 mSv; three-level concept does not apply. Estimate dose from tables. Promote nuclide excretion to limit dose (e.g., forced diuresis). Potassium iodide can be administered within 12 hours to saturate thyroid gland.[13]
- **Radiotherapy:** dose estimated from treatment plan.

Legal Provisions for Radiation Protection, Disclosure and Communication

Legal Provisions for Pediatric Radiation Protection

Based on United Nations Scientific Committee on Effects of Atomic Radiation (UNSCEAR) assessments of levels and effects of exposure to ionizing radiation, ICRP provides recommendations, and International Atomic Energy Agency developed Basic Safety Standards (BSS),[14] which have been adopted worldwide as basis for radiation protection legislation, e.g., Medical Exposure Directive 97/43 of the

European Union (EU) (then transposed to legislation of member countries).

Basic principles concerning exposures of medical patients are **justification, responsibility**, and **optimization**.

- **Justification:** Radiation exposures must be doubly justified, on general grounds and for specific case at hand. May be supported by **referral criteria** issued by several scientific and/or public corporations (e.g., "How to make use of a department of Radiology" from Royal College of Radiologists in U.K., Appropriateness Criteria by American College of Radiology in U.S.)
- **Responsibility:** Both **referring physician** and **imaging specialists** are responsible for justification of medical exposures. To avoid unnecessary exposures, both must make sure that relevant information from prior imaging studies and case history are taken into account and unnecessary duplication of tests is avoided. Imaging personnel are responsible for properly conducting examination (radiologist, technologist, etc.).
- **Optimization:** Legislation in most countries expressly states need for **quality assurance and quality control programs** in pediatric radiology —e.g., routine quality testing, **use of suitable devices, accessory equipment,** and **specific radiation protection measures, documentation of patient doses** or technical parameters needed to calculate them (e.g., nuclear medicine: administered activities), and their evaluation and optimization in relation to **diagnostic reference levels**.
- **Appropriate training** required for staff who expose children to diagnostic radiation.
- **Holding of patients or imaging materials:** should be done by persons not occupationally exposed to radiation. These helpers should use holding devices whenever possible, should be protected by appropriate measures, and should be informed about radiation risks. Except in extremely high dose examinations, radiation exposure of helpers is generally much lower than dose limit of 3 mGy/annum prescribed by legislation in most countries.

In some countries, X-ray record card issued on request of patient or guardian. Radiation exposure parameters and doses (not necessarily effective or organ doses or their calculated values) are entered and updated on card.

Disclosure and Informed Consent

In most countries, patients over 18 years of age are considered adult. While younger patients may have reached legal age of consent for certain matters (usually 14 years), parents or guardians should still be included in disclosure and informed consent, especially for medical procedures that involve significant risk (angiography, interventional radiology). In addition, physicians should seek **informed consent** also from younger patients directly if emancipated or mature enough.[15]

- Diagnostic or therapeutic procedures may be undertaken legally in life-threatening situations, even against parental objections, because in most countries jurisdiction authorizes state intervention in favor of children who require medical care against e.g., religion-based objections of parents.[16]
- The less urgent an indication, the greater the obligation for disclosure and informed consent. For planned procedures, disclosure advisable at time of making appointment, at least 24 hours prior to procedure.
- In other medical specialties, risk disclosure essential even for procedures considered safe (anesthesia risk for non–high-risk patients 1 : 250,000, maximum of 1 : 10,000). Disclosure of radiation risk is far less routine. However, although not yet prescribed in most countries, documented disclosure and informed consent specifying degree of radiation risk for noninvasive X-ray examinations is increasingly advocated[17] and successfully practiced[18,19] at least for high-dose examinations (CT, FL).
- Disclosure should be given personally (physician performing test = ultimately responsible); should be documented on preprinted information and consent forms (= aids to disclosure, not sole means).

Communication with Children and Family Members

Sick children and their family members are often subjected to high stress levels, making communication more difficult. Not only is the hospital environment frightening for children, but parents unconsciously may transfer their own concerns and anxieties to children. Pediatric medicine is impossible without understanding, empathy, patience, professional demeanor, and skilled communication.

Children can be made much more cooperative by tailoring design of waiting rooms and examination rooms to their needs and providing distractions during imaging procedures (age-appropriate toys, books, and audiovisual media, e.g., video projection in MRI or CT gantry, video goggles, headphones); such measures may significantly reduce sedation rate.[12]

Communication with children must be age-appropriate. Up to about 5 years of age, sensitive approach can sometimes but not always improve child's capacity for understanding and cooperation. The procedure should be always conducted as quickly and painlessly as possible (e.g., use anesthetic paste before venipuncture!).

Whenever possible, schedule the most unpleasant diagnostic/therapeutic procedure till last.

Firm restraint accepted in brief examinations of newborns, still tolerable for small children and family members. Prolonged, relatively invasive tests (e.g., voiding cystourethrography—VCUG) often physically and emotionally stressful, even in small children → consider sedation.

Interdisciplinary Communication

Joint responsibility of referring physicians and radiologists prescribed by law and should be operative from planning the examination to reporting findings. Even in age of electronic data transfer, personal communication is often the most valuable information source and safest "fallback solution."

- What specific question should examination answer?
- What specific therapeutic decisions will be based on examination?
- What prior examinations, if any, were performed elsewhere? How can prior images or written findings be accessed?
- **Important**: therapeutically relevant findings should be promptly conveyed to ensure **documented** delivery to clinically responsible colleague.
- Regular interdisciplinary image consultations are standard in most fields (including pediatric radiology) and should not interfere with regular clinical activities, teaching, or training.

References

1 Wrixon AD. New ICRP recommendations. J Radiol Prot 2008; 28(2): 161–168
2 Stamm G, Nagel HD. CT-expo—a novel program for dose evaluation in CT. [Article in German]. Rofo 2002; 174(12): 1570–1576
3 Tapiovaara M, Lakkisto M, Servomaa A. PCXMC: A PC-based Monte Carlo program for calculating patient doses in medical x-ray examinations. Report STUK-A139. Helsinki: Finnish Centre for Radiation and Nuclear Safety; 1997. Website: http://www.stuk.fi/sateilyn_kaytto/ohjelmat/PCXMC/en_GB/pcxmc/(status: August 12, 2012)
4 Sodickson A, Baeyens PF, Andriole KP, et al. Recurrent CT, cumulative radiation exposure, and associated radiation-induced cancer risks from CT of adults. Radiology 2009; 251(1): 175–184
5 Doll R, Wakeford R. Risk of childhood cancer from fetal irradiation. Br J Radiol 1997; 70: 130–139
6 Rajaraman P, Simpson J, Neta G, et al. Early life exposure to diagnostic radiation and ultrasound scans and risk of childhood cancer: case–control study. BMJ 2011; 342: d472
7 Brody AS, Frush DP, Huda W, Brent RL; American Academy of Pediatrics Section on Radiology. Radiation risk to children from computed tomography. Pediatrics 2007; 120(3): 677–682
8 American College of Radiology. ACR Practice Guideline for Imaging Pregnant or Potentially Pregnant Adolescents and Women with Ionizing Radiation. Resolution 26, 2008. http://www.acr.org/~/media/ACR/Documents/PGTS/guidelines/Pregnant_Patients.pdf (status: August 12, 2012)
9 DGMP (German Society of Medical Physics). Report Nr. 7 Prenatal Radiation Exposure from Medical Indications 2002 http://www.dgmp.de/oeffentlichkeitsarbeit/papiere/Bericht7_Neuauflage2002.pdf [in German] (status: August 12, 2012)
10 Schull WJ, Otake M. Cognitive function and prenatal exposure to ionizing radiation. Teratology 1999; 59 (4): 222–226
11 European Commission. Radiation protection publication 100: Guidance for protection of unborn children and infants irradiated due to parental medical exposures. Directorate-General Environment, Nuclear Safety and Civil Protection 1998. http://ec.europa.eu/energy/nuclear/radiation_protection/doc/publication/100_en.pdf (status: August 12, 2012)
12 Donnelly LF. Introduction to Pediatrics—Pediatric Imaging. In: Donnelly LF, ed. Diagnostic Imaging Pediatrics (2nd ed.). Salt Lake City: Amirsys; 2011
13 National Council on Radiological Protection and Measurements. Report No. 128—Radionuclide Exposure of the Embryo/Fetus; Bethesda 1998

14 Safety Series No IAEA. 115: International Basic Safety Standards for Protection against Ionizing Radiation and for the Safety of Radiation Sources; jointly sponsored by FAO, IAEA, ILO, OECD/NEA, PAHO, WHO. Vienna: International Atomic Energy Agency; 1996
15 [No authors listed] Informed consent, parental permission, and assent in pediatric practice. Committee on Bioethics, American Academy of Pediatrics. Pediatrics 1995; 95(2): 314–317
16 Paul SR. Child welfare vs. parental religious views: What do pediatricians do when parents refuse life-saving care for their child? AAP News 2011; 32: 20

17 Semelka RC, Armao DM, Elias J Jr, Picano E. The information imperative: is it time for an informed consent process explaining the risks of medical radiation? Radiology 2012; 262(1): 15–18
18 Larson DB, Rader SB, Forman HP, Fenton LZ. Informing parents about CT radiation exposure in children: it's OK to tell them. AJR Am J Roentgenol 2007; 189(2): 271–275
19 Brenner DJ. Effective dose: a flawed concept that could and should be replaced. Br J Radiol 2008; 81(967): 521–523

1.3   Radiography and Fluoroscopy

Gerald Paertan

Radiography

High performance X-ray tubes provide shortest possible exposure times (< 5 ms; allows for faster respiratory rate and uncontrolled body movements in children). Because children generally have higher water content and less fat, radiographic contrast tends to be poorer than in adults.

Analogue Systems (Screen–Film Radiography, "Plain Film")

Basic requirement: automatic processing with carefully controlled temperature, densitometry, and regular maintenance. A minimum 200-speed image receptor prescribed, e.g., ACR–SPR Practice Guideline for Performance of Pediatric and Adult Chest Radiography.[1] Some countries have more rigorous standards, e.g., quality criteria of German Medical Association, which requires screen–film systems with speed rating of at least 400 (image receptor dose: 2.5 µGy) for imaging of extremities and preferably 800 or higher (image receptor dose: 1.25 µGy) for trunk imaging.[2]

Digital Radiography Systems

■ As in all digital imaging systems, **brightness and contrast independent of dose!** Main image quality parameter is **noise**, which declines (relative to image signal) with increasing dose, creating potential for "*exposure creep*" to avoid noisy images.[3]

■ Image noise quantified by signal-to-noise ratio (SNR). Detectors that are highly efficient in converting X-ray quanta into image signal (detective quantum efficiency—DQE) have better SNR and lower dose requirement.

■ SNR varies with square root of image receptor dose. **Dose must be quadrupled to reduce image noise by half!** Conversely, **halving dose increases noise by only one-fourth.** Therefore, reasonable amount of image noise acceptable and unavoidable for radiation protection (ALARA principle).

Digital Storage Phosphor Plates (Computed Radiography)

■ Older systems with amorphous luminescent screens and single-side readout: with dose not exceeding level of conventional screen–film systems, SNR only marginally acceptable, especially for preterm infant chest and peripheral skeleton imaging.

■ Recent systems with dual-side readout image plates or needle crystal coating instead of amorphous luminescent layer yield higher DQE and image quality (close to solid-state detectors).

■ Spatial resolution in many systems depends on cassette format. Image matrix of about 2000 × 2000 pixels (up to 4000 × 4000 pixels) distributed over available cassette area; pixel size varies accordingly → use of smallest cassettes (18 × 24 cm) for imaging individually targeted body areas (e.g., forearm, hand, preterm chest).

Digital Direct Radiography (Solid-State/Flat Detectors)

- Digital direct radiography has higher DQE than screen–film or computed radiography. Higher DQE requires less radiation dose for comparable image quality or provides higher image quality for same radiation dose.[4]
- Higher DQE probably offsets limited spatial resolution (pixel size ≥ 140 µm/detail resolution ≤ 3.5 line pairs/mm of currently available systems).

Besides stationary systems (bucky table, wall cassette holder), mobile systems/detectors increasingly used, image transmission by cable or, most recently, wireless.

Fluoroscopy

Image-intensifier–television chain (with conventional or digital detector system) or digital solid-state detector. Tube placed below or above table:

- **Below-table design** (advantage: shielding of scattered radiation easy; disadvantage: limited tube-to-patient distance)
- **Above-table design** (advantage: adjustable tube position; disadvantage: difficult to shield against scattered radiation)

> **!** Distance from patient to detector always as close as possible, tube-to-patient distance as wide as possible—especially important with C-arm systems.

Image Intensifier Technology (Conventional, Digital)

Detectors with image intensifier (I.I.) have cylindrical housing, resulting in geometric image distortion, especially at image periphery. **Zooming**, which is set by using smaller **I.I. diameters**, increases necessary dose → **avoid zooming**, whenever possible, even if tempting due to small patient size.

Digital Solid-State Detector Fluoroscopy

No geometric image distortion. **Zooming does not increase radiation dose.** Sharper image outlines than with I.I. technology. Quality of stored fluoroscopic image often adequate for dose-sparing documentation, eliminating need for extra radiographs (spot films).

Image Processing

Digital systems have linear image–signal properties over very wide dose ranges. Raw image data processed for monitor display, hardcopy, and human visual perception. Goal: simultaneous display of all relevant image area.

- Basically, all systems try to exclude areas with diagnostically irrelevant density (surrounding air, metal implants, collimation), then assign optimum contrast and brightness values to diagnostically relevant structures (bone, soft tissues).
- Contrast is reduced in image areas with pronounced light–dark differences and enhanced ("harmonized") in areas of more uniform brightness.
- Image outlines are sharpened by edge enhancement. Excessive or indiscriminate edge enhancement will mask structures with indistinct margins and increase image noise and may create artificial borders, potentially leading to misinterpretation—particularly important in small children.
- Modern multifrequency processing subdivides images into different spatial frequency spectra (= detail size spectra), which are individually contrast-enhanced in varying, optimum degrees.
- Further contrast/brightness optimization, for uniform image appearance on different display media, and to adapt to nonlinearity of human visual system.
- **Important to know:** nature and location of these processing steps within imaging chain to pinpoint errors and **avoid unnecessary repetition of images due to correctable errors or misreadings.**

Image Display Devices

Viewboxes for Plain Film Radiographs

Require periodic quality testing, especially for uniform illumination. Portions of the image outside the collimated field should be masked to eliminate glare.

Monitors

- Require periodic quality testing in accordance with law, regulations, and technical standards. Avoid direct illumination of monitors by external light sources.
- Make initial evaluation only on monitors approved for this specific purpose. Highest performance class (B/W monitor if necessary) should be used for (pediatric) radiography.
- Important to reading images from monitors:
  - **Zoom/magnification functions:** Many monitors have smaller pixel matrix than radiographs displayed on them. Without magnified view, image would be small and details could be missed. Monitors with dense image matrix (but standard format): pixels and image details sometimes so small that zooming must be used (comparable to magnifying loupe in screen–film radiography).
  - **High-contrast image display:** suboptimal settings of pre- and postprocessing options often yield low-contrast images → may cause pathology to be missed (e.g., retrodiaphragmatic infiltrates) → need for manual windowing. Practice with and knowledge of computer tools required.
  - **Attention to soft-tissue structures:** keying image quality to skeletal structures alone ignores inherent advantages of digital systems → critical findings may be missed (e.g., inflammatory or traumatic soft-tissue swelling).

Techniques for Dose Reduction in Radiography and Fluoroscopy

First step in radiation dose reduction: follow established referral criteria and avoid improper examinations/examination techniques—see also Sect. 1.2 (**Table 1.3**).

Preparations and Practice Guidelines

- In some countries, adherence to practice guidelines, definitions, and use of Standard Operating Procedures (SOPs) for most common radiological examinations are compulsory, e.g., standard guidelines of American College of Radiology (www.acr.org), educational material from "Image Gently" campaign (www.imagegently.org).
- Pause and plan before X-rays switched on: all preparations must be completed, all "homework" done, and X-ray equipment "ready for take-off"!
- Accurate patient identification and R/L side labeling are important issues. To reduce errors, expose L and R markers onto image (don't insert them digitally in retrospect!).
- Generally, parents or family members may be present during examination (except for examinations under anesthesia and interventional procedures); provide radiation risk disclosure—at least, if requested to.
- Instruct patient and helpers *before* examination (breath-hold commands, practice position changes, pre-examination visit to FL room, etc.).

Optimum Patient Positioning, Calming, Distraction, and Immobilization

- Medical staff in white garb may scare infants. Some children need time to develop trust, so approach them gently rather than abruptly. Some children are distractable by humorous approach.
- Unless contraindicated, children should be well hydrated and not fasted for examination.
- Pacifier (if accepted), drinking bottle, favorite plush animal, or other toy.
- Use music/TV/video player.
- Use patient restraints and positioning pads liberally; preterm and newborn infants often perceive constraints as physiologic (recalls intra-uterine environment).
- PA views generally preferred over AP views: reduce exposure to radiosensitive anterior tissues (thyroid gland, breast) by 3–5 times. Avoid eyes, thyroid, breast, gonads when possible.
- Avoid temperature loss, especially in preterm and newborn infants → use radiant heater during long examinations, room temperature slightly higher than usual.

Table 1.3 Examples of radiographic and fluoroscopic examinations not indicated in children

Examination	Clinical problem not requiring X-rays	Comments
Radiography		
Skull	Trivial injury (low-risk group)	Indications increasingly rare; most common = suspected child abuse; also ventricular shunt evaluation
	Growing fracture	= Herniating leptomeningeal cyst, not fracture margins "drifting apart"; diagnosis by palpation, eventually pre-OP MRI
Paranasal sinuses	Sinusitis before school age	Sinuses not yet developed in early childhood
Chest	Routine lateral radiograph	Besides increasing radiation exposure, most lateral radiographs in children add no diagnostic information for anatomical reasons
	Routine preoperative chest films	
	Follow-up of pneumonia	Only in selected cases or if findings will have therapeutic implications
		MRI promising; US should be tried for lesions on or near pleura; US better than CT for revealing septa in effusions
	Incidentally detected heart murmur	If necessary: echocardiography
Spinal column	Trivial injury	
Abdomen	Nonspecific abdominal pain	Initial imaging study is US, even with suspected bowel obstruction; X-ray for suspected perforation or volvulus
Pelvis	Hip dysplasia before 6th month	Define cartilage structures with US
	Hip arthritis with no clinical evidence of severe course	"Irritable hip" is common; effusion detected by US
Intravenous pyelography		US (dynamic), MR urography; in selected cases CT usually obsolete
Fluoroscopy		
Upper GI series, double-contrast X-rays	"Gastritis"	Basically not an indication for imaging (initial study = endoscopy); US to exclude other causes of pain; radiography may be appropriate for suspected perforation
		Selective contrast study for suspected intestinal rotation anomaly
Irrigoscopy	Abdominal pain, constipation, bloody stool	Dedicated "unprepared barium irrigoscopy" for suspected Hirschsprung disease
		US; MR enteroclysis for suspected chronic inflammatory bowel disease
MCU/VCUG	Enuresis	

Abbreviations: MCU, micturating cystourethrogram; VCUG, voiding cystourethrography.

Correct Placement of Patient Shielding

Avoid placing shields within exposure field, especially not in measuring areas of automatic exposure control (see below). Readjust shielding when child repositioned. Use thyroid and gonadal shields.

Accurate Collimation

Collimate with light field before exposure, avoid fluoroscopic guidance. Collimation margins from exposure should be visible on image, not digitally added later (**Figs. 1.3a, b**).

In small children, minimal change in collimator and patient position can have significant effects → undesired exposure of structures outside image field (e.g., thyroid gland, tubular bones in chest). Good patient restraint eliminates need for "prophylactic" widening of collimation field.

Selective Use of Scatter-Reduction Grid

Scattered radiation is less in smaller children, reducing the benefit of scatter-reduction grid, which should be used only for chest/abdomen examinations in children over about 9 years of age. Grid increases exposure dose by a factor of 2–6 (for same image receptor dose as without grid). Therefore,

X-ray and FL machines for pediatric imaging should be equipped with (electro)mechanically removable scatter-reduction grid.

Additional Filtration

Removes soft portions of X-ray spectrum that are absorbed in patient's body and do not contribute to image production.

- For trunk examinations: additional filtration of at least 0.1 mm Cu (or equivalent) must be added to inherent tube filtration (2 mm aluminum).
- In FL examinations of gastrointestinal (GI) and urogenital tracts: filtration may be increased by 0.2 to 0.3 mm Cu without appreciable loss of image quality.
- For radiography of peripheral skeleton: 0 to max. 0.1 mm Cu is recommended to avoid degradation of image quality.

Optimum Tube Voltage

Under discussion for digital radiography. Unlike screen–film radiography, high-kilovoltage (kV) technique is not so crucial for better visualization of mediastinal structures. Reduced entrance surface/skin dose due to higher kV (with same image receptor dose and lower milliamperage) does not

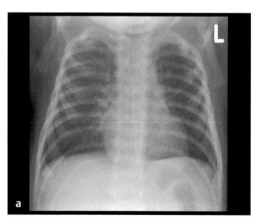
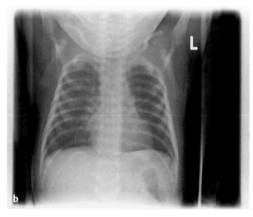

Fig. 1.3a, b   Example of incorrect collimation masked by digital image postprocessing. Six-day-old full-term infant; chest X-ray because of bradycardia and O_2 desaturation; subtle perihilar, radiating interstitial infiltrates are in keeping with aspiration during birth.

a Image is displayed with 11.3 × 10.6 cm = 119.8 cm² field size, with apparently ideal collimation.
b Raw image after removing postprocessed shutter shows that "true" beam collimation was considerably

worse with a radiation field of 17.4 × 14.4 cm = 250.6 cm², which is more than double of the apparent field size → original X-ray beam collimation has always to be displayed on images ("white frame").

necessarily mean reduced organ or effective dose throughout body cross-section; it may even be increased due to greater biological efficacy of harder radiation. Also consider kV response of digital detector media (change in sensitivity with change in radiation quality). For imaging of trunk, optimum may be mid-range kV (compare established reduction to 80 kV for pulmonary artery CT and pediatric CT studies) in combination with strong (0.2–0.3 mm Cu) additional beam filtration. Exposure times should remain short, so that image quality–dose relationship is not improved at cost of motion unsharpness.[4]

Optimum Fluoroscopy Dose Rate

Try to fall well below FL exposure dose rate of 25 mGy/min recommended by IAEA BSS for "normal dose mode" in adults. Avoid "high contrast" or "high dose" modes; try to find out which dose rate is used by FL equipment for specific procedure.

Dedicated pediatric Automatic Exposure Control (AEC) kV/mA curves should be used in fluoroscopic systems for children. Often, AEC preferred—gives pre-set controlled tube potential (kV) and variable tube current (mA) and allows "dose hold."

Selection of Correct Measuring Chamber, AEC "Freezing"

The AEC measuring chamber should measure radiographic exposure in relevant image areas (no air next to patient, no lead shielding, contrast pools, or metal implants). With most FL equipment, AEC can be "frozen" (e.g., between plain and contrast views for irrigoscopy or VCUG).

Pulsed Fluoroscopy

In pulsed FL, decreasing frame rate by one-half will generally reduce entrance dose by one-half (−50% at 15 pulses/s relative to continuous FL, −75% at 7.5 pulses/s, etc.).

Limiting Number of Spot Films

Digital FL may tempt examiner to obtain numerous spot views within short time. Whenever possible, FL sequences should be stored instead of spot views. Frame rate and series numbers should be limited in angiographic and cardiologic studies.

Digital Collimation Indicator

Digital collimation preview without FL on helps to shorten FL time. May need to be reset after patient's position changes during examination.

Avoidance of Zooming in Fluoroscopy

I.I. technology usually has multiple zoom levels, or multiple I.I. input formats that can be selected. The smaller the I.I. input format or higher the zoom level, the better the spatial resolution (detail sharpness) but the higher the necessary dose (does not apply to digital solid-state detector systems).

Minimization of Fluoroscopy Time

As rule of thumb, exposure dose for one spot view is equivalent to FL time of about 10 to 20 seconds, so FL is basically a high-dose procedure → importance to reduce FL time (depending on intensity level of FL usage):

- **FL memory for documentation:** with limited image quality requirements (e.g., single-contrast GI study, VCUG filling phase), FL study can be documented by **last image hold** (LIH) ("fluoro grab") rather than exposed spot views. Using fine motor skills, operator activates FL switch only for fraction of second—just long enough to generate documentable FL image ("step lightly!").
- **Patient positioning for FL-guided radiographic images:** standard radiographic projections generally set with collimator light, but FL may be used for **few seconds** in selected cases (e.g., double-contrast studies of GI tract).
- **Intermittent or continuous surveillance/documentation of contrast inflow or catheter positioning:** e.g., video swallowing study, observation of contrast transit through GI tract, contrast enemas, monitoring of catheter placement for angiography or interventional radiology procedures. Try for short FL times **less than one minute** and no longer than a few minutes.

Quality Assurance

In addition to periodic quality/constancy testing of whole imaging chain:

- Do not delete or discharge failed images—should be collected and regularly **analyzed** to determine reasons for failure (image repeat/reject analysis).[5,6]
- **Image receptor exposure indicators** (manufacturer-specific) should be displayed and evaluated on monitor/hardcopy images (**Table 1.4**).
- Acknowledge fluoroscopy timing alerts during procedure.
- Record and review dose: calibrated dose-measuring device should be available—or rather, legally prescribed—in many countries.

Free educational downloads on these and other radiation protection topics are provided by Radiation Protection of Patients (RpoP) section of IAEA (http://rpop.iaea.org) and by ICRP (http://www.icrp.org/page.asp?id=35) (status: August 12, 2012).

! In Digital X-ray imaging, radiation dose can by no means be estimated by contrast or brightness—attention to image noise is fundamental.

Diagnostic Dose Reference Levels

Not to be used as individual dose constraints, but if consistently exceeded under standard conditions in standard patients, corrective action is mandated. National and international diagnostic dose reference levels (DRLs) can (and should) be supplemented by lower local DRLs, as shown in **Table 1.5**. To confirm compliance with DRL, recording of individual patient doses (e.g., DAP) or exposure parameters (from which dose can be calculated) are recommended (legally mandatory e.g., within Europe and most states in the United States).

Contrast Media

- **Barium suspensions:** for antegrade (oral, via gastric or duodenal tube) and retrograde visualization of GI tract; no intravascular or intracavitary use.
  Advantages: relatively low cost, high inherent contrast, coat GI wall.
  Disadvantages: may cause constipation; intraperitoneal barium is devastating; contraindicated in patients with bowel obstruction, perforation risk, or significant aspiration risk.
- **Iodinated water-soluble:** generally safe for intravascular, intracavitary (fistulography), and GI use.
  Use only low-osmolar, low-viscosity nonionic contrast medium (CM) in pediatric radiology.
  CM should be warmed to body temperature for intravenous (IV) use.
  Advantages: metabolically neutral for most parts, even with aspiration or perforation; have mild laxative effect.
  Disadvantages: relatively high cost, less contrast than barium, do not coat GI wall.

Table 1.4 Comparison of manufacturer-specific exposure indicators (after Uffmann 2008[7])

Image receptor dose (µGy)	Standard recommended by IEC	EXI (Siemens)	EI (Philips)	S (Fuji)	EI (Kodak/Carestream)	logM (Agfa)
1.25	125	190	800	1600	1100	1.6
2.5	250	380	400	800	1400	1.9
5	500	760	200	400	1700	2.2
10	1000	1520	100	200	2000	2.5
Comment	Linear	Linear	Linear	Linear	Logarithmic	Logarithmic for 400 rating

Abbreviations: IEC, International Electrotechnical Commission; EXI, EI, exposure index; S, sensitivity; logM, logarithmic expression of median exposure.

Table 1.5 Diagnostic dose reference levels (in cGy cm²) for selected pediatric fluoroscopy examinations: national reference doses in the UK (from 2005) versus local dose levels of Great Ormond Street Hospital (GOSH), London (from 2006)[a]

Examination	Age group (years)	UK 2005[8]	GOSH 2006[9]
MCU/VCUG	0	30	5
	1	70	5
	5	80	10
	10	150	42
	15	250	42
Barium swallow (pharynx, esophagus)	0	40	8
	1	120	8
	5	130	12
	10	240	32
	15	350	32
Barium meal (small bowel follow through)	0	40	8
	1	110	8
	5	130	12
	10	240	32
	15	640	32

[a] Note the large differences between the relatively high national and the lower local dose levels—by almost an order of magnitude—the latter resulting from optimized, dedicated examination technique from a large pediatric tertiary care hospital.
Abbreviations: MCU, micturating cystourethrogram; VCUG, voiding cystourethrography.

Aside from flavor-enhanced products specially made for oral use, some IV products have acceptable taste.

During pregnancy, iodinated CM should only be applied for vital indications; thyroid function of neonate must be checked in first week after birth.

Breast-feeding may continue after maternal application of iodinated CM.

Especially in preterm neonates and during first 1 to 3 months of life, due to renal immaturity, IV application only for vital indications; age adjusted creatinine and glomerular filtration rate values have to be used for assessment of renal function in children.

! Ionic, strongly hyperosmolar amidotrizoate–salt mixtures (e.g., Gastrografin) generally contraindicated in children in undiluted form. Risk: life-threatening alteration of electrolyte and fluid balance! Possible exception: diluted 3 : 1 and used as therapeutic enema for meconium plug syndrome.

- **Negative contrast media (air, CO_2):** used in pediatric radiology either for intestinal double-contrast studies (almost obsolete today) or for pneumatic reduction of intussusception (advantages include lower radiation dose requirement than positive media).
- **Gadolinium (Gd) and other contrast media for MRI:** see Sect.1.6.

See also Manual on Contrast Media of the American College of Radiology[10] and guidelines on Contrast Media of the European Society of Urogenital Radiology (www.esur.org).

References

1 American College of Radiology. ACR–SPR Practice Guideline for the Performance of Pediatric and Adult Chest Radiography, revised version 2011 (Res. 56). Reston, VA: ACR; 2011 http://www.acr.org/~/media/ACR/Documents/PGTS/guidelines/Chest_Radiography.pdf (status: August 12, 2012)

2 Bundesärztekammer. Leitlinie der BÄK zur Qualitätssicherung in der Röntgendiagnostik: Qualitätskriterien 2008 [German Medical Association: Guidance on Quality Assurance in X-ray diagnostics – quality criteria for radiography]. Website: http://www.baek.de/downloads/LeitRoentgen2008Korr2.pdf (status: August 12, 2012) [in German]

3 Warren-Forward H, Arthur L, Hobson L, et al. An assessment of exposure indices in computed radiography for the posterior-anterior chest and the lateral lumbar spine. Br J Radiol 2007; 80(949): 26–31

4 Schaefer-Prokop C, Neitzel U, Venema HW, Uffmann M, Prokop M. Digital chest radiography: an update on modern technology, dose containment and control of image quality. Eur Radiol 2008; 18(9): 1818–1830

5 Nol J, Isouard G, Mirecki J. Digital repeat analysis; setup and operation. J Digit Imaging 2006; 19(2): 159–166

6 Waaler D, Hofmann B. Image rejects/retakes—radiographic challenges. Radiat Prot Dosimetry 2010; 139 (1–3): 375–379

7 Uffmann M, Schaefer-Prokop C, Neitzel U. Balance of required dose and image quality in digital radiography. [Article in German] Radiologe 2008; 48(3): 249–257

8 Hart D, Hillier MC, Wall BF. National reference doses for common radiographic, fluoroscopic and dental X-ray examinations in the UK. Br J Radiol 2009; 82 (973): 1–12

9 Hiorns MP, Saini A, Marsden PJ. A review of current local dose-area product levels for paediatric fluoroscopy in a tertiary referral centre compared with national standards. Why are they so different? Br J Radiol 2006; 79(940): 326–330

10 American College of Radiology. ACR Manual on Contrast Media Version 8. Reston, VA: ACR; 2012. http://www.nxtbook.com/nxtbooks/acr/contrastmediamanual2012 (status: August 12, 2012)

1.4 Technique and Clinical Value of Ultrasound in Pediatric Radiology

Michael Riccabona

General Aspects of Pediatric Ultrasound

In pediatric age group, the US capabilities are intrinsically better, with dedicated training, adapted handling, and (high-resolution) transducers essential, as compared to adults.

- Superficial structures and less fat → high-frequency and high-resolution transducers (less tissue penetration depth) can be used = accurate evaluation of small(er) pediatric structures.
- US generally repeatable without risk → ideal for functional evaluation, growth monitoring, screening (detection of malformations before manifestation of severe organ damage), follow-up.
- Sonopalpation (= applying gentle, localized transducer pressure during imaging) → easier to classify pain and complaints, investigate cause, correlate imaging findings with origin of clinical symptoms.

Many adult applications of US (e.g., liver, spleen, pancreas, heart, urinary tract, thyroid gland, lymph nodes, etc.) also valid in children. Child-specific applications include, among others:

- Cerebral US through nonossified fontanelle(s)
- Spinal cord US through nonossified spinal canal wall in newborns
- Intussusception, volvulus, hypertrophic pyloric stenosis, gastroesophageal reflux (GER), etc.
- Neonatal US of cartilaginous femoral head: immaturity, dysplasia, and developmental dysplasia of the hip, including (sub)luxation (hip screening)
- Subperiosteal abscess (early childhood osteomyelitis), slipped epiphysis, etc.
- US evaluation of thymus and diaphragm (diaphragm palsy, DD of mediastinal opacities on chest radiographs)
- US evaluation of VUR ("contrast-enhanced voiding urosonography = ce-VUS")

Examination procedure and standardized documentation (of normal findings) established for most US applications in children and newborns (see, e.g., German recommendations at www. OEGUM.at → pediatrics → standards and guidelines).

- Goals: improve quality of examination, standardization, and comparability; meet forensic requirements (increasingly important).
- Not all aspects of pediatric US, diseases, and possible applications covered in this book → seek additional references on pediatric US.

Risks of Ultrasound

Theoretical possibility of tissue alterations (mechanical and thermal effects) due to US:

- Use of excessive acoustic energy and prolonged exposure times.
- Use of US contrast agents (cavitation effects):
  - Especially in preterm infants (brain), genitalia, lung, and bowel (air as cavitation nucleus).
- Note power output (watts/joules) or MI (mechanical index) and TI (thermal index) as measures of relative tissue exposure; should be > 1; keep as low as possible.

- Potential for microorganism transfer by US probe → hygiene is important.
  - Always clean transducer and examination couch, regularly clean equipment (keyboard, air filter, etc.).

> ! Adequate usage essential → minimize risks by careful handling and equipment settings → train in child-specific aspects of diagnostic US.

Basic Rules in Pediatric Ultrasound

US anatomy, morphology, and image patterns often differ from adults, especially in newborns. Examples:

- Preterm infants: physiologically large lateral ventricles; less gyration and less parenchymal differentiation
- Renal parenchymal pattern and renal outlines
  - Normal renal appearance for adults = suspicious for renal pathology in newborns
- Newborns: disproportionately large hepatic left lobe
- Different disorders and therapeutic approaches → different indications/referrals/clinical questions
  - Frequent query = detection of congenital anomalies, oncologic issues much less common → different imaging algorithms, different use of modalities, etc.

Special aspects of pediatric US and practical tips:

- Child-appropriate setting (radiant heater, blankets, pacifier, bottle, towels, suitable couch, toys, pictures, books, distracting videos, etc.).
- Means for warming US gel (use sufficient amount, change regularly).
- Space for accompanying adults, persons holding the child.
- Longer examination time (allow more time for playful introduction and interactive routine).
- Start scanning in painless area (= familiarize child with US probe and examination), then proceed carefully to affected area(s).
- Distract child, announce next step in examination.
- Careful with positioning maneuvers—often not tolerated:

  - If necessary → say what will happen next; maintain sensitive, playful demeanor
  - Give instructions in child-appropriate language (e.g., "make a big tummy," "hold your breath like a diver," etc.)
- Always use transducer with highest possible resolution (that still gives necessary penetration depth); select transducer appropriate for region and conditions (change transducer several times during examination if needed):
  - Abdomen: curved-array and linear transducers (sector transducer rarely used)
  - Musculoskeletal and articular US: linear transducer
  - Cerebral US and thoracic US applications: start with sector transducer, then add high-resolution linear scans (potentially with virtual convex mode) as needed.
- Detailed knowledge of the US scanner and examination requirements (**Fig. 1.4**):
  - Constant scanner adjustments required (focus, penetration depth, image size, TGC, etc.).
  - Examiner concentrates less on scanner operation than on examination and child.
  - Use physiologic US windows (or create them, e.g., by having child drink some tea or other liquid).
- Prerequisite: knowledge of common pediatric disorders and their US appearance.
- Goals: supply information relevant for diagnosis, treatment, and follow-up; do not miss other essential findings; recommend further tests; communicate content and quality of examination:
  - Initial sweep or "sonocope" = basic initial evaluation (e.g., in an emergency = *FAST* [focused abdominal sonography for trauma]).
  - Thorough detailed examination = precise visualization and analysis of all structures (time-consuming).
  - State limits of US → good interaction with clinicians/referring physicians is important.
  - Suggest additional imaging if deemed helpful or mandatory.

■■■■ **Case Study 1.1** ■■■■

Illustrates importance of knowledge and expertise in pediatric US, especially correct device settings, e.g., for lower abdominal transverse scan through urinary bladder.
History: infant with mild hydronephrosis diagnosed in utero.
Initial postpartum examination: what and when? US, 1 week after birth, infant well hydrated.

Findings: Bladder appears normal. Large retrovesical ureter, visible only with correct scan parameters **(b)**.

a) Initial scan: cannot be evaluated. What should be corrected to obtain good image and useful measurements?

b) Image after **changing transducer** (replacing sector probe with higher-resolution linear probe), correcting **frequency** (high-frequency probe), reducing **gain** (lower power setting to decrease reverberations), and making several other adjustments: **focal spot** (deeper placement, multiple focal zones if needed), **image size** (adjusted to target organ and surroundings), **TGC curve** (time gain compensation to reduce/adapt for acoustic enhancement behind bladder → better evaluation of distal ureters, internal genitalia and other lower abdominal structures/ascites), **scan plane** (transverse scan angled slightly away from head), and **measurement** (aligning cursors along geometric organ axes to permit use of volume approximation formula).

Correction factor for approximation formula varies with bladder shape, e.g., spherical or rotational ellipsoid = 0.5, squared off = 1.

May need to activate **harmonic imaging** and **image compounding** (less internal echoes and cleaner borders, better bladder-wall delineation and detail sharpness).

Diagnosis: large distal left ureter—megaureter (obstruction? reflux?).

Further tests: (sonographic) VCUG, US follow-up; may be monitored later, if needed, by scintigraphy and/or magnetic resonance urography.

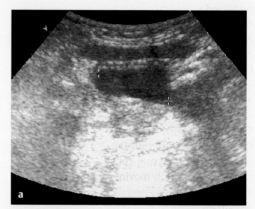
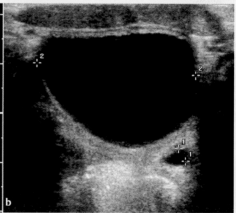

Fig. 1.4a, b

Capabilities of Modern Ultrasound Methods and Applications in Children

Many modern US techniques have become standard in routine pediatric US = improved utilization of US potential in children and newborns (radiation hygiene, ALARA principle):

- Harmonic imaging (HI): receives and processes higher frequency harmonics instead of reflected fundamental frequencies → improved image, fewer artifacts, etc.
- Panoramic US ("extended field of view"): combines consecutive single scans by vector analysis → large survey image, measurement of large structures, conspicuous overview, etc.
- Image compounding ("Sono-CT," cross-beam imaging): multiple single scans acquired at different angles and/or frequencies with stationary transducer and/or averaged from different beam

directions; monitor image → better image details and tissue differentiation, less artifacts, improved penetration with good resolution, etc.

- (Color) Doppler sonography (CDS): Doppler principle = frequency shift of sound waves reflected from moving particles → frequency shift measured to calculate and display flow direction and velocity.
- Power Doppler (amplitude-coded CDS = aCDS): calculates and employs integral of Doppler envelope curve → flow-volume-weighted, less angle-dependent imaging, even at low flow velocities, no directional information; higher acoustic energy can (and must) be used.
- B-flow (and similar non-Doppler flow visualization techniques): non-Doppler-based flow imaging by subtracting consecutive images at same location (= only moving pixels used for image rendering) → good, angle-independent flow visualization with less acoustic energy exposure than in Doppler techniques.
- Contrast-enhanced US (ce-US): enhancement produced by microbubbles that reflect and emit strong, specific (resonance effects) acoustic signals.
  - Can be administered intraluminally or intravenously.
  - Use in children (see also Claudon et al. 2008[1]):
    - VUR diagnosed without radiation ("ce-VUS," see Chapter 5, Riccabona et al. 2008).
    - US for investigating blunt abdominal trauma, determination of brain death (transcranial CDS), liver imaging (usually for oncologic indications as in adults), etc.

> Currently no commercially available ultrasound contrast agent is approved for use in children!

- Three- or four-dimensional US (3D/4D US): can also be used in children—e.g., for imaging head and brain, various small parts, urogenital tract, accurate volumetry, option for image fusion, etc.
- Interventional US: ideal as it allows for continuous, non–radiation-producing real-time guidance of interventional procedures (e.g., catheter placement, US-guided hydrostatic reduction of intussusception, percutaneous aspiration and biopsy, foreign body removal, preoperative localization, etc.).

> Interventional US requires expertise, reserved for specialized centers (knowledge/experience, equipment, devices and instruments, pediatric anesthesia, surgical backup for managing complications, etc.).

- Other new and creative applications helpful for reduction or more selective utilization of radiation-producing tests, e.g., perineal US, hydrocolon ("US enema"), US genitography, ce-VUS and ce-US, sonoelastography, etc.

Other Considerations

Technically proficient, detailed US examination poses no significant risks and is, or should be, easily available.

- Helps to contain rising health care costs, reduces population exposure to ionizing radiation, etc.
- Not cheap in terms of real costs (time-consuming, requires prolonged physician activity, which is relatively costly).

Growing limitation of resources over time → increasingly limited capacities → only guarantee for quality US is selective utilization reducing the total number of (nonindicated or unnecessary) examinations. Reserve detailed scanning for most abdominal and many musculoskeletal indications in children and for neonatal CNS. CT/MRI far less necessary than in adults—increase US use in pediatric age group:

- Promotes radiation hygiene by reducing need for CT/MRI with attendant risks and costs.
- Aids better and more accurate planning of further tests with less radiation exposure.
  - Less unnecessary, stressful, invasive, radiation-producing tests.
- Specific requirements:
  - Detailed knowledge of US capabilities in children.
  - Well-equipped US system with wide range of transducers.
  - Knowledge, training, and sufficient practical experience; may be reinforced by specialized courses or visiting physician programs.

Bibliography

1 Bruyn, de R. Pediatric Ultrasound: How, Why and When. Edinburgh: Churchill Livingstone; 2010, ISBN 978-0443069178

2 Claudon M, Cosgrove D, Albrecht T, et al. Guidelines and good clinical practice recommendations for contrast enhanced ultrasound (CEUS)—update 2008. Ultraschall Med 2008; 29(1): 28–44

3 Internetseiten für Dokumentationsempfehlungen sowie Empfehlungen für Untersuchungsstandards und Bildgebungsalgorithmen: http://www.esur.org; http://www.espr.com; http://www.oegum.at

4 Pilhatsch A, Riccabona M. Role and potential of modern ultrasound in pediatric abdominal imaging. Imaging in Medicine 2011; 3: 393–410(18)

5 Riccabona M. Pediatric Ultrasound, Requisites, and Applications. Heidelberg: Springer; 2014

6 Riccabona M. Pediatric three-dimensional ultrasound: basics and potential clinical value. Clin Imaging 2005; 29(1): 1–5

7 Riccabona M. Modern pediatric ultrasound: potential applications and clinical significance. A review. Clin Imaging 2006; 30(2): 77–86

8 Riccabona M, Avni FE, Blickman JG, et al. Imaging recommendations in paediatric uroradiology: minutes of the ESPR workgroup session on urinary tract infection, fetal hydronephrosis, urinary tract ultrasonography and voiding cystourethrography, Barcelona, Spain, June 2007. Pediatr Radiol 2008; 38(2): 138–145

9 Siegel MJ. Pediatric Sonography, 4th ed. Philadelphia: Lippincott Williams & Wilkins; 2010

1.5   Special Aspects of Computed Tomography in Children

Erich Sorantin

Introduction

CT has become an integral part of pediatric imaging. Usage increased dramatically in recent years due to technical advances and improved diagnostic capabilities. CT scans → significant radiation exposure.

In Great Britain in 1989: number of CT scans = 4% of all X-ray examinations and ≈ 40% of collective medical radiation exposure. Today: CT = 17% of all X-ray examinations and ≈ 75% of medical radiation exposure. CT = high-dose modality.

In 1989, pediatric CT = 4% of all CT; by 1999, rose to > 63%, even 92% for abdominal CT (including scans to exclude appendicitis).

"Children Are Not Small Adults"

Consider differences from adults when imaging: psychology, anatomy and proportions, body composition, radiosensitivity, physiology—imaging has to cover large range of body sizes and dimensions.

Example: body weights in **adult medicine** range from 40 kg (very slender woman, emaciated patient) to 160 kg (wrestler) = **mass factor of 4**.

Pediatric radiology serves patients ranging from preterm infants to 18-year-olds = body weight ranges from 300 g (extreme prematurity) to 120 kg (obese adolescent) = **mass factor of about 300**. This means:

> The right for high quality imaging does not depend on body weight.

Task for pediatric radiology: consider all of these facts in adapting equipment, imaging protocols, and image interpretation for pediatric patients.

Differences between Children and Adults

Psychology

The world experienced by children differs considerably from the adult world.

Many things are difficult for children to understand: "Why do I have to miss kindergarten and go to a building where people run around in strange clothes and you have to wait all the time? You take your clothes off, and they put you in big scary machines with screens that display boring shows (and usually aren't even in color). You have to lie still, and you may even have to go to sleep when they tell you to."

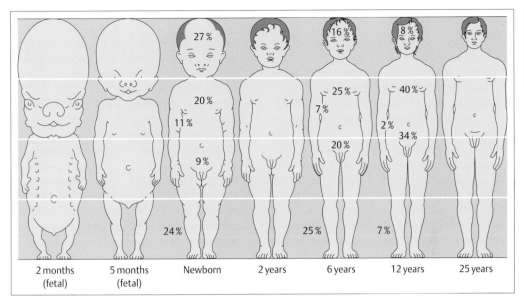

| 2 months (fetal) | 5 months (fetal) | Newborn | 2 years | 6 years | 12 years | 25 years |

Fig. 1.5 Body proportions normalized to body length. Demonstrates dominance of head in first years → many head injuries during first years of life—in combination with bad head control responsible for severe spinal injuries in "whiplash" road accidents. Numbers with gray background indicate radiation sensitivity. (Modified after Kempe et al. 1987, and Schneider 2005.)

Admittedly, caricature lives by exaggeration—but there is much truth in this depiction. Complicating factor: parents' fears transmitted to child ("children are mirrors of their environment").

Anatomy and Proportions

Disproportion between head and body size: Head of younger children larger (than in adults) relative to rest of body (**Fig. 1.5**):

→ High incidence of head injuries in small children.

→ SCIWORA (spinal cervical injury without radiographic abnormality): greater elasticity of bones (more cartilage) and paraspinal soft tissues (especially ligaments) allow compartment to undergo greater length changes than spinal cord. Result = cord lesion without associated bone injury.

→ Smaller children: injuries to upper cervical spine (cranial—C4) more common than in later life.

→ With pediatric craniocerebral trauma: always include C4 in CT scans (see also Chapter 6)

Chest shorter in children → upper abdominal organs less protected, more commonly injured, e.g., by non-age-appropriate child car seat—lap belt across upper abdomen causes mesenteric and intestinal tears.

Chest more elastic and compressible in children → serial rib fractures rare, increased risk of vascular rupture (aorta at ligamentum arteriosum).

Nonlinear growth in children—infant triples body weight during first 12 months but grows by only 50%. Meanwhile, body surface area doubles → change in body proportions. Further growth occurs in spurts, mainly during puberty.

Self-perception poorer during growth periods → problems in coordination and spatial orientation. All this plus disproportionate growth of bones and muscles (= altered mechanical leverage) → typical injuries.

Body Composition

Density differences in various organ systems are age-dependent: bones more cartilaginous than in adults, limb bones contain hematopoietic marrow, less overlying muscle and structural fat.

Result: absolute decrease in radiographic density, less pronounced density differences = decrease in relative contrast.

Chest: air content also affects absorption characteristics. Development of new alveoli not complete until kindergarten age → infant lungs contain less air → baby chest has same overall density as kindergarten child despite larger proportion of skeletal cartilage (due to decreased air content of lungs and thymus). Consider these factors also when developing imaging protocols.

Bones in children are weaker than ligaments → high incidence of bony ligament avulsions. Epiphyses = sites of predilection for various transitional fractures.

Radiosensitivity

See Sect. 1.2. Task of radiology: translate all these factors into imaging protocols tailored to specific equipment and clinical question. Always follow ALARA principle.

Hardware Requirements

All spiral CT scanners have two drawbacks: **overranging** and **overbeaming**.

Overranging: one-half detector rotation at start and end of scan field—necessary to acquire enough data to reconstruct first and last slice. The wider the detector and narrower the scan field, the greater the total dose increase—a particular problem in children.

Overbeaming: more pronounced in scanners with fewer detector rows. "Penumbra" (= edge radiation not useful for image reconstruction) forms at edge of each slice = nondiagnostic portion of radiation → increased exposure; therefore, advantageous to scan children with more detector rows and with capability for "volume CT."

Other key device-specific determinants of pediatric CT:

- **Scanning speed:** high scan speeds (= short rotation times, significantly < 1 second) reduce need for sedation and anesthesia; shorter scan times = higher acquisition cost.
- **Soft-tissue resolution:** particularly important due to difference between children and adults— should be significantly > 3 HU/3 mm; need for large, flexible range of mA and kV settings (80–140 kV, preferably in increments of 10; 10–400 mA, minimum of 5–10-mA increments).
- **Examination time:** main determinant = handling of child; inverse correlation between patient compliance and length of examination; most motivated child becomes less cooperative as scan time increases → need to expedite scan when child on CT table.
- **Automatic dose monitoring systems:** desirable; consider combining with other radiation protection measures (e.g., bismuth shielding) → potential for unwanted dose increase.
- **Check child compatibility** of all other add-ons: monitoring options, contrast injector due to smaller volumes, respiratory and ECG gating, etc.

Contrast Media

Oral

Abdomen: bowel opacification with oral contrast medium, e.g., 2% iopamidol diluted for enteric use. One hour before start of examination, patient starts drinking mixture—last 25% of total volume ingested 15 minutes before CT begins. Total volumes age-dependent (**Table 1.6**).

Intravascular

Due to physiologic renal immaturity: avoid intravenous contrast injection during first 3 months of life—adequate US answers almost all questions in this age group.

Avoid **contrast-induced nephropathy:** follow guidelines of European Society of Urogenital Radiology (ESUR Guidelines on Contrast Media; www.esur.org).

Table 1.6 Age-dependent contrast doses for oral bowel opacification

Age	Dose
Up to 6 months	100 mL
6 months to 1 year	200 mL
1–3 years	300 mL
3–10 years	700 mL
Older children	1000 mL

Table 1.7 Weight- and age-dependent doses of intravenous contrast media. Do not administer > 100 mL

Age	Dose
Less than 1 year	2.5 mL/kg b.w.
Between 1 and 2 years	2.0 mL/kg b.w.
Older than 2 years	1.5 mL/kg b.w.

Contrast dose: adjust for age (**Table 1.7**), maximum 100 mL.

Injection: preferably into ante cubital vein with motorized syringe.

! Venous access in head problematic—risk of superficial temporal artery compression leading to thrombosis and appositional thrombus extension into common carotid artery.

Other venous access sites less than optimal (dorsum of hand or foot) due to difficulty of controlling scan delay.

Usual maximum flow rate = 2.0 mL/s—higher rates often not possible due to small needle lumina. Manual injection may be an option in selected cases (depending on available motor pump, access, age, clinical question, etc.).

Scan delay setting (= time from start of contrast injection to scan initiation): difficult due to highly variable hemodynamics. Bolus tracking recommended for CT angiography (CTA) or thoracic CT (ROI placed over aortic arch or main pulmonary artery trunk).

Table 1.8 Organ factors for contrast injection. For CT scanners with few detector rows: 2 stated values = factors for early and late phase. For 64-slice scanners: increase factors for arterial phase by about 20 to 30%

Organ or region	Factor
Neck	1.0
Chest	0.8
Abdomen	1.4
Liver	0.6 and 1.8
Pelvis	1.8
Kidney	0.8 and 4.8

For threshhold selection, note how long gantry takes to reach starting position for diagnostic scans (= effective scan start): when bolus tracking position and scan starting position identical—contrast threshold about 150–180 HU. Threshold reduction in case of longer scan delay by detector (re)positioning, etc. Example: 80 HU for pulmonary artery CTA.

Bolus tracking systems → increase contrast and radiation dose! In our experience, total dose increased by about 10% (up to 20%).

Timing of initial scan: early (~ 5 s in [small] children due to short distances and rapid blood flow, even earlier [1 s] in infants). Acquire subsequent scans at 1-second intervals.

Calculating scan delay
Injection time = contrast volume/flow rate (usually 2 mL/s);
scan delay = injection time × organ factor
(use departmental organ factors for different examinations; valid for scanners with few detector rows [**Table 1.8**])

Modern **64-slice spiral CT**: increase factor for arterial phase by about 20–30%. Due to short scan times of these systems—replace ⅓ of contrast volume with physiologic saline solution in arterial phases (not for later phases, otherwise contrast enhancement would be too low). Saline push (= NaCl bolus injected immediately after contrast medium) prevents artifacts due to contrast pooling in superior vena cava = better utilization of contrast medium (guideline = ~ 3–5 mL/kg b. w., same flow rate as contrast medium).

With **volume CT** scanners that cover up to 16-cm scan volume with one rotation in < 0.5 second, calculate scan delay as in 64-slice system, then adjust calculated scan delay for actual contrast volume to be injected (pointless to inject contrast after the scan is completed!).

Dose Adjustments

Factors that Influence Dose

(Most) important image quality parameter: **noise** (signal-to-noise ratio—SNR).

Image noise shows inversely portional, nonlinear dependence on following quantities:

- Noise = $1/\sqrt{mA}$
- Noise = $1/\sqrt{rotationtime}$
- Noise = $1/\sqrt{slicethickness}$

Both **tube current** (in mA) and **rotation time** linearly increase radiation dose → doubling mAs (= mA × rotation time) doubles dose. When **slice thickness** decreased by half, tube current must be doubled to get same image quality or SNR (**Fig. 1.6**). When **patient diameter** increases by 4.0 cm, tube current should be approximately doubled. Collimation can provide greatest dose efficiency, depending on manufacturer—this would be the collimation that gives highest resolution for lowest dose requirement. Knowing this value, consider whether reducing slice thickness, thereby increasing dose, would also produce desired information gain.

"Sampling theorem" states that lesion detection requires twice the resolution: therefore, in CT, slice thickness should be less than thickness of imaged lesion.

> Acquisition of overlapping slices can increase spatial resolution without adding to radiation exposure.

Relationship of **tube voltage** (in kV) to dose exponential: when tube voltage is reduced from 120 to 100 kV (= ⅚ of 120 kV), dose falls to 66% ([⅚]² = $^{25}/_{36}$ = ~ ⅔) of initial dose. Reduction from 120 to 80 kV (= ⅔ of 120 kV) decreases dose to less than 50% ([⅔]² = $^{4}/_{9}$) of initial dose. Meanwhile decreased tube voltage → higher contrast.

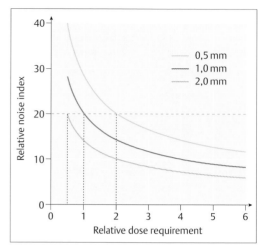

Fig. 1.6   Chart for demonstration of relationship between image noise (y-axis) and relative dose requirements (x-axis). If a relative noise index of 20 is chosen (horizontal dashed line) at slice thickness of 1.0 mm, then at slice thickness of 0.5 mm double the dose, and at 2.0 mm (vertical dotted lines) only half the dose, is needed for same image noise.

Pitch = table feed per rotation (in mm)/(number of detector rows × detector row width) affects dose too—pitch of 1–1.5 theoretically reduces dose by ⅓, pitch of 2.0 by 50%. Slice sensitivity profile widens at higher pitch → less actual dose reduction. Avoid pitch < 1.0 in pediatric imaging (often called "high-quality pitch" by equipment manufacturers). Exceptions: cranial and cardiac CT.

Dose modulation systems (automatic exposure control—AEC) adjust radiation dose according to local factors in scanned body section (different manufacturers offer different options) → tube current adjustment and reduction if possible → should decreases radiation dose without degrading image quality.

> Do not use edge-enhancing kernels when planning examinations, as they increase noise level → dose modulation would even increase dose to maintain constant noise level → use standard kernel for planning, then reconstruct images with an edge-enhancing kernel (as separate series).

For imaging small regions (e.g., cranial CT in infants): **reduce number of slices to 32** in 64-slice scanners → prevents dose increase due to unfavorable imaging geometry.

Table 1.9 SPR (Society of Pediatric Radiology) reduction factors for abdominal and thoracic CT. All databased on 120 kV, converted

AP thickness (cm)	Approximate age	mAs reduction factor Abdomen	Chest[a]
9	Newborn	0.43	0.42
12	1 year	0.51	0.49
14	5 years	0.59	0.47
16	10 years	0.66	0.64
19	15 years	0.76	0.73
22	Thin adult	0.90	0.82
25	Normal adult	Reference value	0.91
31	Overweight adult	1.27	1.16

[a]Reduction factors for chest too low; tube current may be around 66% of abdominal value.

Bismuth shielding for eyes, thyroid gland, breast, gonads → up to 57% dose reduction. Avoid small streak artifacts from bismuth shielding by increasing distance between bismuth and skin (e.g., with 2-cm foam rubber insert). Careful when using bismuth shields in conjunction with AEC systems: indiscriminate use may increase dose by modulation, e.g., when using z-axis modulation (based on scout image). Avoid this effect by acquiring scout image without bismuth shielding, then place shield.

Tube filtration important—especially use of asymmetric shaped filters, usually based on scan field of view (e.g., small, medium, large).

Reconstruction filter (kernel) affects dose: edge-enhancing kernels increase noise while "soft kernels" reduce noise at expense of spatial resolution. Find best tradeoff: representative scans reconstructed with various kernels, followed by semi-quantitative visual evaluation.

Dose Protocols

Recommendations for **scanner settings** (Rogalla and Stoever, Society of Pediatric Radiology—SPR; www.pedrad.org):

- Rogalla and Stoever: adjust tube current mAs = (weight in kg +5) × f
  Factor f: chest = 1, abdomen/pelvis = 1.5, skull = 2–5

Table 1.10 SPR (Society of Pediatric Radiology) reduction factors for cranial CT. All databased on 120 kV, converted

AP thickness (cm)	Approximate age	MAs reduction factor
12	Newborn	0.74
16	1 year	0.86
17	5 years	0.93
19	Normal adult	Reference value

Note empirical fact that abdominal CT usually requires about 1.5 times higher dose than thoracic CT—changes in tube voltage disregarded.

- SPR: starting with ideal parameters for adult scan, adjust mAs product using reduction factors; databased on tube voltage of 120 kV (**Tables 1.9** and **1.10**). Reduction factors for chest (too) low, however—tube current may be about 66% of value for abdomen.

Children = different body structure, so different contrast characteristics → recommended tube voltages < 120 kV; decreasing tube voltage from 120 to 80 kV can reduce dose by up to 50%. For information and tips, visit SPR homepage and link to "Image Gently Campaign."

Tube voltage: 80 kV for infants, 100 kV for small children, 120 kV (= adult value) for children of 9 years or older (or > 30 kg b.w.). With edge-enhancing reconstruction kernel: use 100 kV or (preferably) 120 kV; otherwise images will be blurry despite "sharp kernel."

Tube current: more difficult to adjust. SPR reduction factors = good starting point. If tube voltage < 120 kV, also correct tube current values in exponential fashion: if using 100 kV instead of 120 kV → increase tube current by 50% (only 66% of dose applied). If using 80 kV instead of 120 kV, double tube current (since only $\frac{2}{3}$ = 66% of dose applied due to lower kV).

Low-Dose Protocols

Stated dose values not absolutes, only suggestions —should be adapted to clinical question. Some examples and suggestions from our practice:

- **Shunt evaluation** (if MRI unavailable): reduce tube current by one-half; if results are equivocal or CSF seepage noted with ventricular enlargement → supplement with single scans at normal dose in relevant areas.
- **Craniosynostosis:** reduce tube current for age-adjusted cranial CT by more than one-half; for 3D reconstruction—reconstruct with standard kernel.
- **Cystic fibrosis follow-up:** tube voltage 120 kV (due to edge-enhancing kernel), tube current 50% of age-adjusted protocol, slice thickness 1–2 mm; careful with dose modulation due to possible upregulation based on small slice thickness —set scanner to accept higher noise level; consider low-dose high-resolution CT (HRCT = single slice every 1.5 cm).
- **Funnel chest:** age-adjusted tube voltage; tube current well below 50% of age-adjusted protocol.
- **Skeleton:** tube voltage 120 kV for trauma imaging (use edge-enhancing kernel). Hip trauma → at least 50% reduction of tube current for age-adjusted pelvic scan. Ankle joint: reduce by 70% —if possible, position with knee elevated; for scanning with foot dorsiflexed (same dose as hip scans).

Summary

Some "take-home" points:
- Safety and justification first → before performing CT, consider whether it could be replaced by another modality that does not produce ionizing radiation.

> Best radiation protection = no CT scan!

- Follow **ALARA** principle, adapt dose to clinical question.
- Avoid multiphase examinations—weight information gain and diagnostic benefit against dose.
- Make scout image as short as possible; select proper scan field of view (FOV).
- Employ concise scan length—avoid unnecessary inclusion of neighboring organs.
- Multidetector scanners and small scan regions: consider using fewer detector rows (e.g., 64 → 32).
- Note correct timing and dose of initial scans in bolus tracking.
- Dose modulation program: do not use edge-enhancing kernel.
- Adjust slice thickness for indication—note "sampling theorem" information from manufacturer on slice thickness with highest dose efficiency (and use that value).
- Pitch should not be much less than 1, except for cranial and cardiac CT.
- Do not increase dose for thinner slices, only for 3D reconstructions—may use greater slice overlap (smaller increment) for reconstructions. Use softer reconstruction filters; they help to reduce noise.
- Slice thickness reduction in dose modulation: adjust noise level—more noise acceptable when scanning bony structures only (noise will not be perceived due to large window width).
- Bismuth shielding combined with dose modulation: make sure that dose is not increased.
- Check regularly documented CT dose index and dose–length product values; do they conform to international recommendations?
- Check periodically to see whether dose reduction possible—especially after hardware updates.

Bibliography

1 Cody DD, Mahesh M. AAPM/RSNA physics tutorial for residents: Technologic advances in multidetector CT with a focus on cardiac imaging. Radiographics 2007; 27(6): 1829–1837

2 Image Gently Campaign—Society of Pediatric Radiology (SPR). Website: http://www.pedrad.org/associations/5364/ig/index.cfm?page=364; status: October 25, 2009

3 Kempe CH, Silver K, O'Brien D, Fulginiti VA. Current Pediatric Diagnosis and Treatment. 9th ed. New York: McGraw-Hill; 1987: 17

4 Lee CH, Goo JM, Ye HJ, et al. Radiation dose modulation techniques in the multidetector CT era: from basics to practice. Radiographics 2008; 28(5): 1451–1459

5 Pang D, Wilberger JEJ Jr. Spinal cord injury without radiographic abnormalities in children. J Neurosurg 1982; 57(1): 114–129

6 Paterson A, Frush DP. Dose reduction in paediatric MDCT: general principles. Clin Radiol 2007; 62(6): 507–517

7 Reilly CW. Pediatric spine trauma. J Bone Joint Surg Am 2007; 89(Suppl 1): 98–107

8 Schneider K. Besonderheiten der Aufnahmetechnik und des Strahlenschutzes. In: Benz-Bohm, ed. Kinderradiologie. Stuttgart, New York: Thieme; 2005: 1–16

9 SPR – Image Gently. How to Develop CT Protocols for Children. Website: http://www.pedrad.org/associations/5364/files/Protocols.pdf (status: October 25, 2009)

10 Stöver B, Rogalla P. CT examinations in children. [Article in German] Radiologe 2008; 48(3): 243–248

11 Tsapaki V, Aldrich JE, Sharma R, et al. Dose reduction in CT while maintaining diagnostic confidence: diagnostic reference levels at routine head, chest, and abdominal CT—IAEA-coordinated research project. Radiology 2006; 240(3): 828–834

12 U.S. National Institute of Heath, National Cancer Institute. Radiation Risks and Pediatric Computed Tomography (CT): A Guide for Health Care Providers. Website: http://www.cancer.gov/cancertopics/causes/radiation-risks-pediatric-CT (status: October 25, 2009)

1.6 Special Aspects of Magnetic Resonance Imaging in Children

Franz Wolfgang Hirsch

Indications for MRI Compared with CT

Today, hardly any limitations on MRI use in pediatric patients:

- All parenchymal organs, soft tissues, spinal column, and all joints can be examined by MRI.
- Brain imaging: morphology, spectroscopy, perfusion-weighted imaging, diffusion-weighted imaging, and diffusion-based fiber tracking.

> Functional imaging (e.g., localization of motor areas, language centers) not feasible in small children due to need to establish specific activities (selective finger movements, language paradigms).

- Bone lesions: can be accurately characterized with respect to soft-tissue component, which is generally present; high diagnostic specificity when combined with conventional radiographs → withholding of CT in most cases in children.

> MRI may miss small (posttraumatic) bone fragments and diffuse micro-calcifications in organs.

- Lung imaging: Pulmonary MRI has broadened spectrum of pediatric MRI applications; it has become standard pediatric imaging tool at many centers. Prerequisite: effective respiratory triggering techniques (**Fig. 1.7**).

> Limited accuracy for detecting mild fibrosis, small (cystic) parenchymal lesions, and metastases < 4 mm.

- Emergency imaging after trauma: high logistical costs for adequate MRI examination. Mortality in multiply injured patients rises sharply with time spent in emergency room → time gained by rapid CT examination justifies CT radiation exposure; MRI = limited role (second-line modality, imaging of complications).

████ **Case Study 1.2** ████

History and clinical presentation: 4-year-old boy with 1-week history of fever, cough, respiratory distress, high level C-reactive protein. Presented now with clinical deterioration and respiratory distress despite antibiotic therapy.
Suitable modalities: chest radiograph, US, CT, MRI.
Available images: radiograph, MRI.

Findings:

a   **Chest radiograph:** PA film shows unilateral opacity of right hemithorax with air–fluid level. Further imaging questions: Extent of infiltration? Abscess formation requiring drainage? Abscess contents?

b, c **Thoracic MRI** (T2-weighted TSE [turbo spin-echo], coronal = b, axial = c): complete infiltration of left lung (lobar pneumonia) with four abscesses (arrows) that contain gas-forming bacteria.

d   **Diffusion-weighted MRI** (axial, ADC map [ADC = apparent diffusion coefficient]): hypointensity in largest, posterior abscess—typical of purulent contents.

Diagnosis: lobar pneumonia (staphylococcal) with dorsal lung abscess.

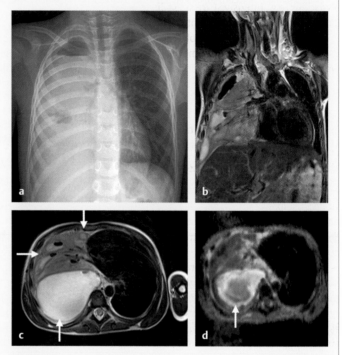

Fig. 1.7a–d

Sedation, General Anesthesia, and Related Problems

Patients < 6 years of age often require sedation for MRI.

Various methods available. No established technique definitely better or worse than others, provided child not jeopardized due to lack of experience or insufficient monitoring.

Common Sedation Methods in Children up to Age 6

- Sedation/general anesthesia by anesthesiologist: when examination time limited—anesthesiologic support essential. Common agent for se-

dation is **propofol 0.5%** IV; may cause respiratory depression, so intubation equipment must be available. Dose: 0.5 to 1.0 mg/kg b.w. IV (followed by continuous infusion at 4–6 mg/kg b.w. per hour as needed, duration of action ~ 5–15 min).

- Sedation with **midazolam** by experienced specialist: 0.1 mg bolus/kg b.w. IV, followed by infusion at 0.1 to 0.2 mg/kg b.w. per hour, onset of action 2 to 3 min, provides 45 to 60 min of sedation.

- Examining radiologist may calm patient. Infants in first months of life may be fed and immobilized in vacuum bag. Other supportive measures: oral sedation with **midazolam juice** (0.4–0.5 mg/kg b.w., duration of action 60–90 min) or

chloral hydrate juice (50–100 mg/kg b.w., duration of action ~ 45–60 min) 20 minutes before imaging. Midazolam can also be administered as intranasal drops in children up to 10 kg b.w.; often acts quickly (10 min) but may cause nasal burning.

Best to have separate examining and sedating physicians (e.g., intensive care specialist, anesthesiologist) for maximum patient safety. "Sine qua non" for all medical sedation of children undergoing MRI: resuscitation equipment and familiarity with pediatric resuscitation.

MRI-compatible ventilator essential, also MRI-compatible monitoring (radio transmission can be used in MRI control room to prevent cable interference with MR examination room).

Monitoring of Children during Sedation

All sedated children require constant monitoring of vital signs; oxygen saturation and heart rate essential (respiratory rate also monitored if needed). All these parameters displayed on modern MRI scanners.

In **first-level controlled operating mode** (see below), additional monitoring of physiologic parameters—even in older children—mandatory (obligatory), owing to higher SAR exposure (SAR = specific absorption rate).

Problem of Lung Evaluation under Sedation

Posterior lung regions hypoventilated in about 40% of sedated children → areas of partial atelectasis that hamper or prevent lung evaluation. Investigation in prone position helps to distinguish atelectasis from pneumonia.

Motion Compensation

Motion compensation essential for imaging structures with physiologic mobility (lung and upper abdomen).

Sequence Architecture

Pediatric examinations require sequences with little motion sensitivity or motion compensation;

e.g., that correct for movements in rotational axis by radial k-space readout (BLADE, PROPELLER sequences [periodically rotated overlapping parallel lines with enhanced reconstruction], etc.).

Note: most of these sequences cannot correct for respiratory (z-axis) motion.

T2-Weighted Single-Shot Sequences (HASTE)

Fast scan times reduce motion artifacts → preferred technique for prenatal imaging (HASTE = half-Fourier acquisition single-shot turbo spin echo).

Respiratory Motion Compensation

Thoracic and abdominal MRI in children require respiratory triggering of sequences so that acquisitions always start in same respiratory position.

With T1-weighted SE (spin-echo) sequences, can greatly prolong scan time because respiratory cycle and T1 acquisition time disproportionate → alternative: pulse triggering alone, at least to eliminate pulsation artifacts.

The technique of respiratory triggering is of minor importance and may be difficult in all methods with shallow breathing:

- Navigator technique: navigator uses diaphragm motion as trigger point for initiating sequence. Relatively simple but susceptible to error due to subjective navigator placement over the diaphragm.
- Respiratory belt triggering: better option in many systems; with slow respiration, best to initiate sequence in early expiration.
- Breath-hold technique with sequential acquisitions: useful only in large children around 10–12 years of age; again, preferred acquisition phase is expiration.

Pulsation Compensation

Pulse triggering can prevent most pulsation artifacts (from large vessels and heart). Combination of pulse and respiratory triggering often leads to excessive scan times → use triggering to eliminate only the artifact expected to be most troublesome.

If pulse triggering omitted: select proper phase-encoding direction to keep pulsation artifacts out of ROI.

Bowel Motion

Helpful to suppress bowel motility with butylscopolamine (e.g., Buscopan, 0.3 mg/kg b.w., max. 20 mg) in abdominal and pelvic examinations, unless contraindicated.

Short half-life → may need to repeat dose after 20 minutes.

SAR Exposure

SAR = rate at which RF energy deposited in body (W/kg b.w.). SAR limits in children regulated by IEC 60601-2-33 standard, which defines three levels of operating modes for MRI:

- **Normal operating mode:** no physiologic stress to patient; suitable routine patient monitoring, not further specified, prescribed.
- **First-level controlled operating mode:** SAR may cause physiologic stress to patient. Change to this mode indicated on unit and must be confirmed by operator → requirement to monitor physiologic parameters (e.g., pulse oximetry).
- **Second-level controlled operating mode:** may pose significant risk to patient (used only in clinical studies with approval of ethics committee; very rarely used in children).

Various reference systems used in describing SAR: whole-body SAR (analogous to effective dose in radiography), partial-body SAR (under transmitter coil), or local SAR (averaged over 10 kg of tissue) (**Table 1.11**).

Imaging in normal mode is desirable, as it does not cause medically significant adverse effects. SAR exposure in children can be reduced by using smaller flip angles, decreasing number of slices, adding intervals between imaging slabs, or increasing TR value (repetition time).

SAR limits also apply to prenatal diagnosis. High SAR values develop near coil in maternal body, so fetal exposure low. Practice on lowest age limit varies—some suggest 18th week of gestation as earliest time for fetal MRI (then organogenesis largely complete). Always weigh risks and benefits. Document that US imaging could not supply desired information—MRI is essential decision-making study (e.g., pregnancy termination? treatment?).

Side Effects

Static Magnetic Field

Dizziness, metallic taste, nausea, tinnitus—actual energy deposition by static magnetic field negligible.

Table 1.11 Radiofrequency exposure limits and specific absorption rate limits for three operating modes of medical MRI[4]

Body region	Normal (W/kg b.w.)	First level controlled (W/kg b.w.)	Second level controlled (W/kg b.w.)
Whole body	2	4	> 4
Partial body	2–10	4–10	> 10
Head	3.2	3.2	> 3.2
Local (trunk)	10	10	> 10
Local (extremities)	10	20	> 20
Temperature rise in torso	0.5°C	1.0°C	> 1.0°C

W/kg b.w. = watts per kilogram body weight.

Radiofrequency Fields

Energy deposited in body by RF fields with changing frequencies (0.1 MHz to 10 GHz). In theory, may cause tissue heating or burns.

! Avoid forming conductive loops (by crossing limbs or contact between skin tissues) → increased risk of burns.

Gradient Fields

Third magnetic field component: low frequencies (30–300 Hz) induce currents that may cause peripheral nerve stimulation (PNS). Myocardial stimulation may also occur. PNS limits for every pulse sequence and gradient system determined in volunteers—normal operating mode may reach no more than 80% of PNS threshold.

Web sites for MRI safety information: www.mri-safety.com and www.ismrm.org.

Small Volumes, Low Signal Intensity

Imaged volumes in children small, and slice thicknesses and voxels must often be smaller than in adults → pediatric examinations do not have same scan times as in adults. Average scan times 1.5 times longer in small children.

General rule of thumb:

- Matrix for typical small field of view in children cannot be arbitrarily increased because selected matrix size and number of voxels must fit small FOV → often smaller matrix size necessary than in adults.
- Conversely, increasing FOV with same matrix yields more signal but only because individual voxel size increases and considerable "air" also sampled → better to reduce matrix size primarily while keeping small FOV.
- Increasing number of acquisitions can compensate for low signal intensity per voxel. Signal to noise ratio ≥ 1. But number of repetitions not linearly proportional to signal yield → more than three repetitive acquisitions not advised, especially due to increased motion artifact.
- Parallel imaging of limited value in children; acceleration factor > 2 rarely attainable with good

image quality and small voxels. With high field strength (3.0 T), however, high signal reserves can shorten imaging time without significant loss of diagnostic quality, especially in T2-weighted sequences.

- Spatial resolution depends on organ and question. Usually should be higher as in adults. Consider using (isotropic) 3D sequences if applicable.

Noise Protection

Changing gradient fields causes significant noise exposure in MRI. Effective sound pressure level of 99 dB or higher requires hearing protection. Headsets and ear plugs difficult to use in infants → better option, viz. temporary adhesive earmuffs (made of disposable material).

Contrast Agents for Bowel and Vascular Imaging, NSF Prevention

Contrast agents are essential for many examinations, but may provide relatively small diagnostic gain. General guidelines for use contrast agents in MRI are set out below.

T1 Contrast Agents

Gd (gadolinium) contrast agents with interstitial distribution pattern = most frequent contrast agents used in pediatric radiology.

Usually administered by intravascular line, occasionally instilled into body cavities or abscess cavities.

Popular contrast agents in traditional or current use:

- Gd-DTPA (diethylene triamine pentaacetic acid) = **Magnevist** (Bayer): a linear, Gd-based agent that belongs to the class which has been attributed a higher risk of nephrogenic systemic fibrosis (NSF, see below), but approved almost universally for children of all ages and for all applications (e.g., magnetic resonance angiography—MRA). Its use is declining in infants and small children—should be carefully considered. Contraindicated in neonates and restricted to minimum recommended dose in infants up to 1 year of age (classified as a "high risk agent" in 2009 by European Medicines Agency—EMA).

Three macrocyclic Gd-based agents available that exhibit higher complex stability belong to group with lower NSF risk, but approval for pediatric use varies in different countries: The U.S. Food and Drug Administration (FDA) classification differentiates T1-contrast agents into high-risk and low-risk agents.

In Europe, a three-stage classification of the NSF risk is used. Three more stable, cyclic T1 contrast agents with lower NSF risk available, but approval for pediatric use varies in different countries:

- Gadubutrol = Gadovist (Bayer)
- Gadoterate Meglumine = Dotarem (Guerbet)
- Gadoteriol = Prohance (Bracco)

In several other regions similar NSF risk classification under discussion and may be implemented in next years. Readers always obliged to inform themselves about approval status and current risk classification of contrast agent in respective country.

T2 Contrast Agents

Iron-containing contrast agents → decreased signal intensity in structures that concentrate iron.

Most familiar: iron uptake in reticuloendothelial system (RES) of healthy liver and healthy lymph nodes. When RES cells replaced by tumor, affected areas appear bright after T2 contrast administration.

To date, not approved for use in children.

Gastrointestinal Contrast Agents

T2-positive and T2-negative bowel contrast agents are in use.

- **T2-positive bowel contrast** with hyperosmolar water or NaCl solutions: methylcellulose, 2.5% mannitol, polyethylene glycol suspension, and many others. Administered by enteroclysis, orally, or by duodenal tube (not usually necessary).
  Can also be used for colon imaging (contrast enema, "MR irrigoscopy") or MR defecography (or with ordinary enema fluid).
- **Negative T2 contrast agents** for stomach and proximal small bowel—recommended for pancreatic imaging and MRCP (magnetic resonance cholangiopancreatography): manganese- or

iron-containing juices (e.g., Mate tea, currant juice, pure pineapple juice).

Contrast Agents for Body Cavities and Fistulas

In principle, duct systems can be visualized on MRI by instillation of sterile water or NaCl solution. Pathology usually associated with perifocal edema → poor results with T2 contrast agents.

T1 contrast agents can delineate duct systems and cavities, but fat suppression also required. Dilute for intrathecal administration.

> Always dilute T1 contrast agents 1 : 100 with distilled water (prevents signal reversal by highly concentrated medium). Off-label use in children → weigh individual risks and benefits.

Intravascular Contrast Agents

Not currently offered or approved for use in children. Example: **Ablavar** (Lantheus).

Nephrogenic Systemic Fibrosis

Isolated cases of NSF reported in children, but only in patients with renal failure. Clinical signs and manifestations of Gd-induced NSF can appear 2 to 3 months to several years after contrast injection—level of knowledge constantly expanding. Possible effects of Gd deposition in pediatric bone marrow uncertain.

Initial symptoms: pain, itching, swelling, erythema. Later: thickening of skin and fibrosis of internal organs.

No treatment options at present → contractures, even cachexia and death → prevention essential, which is sole viable option.

- Renal function assessment (calculated glomerular filtration rate = cGFR), at least in patients with possible overt renal dysfunction.

> Note physiologic immaturity of kidneys in newborns.

- Use Gd-based agents only if they can establish a diagnosis that cannot be made with other modalities (e.g., good-quality, repeatable US scans).
- Keep contrast doses as low as possible (avoid "double dose" in children).

- Avoid repetitive dosing.
- Use agent with high relaxivity.
- Higher field strengths preferred (reduce necessary contrast dose).
- Use agent with lower NSF risk (i.e., macrocyclic compounds, e.g., Dotarem, Gadovist, Prohance), especially in risk patients (renal failure). See also FDA, EMA, or ESUR recommendations. Other measures: correct acidosis, hydrate, seek nephrology consultant.
- Secure written informed consent.

Current guidelines for contrast administration: www.fda.gov and www.ESUR.org.

Special Modalities: 3.0-Tesla Imaging, Whole-Body Magnetic Resonance Imaging

3.0-Tesla Imaging

MRI at 3.0 Tesla (T) is possible without problems even in small children, although SAR burden increases exponentially with magnetic field strength. No problems with (now optimized) sequences in routine imaging except when repetitive GRE (gradient echo) sequences acquired in contrast-enhanced MRA. **First-level controlled operating mode** (see above) occasionally necessary and requires adequate monitoring. SAR can be reduced by decreasing flip angle, acquiring fewer slices, or lengthening TR.

Abdominal imaging at 3.0 T more successful in children than adults: shorter wavelength good match for smaller body size and eliminates typical 3.0 T interference artifacts.

Note on brain imaging: poorer T1-contrast in SE sequences, not a limiting factor in practical operation → unlike 1.5-T imaging, T1-weighted GRE sequences good alternative even in brain with 3.0 T.

Whole-Body Magnetic Resonance Imaging

Does not overcome known limitations of MRI. But, diseases with generalized distribution pattern can be characterized in one examination without radiation exposure.

Applications: neoplastic diseases (Hodgkin lymphoma, Ewing sarcoma, eosinophilic granuloma, etc.), child abuse, virtual autopsy for sudden infant death (**Fig. 1.8**).

Appropriate in children, based on current knowledge: scan whole body with axial and coronal T2 fat-saturated sequences. Then selectively scan regions with unexplained hyperintensity → reduce need for exposure-intensive PET (positron emission tomography) examinations.

> MRI detects more false-positive lesions than PET after chemotherapy. Equivocal findings for rib infiltration.

Bibliography

1 Chavhan GB, Babyn PS. Whole-body MR imaging in children: principles, technique, current applications, and future directions. Radiographics 2011; 31(6): 1757–1772

2 Darge K, Jaramillo D, Siegel MJ. Whole-body MRI in children: current status and future applications. Eur J Radiol 2008; 68(2): 289–298

3 Hirsch W, Sorge I, Krohmer S, Weber D, Meier K, Till H. MRI of the lungs in children. Eur J Radiol 2008; 68(2): 278–288

4 IEC. (2010). Medical electrical equipment—Part 2-33: Particular requirements for the basic safety and essential performance of magnetic resonance equipment for medical diagnosis. (IEC 60601-2-33). Geneva: International Electrotechnical Commission

5 Krauss B, Green SM. Procedural sedation and analgesia in children. Lancet 2006; 367(9512): 766–780

6 Mendichovszky IA, Marks SD, Simcock CM, Olsen OE. Gadolinium and nephrogenic systemic fibrosis: time to tighten practice. Pediatr Radiol 2008; 38(5): 489–496, quiz 602–603

7 Olsen OE. Practical body MRI—A paediatric perspective. Eur J Radiol 2008; 68(2): 299–308

8 Riccabona M. Potential of MR-imaging in the paediatric abdomen. Eur J Radiol 2008; 68(2): 235–244

9 Riccabona M, Olsen OE, Claudon M, Dacher JN, Fotter R. Gadolinium and nephrogenic systemic fibrosis. In: Fotter R. Pediatric Uroradiology, 2nd ed. Berlin, Heidelberg: Springer; 2008

━━━━ **Case Study 1.3** ━━━━

History and clinical presentation: 12-year-old girl with mandibular swelling, identified histologically as chronic granulating inflammation with no signs of malignancy. Patient had sustained minor injury with pain in pelvic region. Inflammatory markers in blood did not support diagnosis of bacterial osteomyelitis → suspicion of chronic recurrent multifocal osteomyelitis (CRMO).
Suitable modalities: skeletal radiographs, scintigraphy, MRI.
Available images: Whole-body MRI (close-up views) and regular focused MRI.

Findings:

a   **T2 TIRM** (turbo inversion recovery magnitude), coronal image (skull and mandible) from whole-body MRI: hyperintense lesions in left mandible (arrow).

b   **T1 TSE**, coronal image (skull and mandible), regular MRI (without contrast): hypointense mass with bone involvement (arrow).

c   **T2 TIRM**, coronal image (abdomen, pelvis and lower limb) from whole-body MRI: hyperintense lesions in right ilium (acetabular roof), left femoral metaphysis and left distal tibial metaphysis (arrows).

d   **T1 TSE**, coronal image (abdomen, pelvis and lower limb), regular MRI (without contrast): bony lesions (arrows). Hypointense to fat-containing bone marrow on unenhanced T1-weighted image.

Whole-body MRI spatial resolution < local MRI, but covers all body regions.
Diagnosis: Chronic recurrent multifocal osteomyelitis (CRMO).

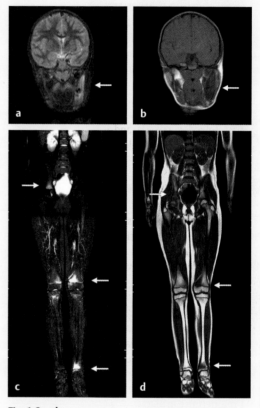

Fig. 1.8a–d

2 Imaging of the Pediatric Chest

2.1 Chest Radiography, Computed Tomography, and Magnetic Resonance Imaging—Lung, Pleura, and Thoracic Cage

Gundula Staatz

Indications

See also Chapter 1.
- Strict selection criteria and child-oriented examination technique; selection of suitable procedures based on Radiation Protection Commission guidelines
- **Chest radiograph** for congenital or acquired thoracic disease: initial examination in one plane. Obtain two planes for suspected tuberculosis (Tb), metastases, cystic fibrosis (CF) scoring, or equivocal findings
- **CT:** dedicated cross-sectional imaging in patients with equivocal pulmonary or thoracic diseases or malignancies
- **MRI:** alternative follow-up method for CF and for tumors of mediastinum or chest wall
- **US:** pleural or pericardial effusion, peripheral pulmonary mass, evaluation of diaphragm motility and mediastinum (early childhood, see Sect. 2.2)

Examination Technique

- **Chest radiograph** with optimum technical factors (1 mm Al +0.1 mm Cu), grid in children > 8 years, 400 to 600 speed film–screen combinations, digital image plates or flat-panel detectors (see Sect. 1.3). Use shutters!
- **Thoracic FL**, inspiratory and expiratory images for suspected foreign body (FB) aspiration, pulsed FL, last image hold (see Sect. 1.3)
- **CT** using low-dose technique (see Sect. 1.5)
- Adherence to **dose reference values** for pediatric examinations (Radiation Protection Agency 2003) (see Sect. 1.2)

- **MRI:** fast T2- and T1-weighted sequences, motion and artifact suppression by sequence selection, respiratory or ECG gating (see Sect. 1.6)
- **US:** high-resolution sector probes (lung) or linear probes (chest wall)

Normal Findings

Normal anatomy varies with age, especially in school-age children:
- At full inspiration, diaphragm leaflets are at level of posterior 8th and 9th ribs on right side
- Lungs more radiolucent than in adults due to smaller thoracic diameter (**Fig. 2.1**)
- Air bronchogram in cardiac silhouette: normal finding in newborns
- Cardiothoracic ratio up to 65%: normal in children < 2 years old

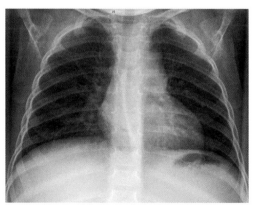

Fig. 2.1 Normal findings in small children. Radiolucent lung and mediastinal widening due to prominent thymus.

- Frequent mediastinal widening due to thymus (no tracheal narrowing!)
- Bowing of trachea in expiration

Stridor

Definition: abnormal breath sound due to obstruction of larynx or tracheobronchial tree. Stridor may be inspiratory or expiratory.

Causes:

- Inspiratory stridor usually due to extrathoracic airway obstruction (pharyngeal, supraglottic, or subglottic level)
- Expiratory stridor may result from intrathoracic tracheal narrowing or narrowing of small airways (bronchi)
- Most frequent cause of inspiratory stridor in infants = laryngomalacia (soft epiglottis)
- Other causes of stridor (see below): tracheomalacia, infection (croup, tracheobronchitis), FB aspiration, and tracheal stenosis due to vascular compression or mass

Imaging:

- Functional disorders usually diagnosed clinically or endoscopically
- Suspicion of extrinsic tracheal compression by vessel or mass: chest radiograph followed by cross-sectional imaging

Tracheal Stenosis

Tracheal stenosis most often results from cervicothoracic anomalies. Cardinal symptom: stridor or respiratory failure. Initial study for neck imaging: US. Further cervical and thoracic imaging → low-dose CT (**Fig. 2.2a**) or MRI.

Intrinsic tracheal stenosis:

- Primary tracheal stenosis, e.g., due to branch anomaly or cartilage rings
- Tracheal wall hemangioma, cyst, or web

Extrinsic tracheal stenosis:

- Mass (lymphangioma, lymphoma, bronchogenic cyst, etc.)
- Extrinsic vascular compression, e.g., by aortic arch anomaly (**Fig. 2.2**), aberrant brachiocephal-

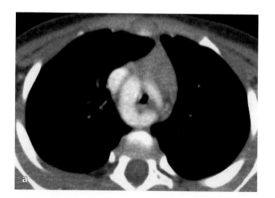

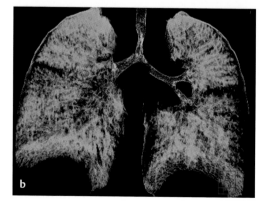

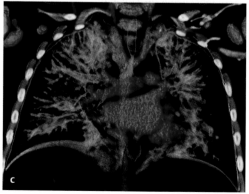

Fig. 2.2a–c Tracheal compression by double aortic arch. Contrast-enhanced low-dose CT (**a**) and virtual bronchographic images without (**b**) and with (**c**) vascular reconstruction show narrowing of trachea by duplicated, circumflex aortic arch.

ic trunk, pulmonary sling, etc. (see Sect. 2.2 and 2.3)

- Postoperative scarring after repair of esophageal atresia

> Suspected vascular compression of tracheobronchial tree → contrast-enhanced (spiral) CT acquisitions in arterial inflow phase (or MRA). Multiplanar reformatting and virtual bronchographic images are very helpful (**Fig. 2.2b, c**).

Malformations of the Tracheobronchial Tree

Heterogeneous group of various congenital malformations. Most common anomalies: branch anomalies, congenital lobar emphysema, bronchogenic cyst, congenital cystic adenomatoid malformation (CCAM), pulmonary sequestration. Usually diagnosed prenatally by fetal US and MRI. Summarized as "foregut malformations."

Congenital Lobar Emphysema

Definition: progressive, irreversible hyperinflation of a pulmonary lobe without destruction of alveolar septa.
Etiology: congenital bronchial stenosis due to bronchial cartilage anomaly, endobronchial obstruction, or bronchial compression. Most common site of occurrence: left upper lobe.
Clinical features: cardinal symptom = diminished breath sounds, cough, dyspnea, expiratory wheeze, intermittent cyanosis.
Imaging:
- Diagnosis: chest radiographs and CT
- Homogeneous opacity in first days of life due to amniotic fluid filling
- Increased lucency of affected lung zone (**Fig. 2.3**)
- Pulmonary herniation and mediastinal shift to opposite side; atelectasis of adjacent lobes
- Depression of ipsilateral hemidiaphragm

DD: pneumothorax, bronchial atresia, pneumatocele, CCAM.

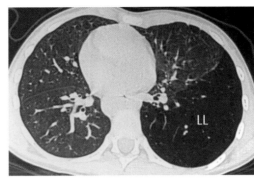

Fig. 2.3 Congenital lobar emphysema. Thoracic CT (lung window) shows marked hyperinflation of left lower lobe (LL). Other findings: areas of mild compression atelectasis in left upper lobe and mediastinal shift to right. (Source: Staatz G. Direct Diagnosis in Radiology: Pediatric Imaging. Stuttgart: Thieme; 2008.)

Bronchogenic Cyst

Definition: cavity lined with respiratory epithelium plus cartilaginous, muscular, and glandular tissue elements in the cyst wall.
Etiology: disturbance of bronchial branching due to abnormal budding of foregut in utero.
Clinical features: often detected incidentally. Compression of trachea and bronchi → possible cough, stridor, dyspnea. Inflammatory symptoms due to superinfection or secondary pneumonia.
Imaging:
- Diagnosis: chest radiographs and CT/MRI
- Location: mediastinal (85%) or in lung parenchyma (15%); often near carina
- Filled with fluid and/or air (**Fig. 2.4**)
- Valve mechanism: hyperinflation of affected lung, contralateral mediastinal shift

DD: gastroenteric cyst, esophageal duplication, neuroenteric cyst, CCAM, pneumatocele, lung abscess.

> Cyst contents may have variable density on CT and MRI. Contrast enhancement of cyst wall suggests superinfection.

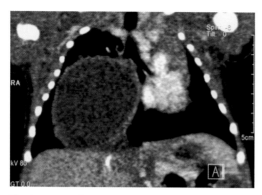

Fig. 2.4   Bronchogenic cyst in 1-day-old newborn.
Coronal reformatted image from low-dose CT shows fluid-filled bronchogenic cyst adjacent to the tracheal bifurcation.

Congenital Cystic Adenomatoid Malformation

Definition and etiology: congenital lung anomaly. A multicystic mass develops in fetal life due to adenomatoid proliferation of bronchioles.
Clinical features: may be asymptomatic or present with respiratory distress and cyanosis, depending on extent. Recurrent pulmonary infections.
Imaging:
- Diagnosis: US/MRI; occasionally low-dose CT
- In utero: polyhydramnios, pulmonary hypoplasia, fetal ascites
- Associated renal, cardiac, intestinal, and skeletal anomalies
- Cystic mass, sometimes with air–fluid level
- Generally unilateral (95%); findings vary with cyst type and morphology:
  – Type I: cyst diameter > 2 cm (50%)
  – Type II: cyst diameter < 2 cm (40%)
  – Type III: solid form with microcysts (10%)

DD: pneumatocele, bronchogenic cyst, sequestration, diaphragmatic hernia, cavitary necrosis in pneumonia, lung abscess.

> Malignant transformation (rhabdomyosarcoma) may occur.

Pulmonary Sequestration

Definition: nonfunctioning lung tissue that does not communicate with tracheobronchial tree; has systemic arterial blood supply.

Classification:
- Intralobar form (within visceral pleura): usually affects posterobasal lower lobe, more common in left lung (**Fig. 2.5**). Usually derives arterial supply from thoracic aorta, less commonly from abdominal aorta. Drained by pulmonary veins.
- Extralobar form (has separate pleura): most common on left side between lower lobe and diaphragm. Arterial supply from systemic circulation, drained by systemic veins (inferior vena cava [IVC], azygos vein).

Clinical features: asymptomatic or recurrent episodes of bronchopneumonia.
Imaging:
- Prenatal: US/MRI; initial postnatal studies: chest radiograph and color Doppler ultrasound (CDU)
- Further sectional imaging: MRA, occasionally CTA
- Constant, homogeneous opacity on chest radiograph; air–fluid level indicates infection
- US usually shows hyperechoic mass
- CDU or MRA/CTA defines feeding and draining systemic vessels

DD: cavitary necrosis in pneumonia, lung abscess, arteriovenous fistula (AVF).

Neonatal Lung Diseases Requiring Intensive Care

Transient Neonatal Tachypnea (Wet Lung)

Definition and etiology: delayed absorption of fetal lung fluid, as in newborns delivered by cesarean section.
Clinical features: tachypnea and dyspnea.
Imaging:
- Increased, symmetrical perihilar interstitial markings with diffuse haziness in both lungs (**Fig. 2.6**)
- Hyperinflation of both lungs, occasionally with mottled pattern
- Regresses within 12 to 24 hours

DD: respiratory distress syndrome, perinatal pneumonia, patent ductus arteriosus (PDA).

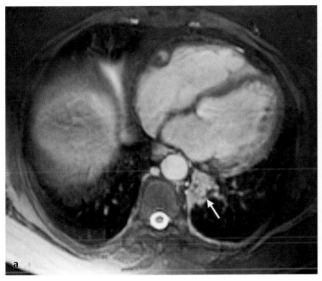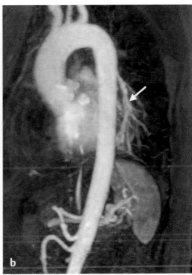

Fig. 2.5a, b   Pulmonary sequestration. (Source: Staatz G. Direct Diagnosis in Radiology: Pediatric Imaging. Stuttgart: Thieme; 2008.)

a MRI (axial gradient-echo sequence). Sequestered segment appears as a hyperintense mass (arrow) at a typical site in the left lower lobe.

b MRI (maximum intensity projection [MIP], contrast-enhanced 3D MRA) shows a rich arterial blood supply to the sequestrum (arrow), in this case via the left coronary artery (origin not visible on MIP).

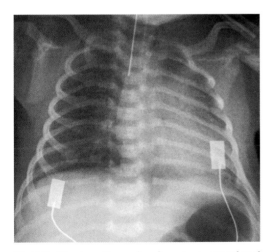

Fig. 2.6   Chest radiograph of mature, ventilated newborn several hours after cesarean delivery. shows diffuse haziness of both lungs due to transient neonatal tachypnea (wet lung). Endotracheal tube, ECG leads.

Neonatal Pneumonia

Definition: any pneumonia acquired in utero or during perinatal or postpartum period.

Etiology: bacterial or viral infection, e.g., due to chorioamnionitis or aspiration of infected amniotic fluid.

Main causative organisms: B-streptococci, staphylococci, *Escherichia coli, Klebsiella* spp., *Pseudomonas*, pneumococci, herpes virus, varicella, respiratory syncytial virus (RSV), adenovirus.

Clinical features: mild inflammatory signs and tachydyspnea, ranging to septic shock with disseminated intravascular coagulation.

Imaging: highly variable findings, often nonspecific. Most cases show increased interstitial lung markings (**Fig. 2.7**) and secondary hyperinflation of noninfiltrated lung areas.

- **B streptococci:** reticulogranular pattern (preterm infants); patchy, confluent opacities; lobar or segmental infiltration; hyperinflation of noninfiltrated areas; cardiomegaly (toxic)

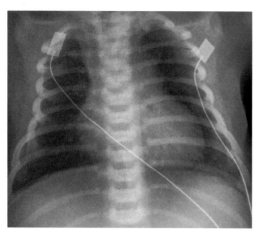

Fig. 2.7   Chest radiograph of septic newborn shows pulmonary hyperinflation and increased, predominantly central perihilar streaks in neonatal pneumonia. ECG leads.

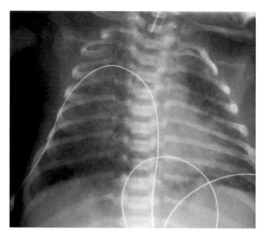

Fig. 2.8   Meconium aspiration syndrome. AP chest radiograph in newborn shows patchy, partially confluent opacities due to meconium aspiration. (Source: Staatz G: Direct Diagnosis in Radiology: Pediatric Imaging. Stuttgart: Thieme; 2008). Endotracheal tubes, lead wires.

- **Staphylococci:** fulminating form with coarse alveolar opacities; infiltrates may coalesce and liquefy; pneumatocele formation

DD: transient tachypnea (wet lung), respiratory distress syndrome, meconium aspiration.

Meconium Aspiration

Definition: aspirating mixture of meconium and amniotic fluid, most common in full-term or post-term infants.

Etiology: intrauterine or intrapartum hypoxia → reflex passage of meconium. Aspirated meconium → obstructs bronchioles, culminating in chemical pneumonitis.

Clinical features: depend on degree of asphyxia → respiratory failure, stridor, cyanosis, bradycardia, shock symptoms.

Imaging:

- Dense, patchy, partially confluent opacities surrounded by cystic lucent zones (**Fig. 2.8**)
- Generally resolves in 2 to 3 days unless infection supervenes

Complication: superinfection, alveolar ruptures occur in aspirate-free lung areas; development of pulmonary interstitial emphysema, pneumothorax, pneumomediastinum.

DD: perinatal pneumonia, pulmonary hemorrhage, congenital pulmonary lymphangiectasia.

Respiratory Distress Syndrome

Definition: functional pulmonary immaturity based on primary surfactant deficiency in preterm infants (< 36 weeks gestation). Synonym: **idiopathic respiratory distress syndrom**e (IRDS).

Etiology: decreased phospholipid synthesis in alveolar type II cells, alveolar instability, secondary alveolar collapse during expiration.

Clinical features: respiratory failure, diminished breath sounds, cyanosis, expiratory stridor, tachypnea.

Imaging: chest radiographs; US in rare cases. Four grades of severity/stages are distinguished based on radiographic findings:

- Grade I: diffuse lung haziness with reticulogranular pattern
- Grade II: above findings plus air bronchogram that transcends cardiac borders
- Grade III: indistinct outlines of heart, mediastinum, and diaphragm (**Fig. 2.9**)
- Grade IV: white lung = homogeneous opacity with no discernible cardiac or mediastinal shadows

DD: transient tachypnea (wet lung), perinatal pneumonia, pulmonary hemorrhage.

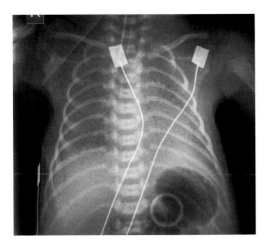

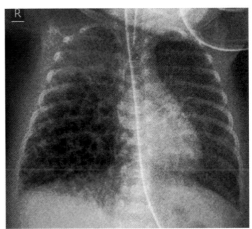

Fig. 2.9 Grades III–IV respiratory distress syndrome in a ventilated preterm infant. Chest radiograph shows diffuse, fine reticulogranular pattern in both lungs with poor delineation of cardiac and mediastinal shadows. Endotracheal tubes, ECG leads, CO_2 sensor.

Fig. 2.10 Pulmonary interstitial emphysema of right lower lobe in small ventilated newborn. Cystlike lucencies, some with bubbly appearance, visible in right lower lobe. Endotracheal tubes, stomach tube.

Barotrauma

Complication of mechanical ventilation with positive end-expiratory pressure (PEEP). Leads to abnormal extra-alveolar air collections → pulmonary interstitial emphysema (PIE), pneumothorax, pneumomediastinum, pneumopericardium, systemic intravascular air embolism, pneumoperitoneum.

Pulmonary Interstitial Emphysema

Most frequent complication of mechanical ventilation, occurs in 30 to 40% of all ventilated preterm infants.

Imaging:
- Alveolar overexpansion: chest radiograph shows round lucencies up to 1.5 mm in diameter
- After rupture of multiple alveoli: diffusely distributed, cystlike, or meandering lucencies in interstitium, about 2 mm in diameter (**Fig. 2.10**)
- Larger pseudocysts may develop over time (first week of life)
- Complications due to pneumothorax, pneumomediastinum, pneumopericardium, pneumoperitoneum, air embolism

Pneumothorax, Pneumomediastinum, Pneumoperitoneum

- Pneumothorax: air collection between parietal and visceral pleural layers; lateral or laterobasal location, most common in pediatric ICU patients
- Pneumomediastinum: air collection usually in upper anterior mediastinum, causing elevation of thymus (spinnaker sign); other possible sites: inferior pulmonary ligament, infra-azygos region, between heart and diaphragm
- Pneumoperitoneum: spread of primary intrathoracic air into peritoneal cavity through openings in diaphragm

> An anterior pneumothorax sometimes is manifested only by increased lucency of affected lung and sharp delineation of cardiac border. DD: Mach band effect—artifact due to edge enhancement by digital image processing filters.

Bronchopulmonary Dysplasia = Long-Term Effects of Neonatal Lung Disease

Definition: chronic lung disease caused by mechanical ventilation at high pressure and high inspiratory oxygen concentration (> 21%) for at least 28 days.
Etiology: barotrauma, oxygen toxicity, other risk factors—lead to bronchoalveolar and intrapulmonary inflammatory reactions → interstitial pulmo-

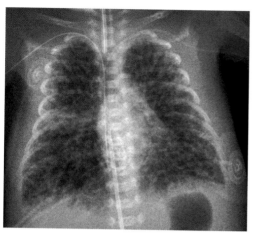

Fig. 2.11   Bronchopulmonary dysplasia in preterm infant on long-term ventilation. Chest radiograph shows massive hyperinflation along with diffuse, bubbly pseudocystic lung lucencies and increased linear and reticular markings (fibrosis). Endotracheal tubes, central venous catheter.

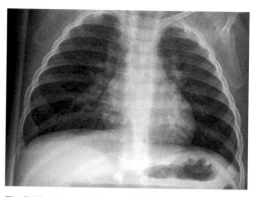

Fig. 2.12   Bronchitis in small child. Radiograph shows increased peribronchial bronchitic markings at center of both lungs and enlarged hila consistent with reactive hilar lymphadenopathy due to infection.

nary edema, necrosis of bronchial mucosa and alveoli, epithelial metaplasia, focal fibrosis, structural changes of intima/media and mostly peripheral pulmonary arteries (PAs).

Clinical features: tachydyspnea, cyanosis, obstructive apnea, signs of pulmonary hypertension with right-heart overload. Later: recurrent lung infections, susceptibility to obstructive bronchitis.

Imaging: Chest radiograph demonstrates stages of progression:

- Diffuse lung haziness with reticulogranular pattern, positive air bronchogram
- Complete opacification of both lungs
- Diffuse, bubbly, pseudocystic lung lucencies (sponge pattern, **Fig. 2.11**)
- Concomitant coarse perihilar opacities (fibrosis), cardiomegaly
- Late finding on HRCT: regional hyperinflation of pseudocystic areas, thickening of intralobar septa (linear and reticular opacities), zones of subsegmental atelectasis, pulmonary fibrosis

DD: respiratory distress syndrome (stage I), PDA, pneumonia, congenital lymphangiectasia, anomalous pulmonary venous drainage.

Diseases of the Bronchi and Small Airways

Bronchitis

Definition and etiology: inflammatory disease of bronchi caused by viral infection (RSV, parainfluenza virus, rhinovirus, etc.).

Clinical features: rhinitis, pharyngitis, cough, dyspnea.

Imaging: chest radiograph.

- Thickened bronchial walls, increased peribronchial markings
- Reactive hilar lymph node enlargement due to infection (**Fig. 2.12**)

DD: bronchopneumonia.

(Early) Childhood Asthma

Definition: chronic inflammation of the lower airways, characterized by recurrent bronchiolitis, reversible bronchial obstruction, bronchial hyperreactivity.

Etiology: extrinsic (allergic/atopic) or intrinsic (no atopy).

Clinical features: persistent cough, expiratory wheeze, inspiratory dyspnea.

Imaging:

- Chest radiograph (for exclusion of complications and other causes of pulmonary symptoms): hyperinflation (**Fig. 2.13**), bronchial wall thickening, increased peribronchial or interstitial markings
- HRCT: hyperinflation (air trapping), mosaic perfusion pattern, bronchial wall thickening, atelectasis
  - especially of middle lobes, central bronchiectasis, sites of mucoid impaction (older patients)

DD: FB aspiration, cystic fibrosis, ciliary dyskinesia, GER.

Bronchiolitis

Definition and etiology:

- Bronchiolitis: inflammatory disease of bronchioles in children < 2 years caused by infection with RSV, adenovirus, or parainfluenza virus
- Bronchiolitis obliterans: necrotizing, fibrosing bronchiolitis leading to obliteration of the bronchioles, especially after cardiac or bone-marrow transplantation. Special form: Swyer–James–McLeod syndrome = unilateral postinfectious bronchiolitis obliterans
- Bronchiolitis obliterans organizing pneumonia (BOOP): granulation tissue and fibrin-rich exudate in lumen of bronchioles, spreading to alveoli

Clinical features: dyspnea, cyanosis, expiratory wheeze.

Imaging:

- **Chest radiograph:** hyperinflation, atelectasis, bronchial wall thickening, streaky perihilar opacities and infiltrates, hilar lymphadenopathy
- **HRCT** in small airways disease (**Fig. 2.14**): air trapping, mosaic perfusion, ground-glass opacity, centrilobar nodules, bronchial wall thickening, central or peripheral bronchiectasis, sites of mucoid impaction

> Swyer–James–McLeod syndrome = unilateral small or normal-sized hyperlucent lung.

DD: bronchopneumonia, cystic fibrosis.

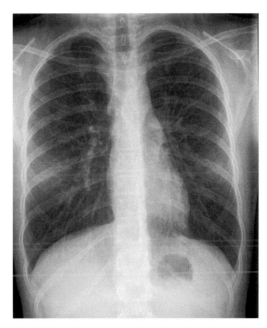

Fig. 2.13 Asthma in adolescent male. Chest radiograph shows marked hyperinflation and predominantly central thickening of bronchial walls.

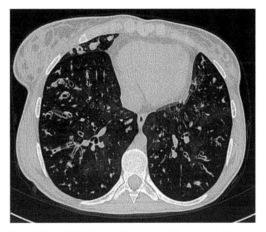

Fig. 2.14 HRCT in small airways disease. Axial scan shows patchy mosaic perfusion pattern, areas of bronchiectasis, and peripheral mucoid impactions.

Pneumonias

Inflammatory lung disease that may involve the alveolar spaces and interstitium. Hematogenous infection in newborns. Pneumonia in older children is usually due to inhalation or aspiration of infectious organisms.

Bronchopneumonia

Definition and etiology: viral pneumonia with diffuse interstitial involvement and secondary alveolar involvement. Starts in perihilar region and spreads peripherally. Age-dependent spectrum of causative organisms; most common pathogens are RSV and enteroviruses.

Clinical features: tachypnea, cough, obstruction with expiratory wheeze.

Imaging: chest radiograph.

- Initial findings: increased streaky peribronchial markings (infiltrates, **Fig. 2.15**), bihilar lymphadenopathy, predominantly laterobasal hyperinflation
- Later: increased focal (alveolar) markings, areas of dystelectasis and infiltration

DD: bronchitis, cystic fibrosis, ciliary dyskinesia.

Lobar Pneumonia

Definition and etiology: bacterial pneumonia involving the alveoli of one pulmonary lobe or segment. Main causative organism = *Streptococcus pneumoniae*. Less common: *Haemophilus influenzae*, mycoplasma pneumonia, *Chlamydia pneumoniae*, *Staphylococcus aureus*.

Clinical features: dyspnea, cyanosis, labored breathing, fever, cough.

Imaging:

- **Chest radiograph:** partially confluent alveolar opacities, homogeneous segmental or lobar opacities (**Fig. 2.16**), positive air bronchogram; may also have a globular appearance and mimic a mass ("round pneumonia"). Increased volume of affected pulmonary lobe with displacement of adjacent interlobar fissure; possible concomitant pleural effusion (see below)
- **US:** hypoechoic, liverlike area in air-filled lung

> Pneumatoceles may develop after staphylococcal pneumonia.

DD: pulmonary sequestration, mass.

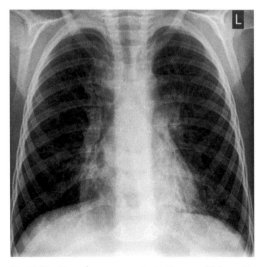

Fig. 2.15 Bronchopneumonia in 5-year-old boy. Bilateral, predominantly central, streaky peribronchial infiltrates extend into lower lung zones, accompanied by bihilar lymphadenopathy.

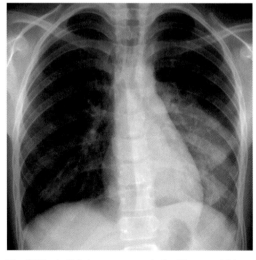

Fig. 2.16 Left lobar pneumonia in 12-year-old boy. Chest radiograph shows patchy, homogeneous opacity in left lower lobe due to pneumococcal infection.

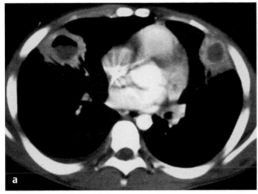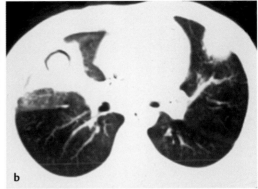

Fig. 2.17a, b   Invasive aspergillosis in immunosuppressed patient with acute lymphoblastic leukemia.

a Postcontrast CT with soft-tissue window.

b Postcontrast CT with lung window. Scans show bilateral wedge-shaped opacities based on pleura (infarctions) with central liquefaction and typical air crescent on right side.

Opportunistic Infections in Immunosuppressed Patients

Etiology: opportunistic infections in immunosuppressed children, usually caused by *Aspergillus* and *Candida* species, *Pneumocystis carinii*, and cytomegalovirus (CMV).

Clinical features: cough, fever, sepsis.

Imaging: initial imaging study is chest radiography, supplemented by CT.

- **Invasive mycosis:** increased bronchopneumonic markings, rounded or oval infiltrates, wedge-shaped opacities based on pleura (infarctions), air crescent sign (**Fig. 2.17**), pleural effusion. Halo sign on CT: focus surrounded by narrow, hypoattenuating rim (hemorrhagic necrosis)

> HRCT is very sensitive for suspected pulmonary mycosis owing to early detection of small infiltrates and foci of liquefaction.

- ***Pneumocystis carinii:*** symmetrical haziness predominantly affecting the lower and middle lung zones, increased reticular interstitial markings Interstitial emphysema may develop later; end stage = "white" lung with bilateral lung haziness
- **CMV:** multiple disseminated pulmonary nodules, bronchial wall thickening, infiltrates; mild pleural effusion

Complications

Pleural Effusion and Pleural Empyema

Definition: fluid in the space between the pleural layers. Purulent effusion = empyema.

Etiology: effusion may have an inflammatory, cardiac, neoplastic, or traumatic cause. Empyema often caused by *Staphylococcus aureus* and pneumococci.

Clinical features: respiration-dependent chest pain, dyspnea, cough. Empyema: elevated inflammatory markers and general malaise.

Imaging: chest radiograph, CT, US.

- Shadowing of the costophrenic angle ranging to complete opacification of one hemithorax
- Massive effusion: contralateral mediastinal shift, compression atelectasis (**Fig. 2.18**)
- Empyema: contrast enhancement and thickening of the pleura; possible septations within effusion
- US: echo-free fluid in pleural space and/or beneath the lung; empyema shows increasing internal echoes and septations with associated pleural thickening

> (US) follow-ups consist of standard examinations in sitting position, for example (septation of pleural empyema often not visible on CT scans).

DD: pleural tumors.

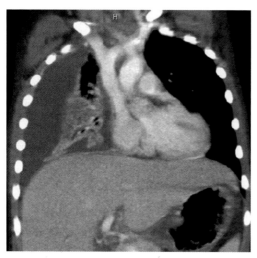

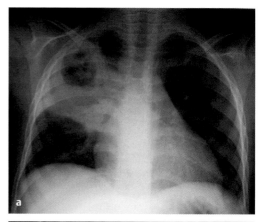

Fig. 2.18   Pleural empyema in right lung of 5-year-old girl with pneumococcal pneumonia. Coronal reformatted image in contrast-enhanced CT shows massive right-sided effusion with contralateral mediastinal shift and almost complete atelectasis of right lung. (Note: Emypema assessment can also be achieved by thoracic US [radiation protection!]; US is better to visualize small septae, may be also used for guiding drainage.)

Cavitary Necrosis

Definition: air- and fluid-filled areas in pneumonic lung without associated wall thickening.

Etiology: thromboembolic occlusion of alveolar capillaries with surrounding inflammatory reaction → ischemia and necrosis of lung parenchyma.

Clinical features: persistent signs of pneumonia with little response to antibiotics.

Imaging: radiographs and CT (**Fig. 2.19**).

- Detection of multiple lucencies in consolidated pneumonic infiltrates
- CT shows thin-walled cavities filled with air or air–fluid mixture. Contrast enhancement decreased in affected lung area

DD: CCAM, pulmonary abscess, Tb, Wegener granulomatosis.

Pulmonary Abscess

Definition: intrapulmonary air- and fluid-filled cavity or purulent collection with a thick wall.

Etiology: main causative organism is *Staphylococcus aureus*.

Clinical features: high inflammatory markers, malaise, shortness of breath.

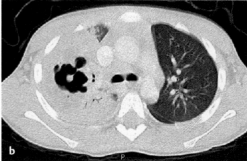

Fig. 2.19a, b   Cavitary necrosis in 6-year-old boy with right upper lobar pneumonia. a Chest radiograph shows rounded lucencies within patchy area of pneumonic consolidation. **b** Axial CT shows corresponding thin-walled air-filled cavities.

Imaging: chest radiograph, sometimes US, usually CT, occasionally MRI.

- Air- and fluid-filled cavity with thick, enhancing wall in preexisting area of consolidated pneumonia.

DD: CCAM, pulmonary sequestration, cavitary necrosis.

Recurrent Infections

Immune status should be investigated in children with recurrent infections. If chest radiograph does not show resolution of pulmonary findings with appropriate therapy → (HR) CT is indicated to confirm or exclude a tracheobronchial anomaly or small airways disease (e.g., allergic alveolitis).

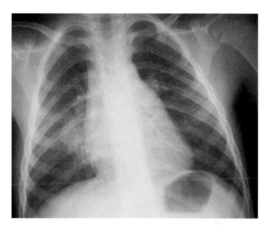

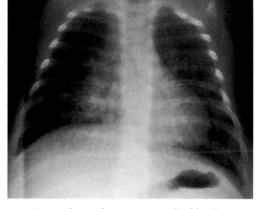

Fig. 2.20   Hilar lymph node tuberculosis in small child. Chest radiograph shows hilar scalloping and enlargement, more pronounced on right side than left, in tuberculous lymphadenitis.

Fig. 2.21   Miliary Tb in a 6-month-old infant. AP chest radiograph shows disseminated micronodular foci in both lungs. Hilar lymph node enlargement more pronounced on right side. (Source: Staatz G: Direct Diagnosis in Radiology: Pediatric Imaging. Stuttgart: Thieme; 2008.)

Pulmonary Tuberculosis

Definition: infection with *Mycobacterium tuberculosis.*

Etiology:

- **Primary Tb** (children): aspiration of bacteria, formation of an inflammatory primary complex (lung parenchyma and hilum). Lymphogenous and hematogenous spread via thoracic duct to the lung (miliary Tb) and whole body may occur in immunosuppressed patients, infants, and small children
- **Postprimary Tb** (adolescents and adults): reactivation of tuberculous foci or reinfection: generalized and organ stage

Clinical features:

- Primary Tb: usually subclinical; mild signs of infection
- Postprimary Tb: night sweats, weight loss, chills, fever, cough, hemoptysis, lymph node swelling

Imaging: chest radiograph, CT, US.

- **Chest radiograph in primary Tb:** isolated infiltrate (midzone), (ipsilateral) hilar lymphadenopathy (**Fig. 2.20**), pleural effusion; primary progressive pneumonia with liquefying infiltrates and massive lymph node swelling
  Fine nodular pattern in miliary Tb (**Fig. 2.21**)

- **Chest radiograph in postprimary Tb:**
  - Exudative stage with infiltrates mainly in upper lobe and apical lower lobe
  - Cavitating stage with thin-walled air-filled cavities within infiltrates
  - Fibrocirrhotic stage with plaque formation, parenchymal opacities due to scarring, and hilar retraction. Later, possible bullous emphysema, bronchiectasis, and loss of lung volume

> Suspected pulmonary Tb → chest radiographs in two planes (hilar evaluation).

- **CT in primary Tb:** analogous to radiographic findings; very sensitive for detecting lymph node enlargement, liquefaction, and calcifications
  Miliary Tb: multiple well-circumscribed intrapulmonary nodules
- **CT in postprimary Tb:** infiltrates, cavities, hilar lymphadenopathy
- **US:** detection and quantification of pleural effusion

DD: pneumonia due to other causes, fungal infection, lymphoma, sarcoidosis, Wegener granulomatosis.

Cystic Fibrosis

Definition and etiology: autosomal recessive genetic defect involving chromosome 7 (cystic fibrosis transmembrane conductance regulator—CFTR). Most common congenital metabolic disease with incidence of 1:2,500. Abnormal chloride transport. Formation of thick, highly viscous glandular secretions. Multiorgan disease with predilection for lung, pancreas, bowel, and liver.

Clinical features: often manifested initially in GI tract (e.g., meconium ileus); recurrent pulmonary infections, obstruction, failure to thrive, sinusitis, gallstones, pancreatic failure, hepatic cirrhosis.

Imaging: chest radiograph, CT. Increasing use of MRI (follow-up).

- **Chest radiograph in early stage:** lung normal or hyperinflated; thickening of bronchial walls
- **Chest radiograph in intermediate stage:** increasing hyperinflation, increased peribronchial markings, infiltrates, atelectasis, bronchiectasis (chiefly in upper lobe), mucus plugging, bihilar lymphadenopathy

- **Chest radiograph in late stage:** pulmonary fibrosis, pronounced foci of cystic bronchiectasis Complications: pneumothorax, hemoptysis (**Fig. 2.22**), pulmonary hypertension and cor pulmonale (right ventricular [RV] hypertrophy)

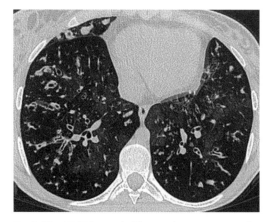

Fig. 2.23 HRCT in cystic fibrosis shows mosaic perfusion, bronchial wall thickening, and sites of bronchiectasis and mucus plugging.

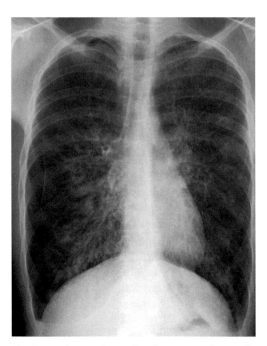

Fig. 2.22 Chest radiograph in late stage of cystic fibrosis: hyperinflation, pulmonary fibrosis, bronchiectasis, and bihilar lymphadenopathy, complicated by right peripheral pneumothorax.

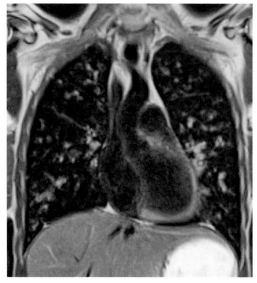

Fig. 2.24 Coronal T2-weighted MRI in cystic fibrosis shows hyperintense mucus plugging and thick-walled areas of bronchiectasis.

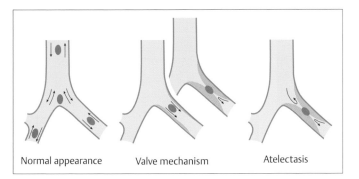

Fig. 2.25 Effects of foreign body aspiration. Appearance varies with size and location of foreign body.

Normal appearance   Valve mechanism   Atelectasis

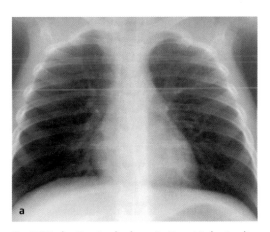

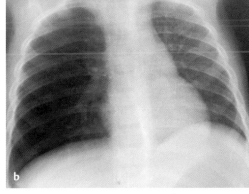

Fig. 2.26a, b   Foreign body aspiration. AP chest radiographs. Spot views under FL control in inspiration (**a**) and expiration (**b**) show marked overinflation of right lung with contralateral mediastinal shifting and paradoxical diaphragm motion on expiration. A peanut had been aspirated into right main bronchus, creating a valve mechanism (Source: Staatz G. Direct Diagnosis in Radiology: Pediatric Imaging. Stuttgart: Thieme; 2008.)

- **HRCT/MRI:** mosaic perfusion, bronchial wall thickening, bronchiectasis (**Figs. 2.23** and **2.24**), mucus plugging, centrilobular nodules ("tree in bud" appearance), consolidation/infiltrates
DD: asthma, ciliary dyskinesia.

Bronchiectasis

Definition and etiology: irreversible dilatation of the bronchial tree. Cylindrical, saccular, and tubular (varicose) forms.

  Clinical features: cough, sputum production.
  Imaging: chest radiograph, HRCT (MRI).
- Bronchial diameter > diameter of adjacent PA (**Fig. 2.23**)
- Bronchial wall thickening and visualization of a bronchus in lung periphery
- Mucus plugging, mosaic perfusion

Foreign Body Aspiration

Definition: inhalation of a FB (e.g., peanut, piece of carrot, toy part) into the tracheobronchial tree.
Clinical features: cough, dyspnea, cyanosis, fever, stridor.
Imaging:
- **Chest radiographs** in inspiration and expiration: obstructive emphysema/hyperinflated lung area, asymmetrical lung lucency, atelectasis
- **FL** (**Figs. 2.25** and **2.26**): valve mechanism, mediastinal flutter (toward healthy side in expiration), paradoxical diaphragm motion (may also be detectable by US)
- **CT/MRI** used only in exceptional cases, demonstrate late sequelae (bronchiectasis, bronchiolitis obliterans)
DD: asthma, bronchiolitis, tracheal stenosis.

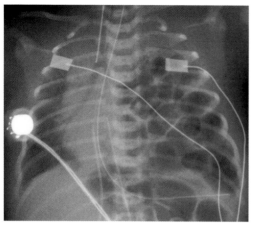

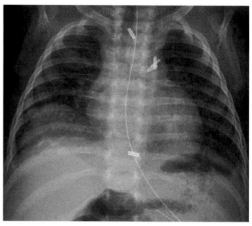

Fig. 2.27   Large, left-sided congenital diaphragmatic hernia in a newborn. AP chest radiograph. Herniated bowel loops have led to pulmonary hypoplasia on left side and mediastinal shift to right side. (Source: Staatz G: Direct Diagnosis in Radiology: Pediatric Imaging. Stuttgart: Thieme; 2008.) Endotracheal tubes, stomach tube, umbilical vein catheter, ECG leads.

Fig. 2.28   Postoperative elevation of right hemi-diaphragm (after cardiac surgery) due to diaphragmatic palsy. Stomach tube, surgical clips.

Diaphragmatic Disorders

Diaphragmatic Hernia

Definition and etiology: herniation of abdominal contents into chest cavity through a congenital or acquired opening in the diaphragm → hiatal hernia (hernial opening: esophageal hiatus), Bochdalek hernia (lumbocostal), Morgagni hernia (anterior parasternal).

Clinical features: congenital diaphragmatic hernia and pulmonary hypoplasia present with respiratory failure. Later: pressure sensation, pain, dyspnea, tachycardia, reflux disease.

Imaging:

- **Chest radiograph:** intrathoracic opacity or, with enterothorax, cystlike areas of air density within the chest (**Fig. 2.27**)

  With pulmonary hypoplasia: include upper abdomen in radiographs!

- **US:** median/paramedian longitudinal scan and subxiphoid transverse scan show intrathoracic abdominal organs and a discontinuity in the diaphragm

DD: relaxation of diaphragm, CCAM.

Diaphragmatic Palsy

Definition: absence or weakness of diaphragmatic motion.

Etiology: congenital or acquired (posttraumatic) phrenic nerve palsy.

Clinical features: paradoxical respiratory pattern.

Imaging:

- **Chest radiograph:** elevation of the diaphragm (**Fig. 2.28**)
- **US:** absent or diminished diaphragm motion; reduced, absent or paradoxical amplitudes of diaphragm motion in M-mode trace. Transverse scan shows greater distance from probe to diaphragmatic line on affected side

DD: relaxation of diaphragm, diaphragmatic hernia.

Bibliography

1 Agrons GA, Courtney SE, Stocker JT, Markowitz RI. From the archives of the AFIP: Lung disease in premature neonates: radiologic-pathologic correlation. Radiographics 2005; 25(4): 1047–1073

2 Berrocal T, Madrid C, Novo S, Gutiérrez J, Arjonilla A, Gómez-León N. Congenital anomalies of the tracheobronchial tree, lung, and mediastinum: embryology, radiology, and pathology. Radiographics 2004; 24(1): e17

3 Bland RD. Neonatal chronic lung disease in the post-surfactant era. Biol Neonate 2005; 88(3): 181–191

Case Study 2.1

History and clinical presentation: 15-year-old boy with fever, cough, and mild dyspnea of several days' duration. Elevated CRP, leukocytosis.

Imaging: chest radiographs in two planes.
Findings: patchy opacity with concave border in lateral segment of right middle lobe.
Diagnosis: middle lobe pneumonia.

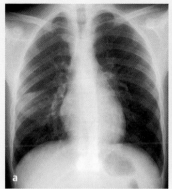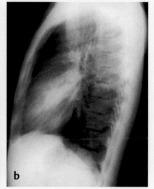

Fig. 2.29a, b

Case Study 2.2

History and clinical presentation: 17-year-old male with cough, productive of sputum in morning. Dyspnea on exertion. Restrictive ventilatory defect. History of measles pneumonia in early childhood.

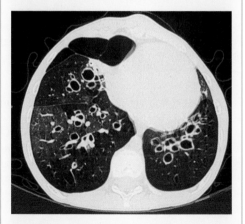

Fig. 2.30

Imaging: HRCT.
Findings: hyperinflation, bullae, mosaic perfusion, areas of cylindrical bronchiectasis.
Diagnosis: small airways disease based on measles bronchiolitis.

Case Study 2.3

History and clinical presentation: preterm infant born at 23 weeks, long-term ventilation.

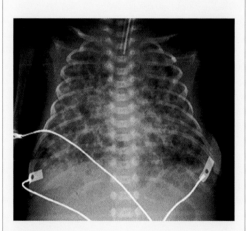

Fig. 2.31

Imaging: AP chest radiograph.
Findings: hyperinflation, coarse honeycomb lung structure with pseudocysts (sponge pattern) and increased interstitial markings. Endotracheal tube, ECG leads.
Diagnosis: bronchopulmonary dysplasia.

History and clinical presentation: 2-year-old child with several months' history of persistent cough and recurrent febrile episodes. Had repeatedly eaten peanuts with older siblings.

Imaging: AP chest radiograph.
Findings: hyperinflation of right lung with mediastinal shift to left, infiltrative dystelectatic changes in left lower lobe; accompanying effusion.
Diagnosis: FB aspiration (peanut) with secondary super-infection of affected lower lobe (aspiration pneumonia). Peanut was removed bronchoscopically.

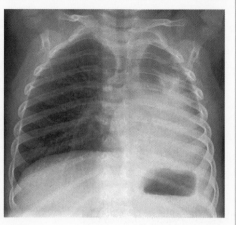

Fig. 2.32

History and clinical presentation: 4-year-old boy with chronic cough and low-grade fever. Grandmother has "chronic" lung disease.

Imaging: AP chest radiograph and CT.
Findings: Chest radiograph (**Fig. 2.33**) shows patchy opacity in middle lobe, mediastinal widening, and bilateral hilar enlargement. CT shows patchy infiltrate with liquefaction in right middle lobe (**Fig. 2.34a**) and conglomerate, cavitating nodal masses in mediastinal and hilar regions (**Fig. 2.34b**).
Diagnosis: Tb.

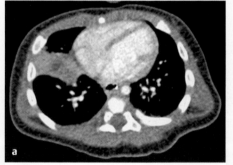

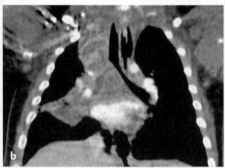

Fig. 2.34a, b

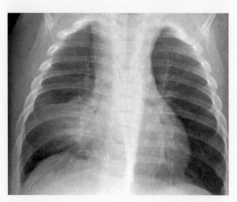

Fig. 2.33

Case Study 2.6

History and clinical presentation: preterm infant born at 31 weeks, ventilated since first day of life. Sudden, massive fall in blood pressure.

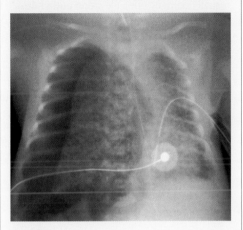

Fig. 2.35

Imaging: AP chest radiograph.
Findings: mediastinal shift to left with small heart silhouette. Cystlike lucencies diffusely distributed in lung. Air in right pleural space. Massive, asymmetric depression of right hemidiaphragm. Endotracheal tube terminates at C7 level. Tip of nasogastric tube not shown. Flow-directed catheter introduced from right side, tip somewhat low. External lead. Chest tube on left side.
Diagnosis: pulmonary interstitial emphysema with right tension pneumothorax.

4 Bundesamt für Strahlenschutz. Bundesanzeiger No. 143 of August 5, 2003: 17503

5 Donnelly LF, Frush DP, Bisset GS III. The multiple presentations of foreign bodies in children. AJR Am J Roentgenol 1998; 170(2): 471–477

6 Donnelly LF, Frush DP. Localized radiolucent chest lesions in neonates: causes and differentiation. AJR Am J Roentgenol 1999; 172(6): 1651–1658

7 Honnef D, Wildberger JE, Das M, et al. Value of virtual tracheobronchoscopy and bronchography from 16-slice multidetector-row spiral computed tomography for assessment of suspected tracheobronchial stenosis in children. Eur Radiol 2006; 16(8): 1684–1691

8 Jobe AH, Bancalari E. Bronchopulmonary dysplasia. Am J Respir Crit Care Med 2001; 163(7): 1723–1729

9 Kilian AK, Büsing KA, Schaible T, Neff KW. Fetal magnetic resonance imaging. Diagnostics in congenital diaphragmatic hernia. [Article in German] Radiologe 2006; 46(2): 128–132

10 Kim WS, Lee KS, Kim IO, et al. Congenital cystic adenomatoid malformation of the lung: CT-pathologic correlation. AJR Am J Roentgenol 1997; 168(1): 47–53

11 Kirks DR. Practical Pediatric Imaging: Diagnostic Radiology of Infants and Children. Philadelphia: Lippincott-Raven; 1998

12 Ley-Zaporozhan J, Ley S, Sommerburg O, Komm N, Müller FM, Schenk JP. Clinical application of MRI in children for the assessment of pulmonary diseases. Rofo 2009; 181(5): 419–432

13 McAdams HP, Kirejczyk WM, Rosado-de-Christenson ML, Matsumoto S. Bronchogenic cyst: imaging features with clinical and histopathologic correlation. Radiology 2000; 217(2): 441–446

14 Marais BJ, Gie RP, Schaaf HS, et al. A proposed radiological classification of childhood intra-thoracic tuberculosis. Pediatr Radiol 2004; 34(11): 886–894

15 Moskowitz SM, Gibson RL, Effmann EL. Cystic fibrosis lung disease: genetic influences, microbial interactions, and radiological assessment. Pediatr Radiol 2005; 35(8): 739–757

16 Ozçelik U, Göçmen A, Kiper N, Doğru D, Dilber E, Yalçin EG. Congenital lobar emphysema: evaluation and long-term follow-up of thirty cases at a single center. Pediatr Pulmonol 2003; 35(5): 384–391

17 Ramnath RR, Heller RM, Ben-Ami T, et al. Implications of early sonographic evaluation of parapneumonic effusions in children with pneumonia. Pediatrics 1998; 101(1 Pt 1): 68–71

18 Rossi UG, Owens CM. The radiology of chronic lung disease in children. Arch Dis Child 2005; 90(6): 601–607

19 Starke JR. Diagnosis of tuberculosis in children. Pediatr Infect Dis J 2000; 19(11): 1095–1096

20 Swischuk LE. Imaging of the Newborn, Infant, and Young Child. Baltimore: Williams & Wilkins; 1997: 111–116

21 Swischuk LE. Emergency Imaging of the Acutely Ill or Injured Children. Baltimore: Williams & Wilkins; 2000: 1–15

22 van Leeuwen K, Teitelbaum DH, Hirschl RB, et al. Prenatal diagnosis of congenital cystic adenomatoid malformation and its postnatal presentation, surgical indications, and natural history. J Pediatr Surg 1999; 34(5): 794–798, discussion 798–799

Gisela Schweigmann, Ingmar Gassner

2.2 Mediastinum

Thymus

Normal Thymus

See **Fig. 2.36**.

General: bilobed lymphoid organ located in anterior mediastinum, variable in size and shape.

- In healthy newborn: usually large. Often visible on chest radiograph up to 2 years of age, sometimes longer. Often rapidly involutes in response to acute physiologic stress, then enlarges due to rebound effect
- Thymus may extend into neck and to posterior mediastinum; indented by ribs (→ wavy lateral border on chest radiograph)

> Normal thymus = soft, never displaces or compresses adjacent structures (trachea, vessels).

Imaging:

- **AP chest radiograph:** bilateral or unilateral mediastinal widening. Often blends with cardiac silhouette, sometimes delineated from it by small notch in lower end; sometimes displays "Sail sign" (horizontal inferior thymic margin, usually on right side). Elevation of thymic lobes in setting of pneumomediastinum
- **Lateral chest radiograph:** retrosternal opacity with curved inferior border
- **US:** see thoracic US (Sect. 2.3)
- **CT/MRI:** homogeneous parenchyma, no calcifications. Configuration in axial plane varies with age. Younger children: quadrangular with convex borders; teenagers: triangular with straight or concave lateral border; after puberty: change in density and signal intensity due to fatty infiltration.

Thymic Hyperplasia

Thymic hyperplasia is usually a rebound effect after chemotherapy or corticosteroid therapy (following therapy, even months thereafter). Diagnostic clue: absence of other active disease and diminishing size over time.

Imaging: diffuse thymic enlargement with normal shape, density, and signal characteristics.

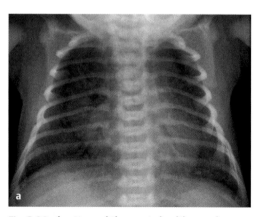
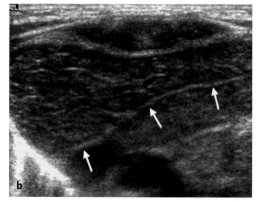

Fig. 2.36a, b   Normal thymus in healthy newborn.

a AP chest radiograph shows bilateral mediastinal widening by thymus. Thymus extends to diaphragm on right side. Wave sign noted on left side.

b Transsternal axial US scan shows hypoechoic thymic tissue with multiple linear and punctate internal echoes. Boundary between the two thymic lobes (arrows).

Thymic Aplasia or Hypoplasia

Occurrence: in children with chromosome abnormalities. Most common in Di George syndrome/CATCH 22 syndrome (defect on chromosome 22q11.2). Hypoplasia/aplasia of thymus and parathyroids (hypocalcemia!) and cardiac anomalies (e.g., truncus arteriosus, interrupted aortic arch). Congenital and other immune deficiencies (including HIV infection).
Imaging: narrow upper mediastinum due to absent or hypoplastic thymus.

Mediastinal Masses

See also Chapter 8.
Sites of **predilection**:
- **Anterior mediastinum:** malignant lymphoma, thymus (benign enlargement), thymoma, teratoma, dermoid, cystic hygroma
- **Middle mediastinum:** lymphadenopathy (inflammatory, neoplastic), bronchogenic cyst, duplication cyst
- **Posterior mediastinum:** most posterior masses have neurogenic cause; arise from sympathetic ganglion cells (neuroblastoma–ganglioneuroblastoma–ganglioneuroma complex). A few arise from peripheral nerves (neurofibroma, schwannoma)

Imaging:
- **Chest radiograph:** usually detects mass initially, localizes it to mediastinum; calcification, chest wall involvement, tracheal narrowing or displacement. Yields little information on morphology or precise extent
- **US:** supra- and parasternal approach; good for evaluating internal structure and therapeutic follow-up
- **CT/MRI:** accurate localization, extent, vascularity, enhancement characteristics, internal structure
- **Scintigraphy:** detects lesions of thyroid origin or gastric mucosa in gastroenteric cysts

Thymic Tumors

Thymic Cysts
- Rare, thin-walled, fluid-filled cysts, may contain sediment layer (intracystic hemorrhage, infection); may be multilocular resembling cystic hygroma
- Usually congenital, may also occur after trauma or thoracotomy
- Multiple cysts may be found in HIV infection and Langerhans cell histiocytosis

Thymic Enlargement due to Infiltration by Leukemia or Lymphoma
- Thymus often enormous; concomitant pleural effusion possible.
Imaging: US shows very hypoechoic mass, may mimic a cyst.

Thymoma
- < 5% of pediatric mediastinal tumors; < 10% associated with myasthenia gravis; usually benign
- Hallmark of **invasive malignant thymoma:** spread to mediastinum or chest wall; metastatic deposits along mediastinal, pleural, and pericardial interfaces
Imaging:
- **Chest radiograph:** disproportionately large "thymus"
- **US/CT/MRI:** complex anterior mediastinal mass with solid elements, cystic areas due to hemorrhage or necrosis, calcifications in up to 25% of cases.

Thymic Lipoma
- Rare. Most cases occur in second decade and are detected incidentally. Tumor contains mature fat and thymic tissue
Imaging:
- **Chest radiograph:** giant mediastinal mass extending to diaphragm
- **CT/MRI:** heterogeneous mass, contains fat. No compression or infiltration of adjacent structures

Germ Cell Tumors

General: 90% of germ cell tumors are benign.

- **Dermoids** (ectodermal elements only), teratomas (elements from all three germ layers), cystic or solid, sharply circumscribed, thick walls
- Mature **teratomas:** typical calcification (amorphous bones/teeth), fluid, fat, also in posterior mediastinum
- 10% of germ cell tumors are **malignant:** soft-tissue mass with ill-defined margins, calcifications only occasionally present, bleeding risk due to marked vascularity

Imaging:

- **Chest radiograph:** tumors within pericardium mimic cardiomegaly

Lymphangioma (Cystic Hygroma)

- Upper anterior mediastinum, almost always extension from cervical hygroma; primary mediastinal lymphangioma extremely rare
- Intralesional hemorrhage—sudden increase in size (sediment layer)
- Infiltration of adjacent soft tissues, encasement of mediastinal structures
- May displace trachea and esophagus, compress adjacent structures
- Calcification secondary to infection or bleeding

Malignant Lymphoma

See **Fig. 2.37**.

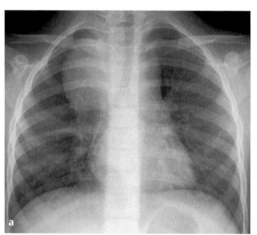
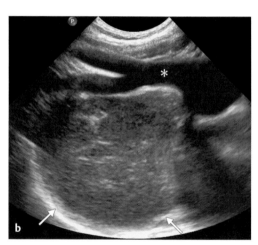
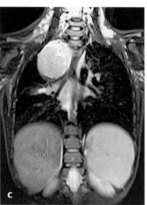

Fig. 2.37a–c   Mediastinal T cell lymphoma in a 6-year-old girl.
a PA chest radiograph shows opacity with sharp, convex lateral margin widening upper mediastinum to the right and displacing trachea to left.
b Suprasternal oblique US scan shows hypoechoic mass (arrows) with scant septa bordering on brachiocephalic trunk (*).
c MRI. Coronal TIRM sequence shows well-circumscribed hyperintense mass in right upper mediastinum displacing trachea to left.

Most common anterior mediastinal mass, accounts for 23% of all mediastinal masses in children. Three main types:

- Hodgkin disease: contiguous spread; 85% initial mediastinal masses, 30% initial hilar lymphadenopathy; occasionally direct intrapulmonary spread
- Non-Hodgkin lymphoma (NHL): hematogenous spread; 50% initial mediastinal masses; lung involvement may occur without lymphadenopathy
- Posttransplant lymphoproliferative disease (PTLD)
- Pleural effusion due to lymphatic or venous stasis; *but*, most pericardial effusions caused by direct tumor spread
- Frequent infiltration of thymus; cysts may form after necrosis

Imaging:

- **Chest radiograph:** widening of upper anterior mediastinum; compression or deviation of trachea; spherical hilar enlargement; cardiac borders enlarged due to pericardial effusion; pleural effusion
- **CT:** mediastinal and hilar lymphadenopathy (without calcification before treatment); thickened pericardium; pericardial effusion; pulmonary nodules and consolidation; airway compression; vascular compression (= high general anesthesia risk)
- **MRI:** mediastinal evaluation; detection of multifocal spread on whole-body MRI
- **PET:** most lymphomas PET-positive; useful for monitoring disease activity over time

Inflammatory Lymph Node Changes

Granulomatous lymphadenopathy (**Tb, histoplasmosis, sarcoidosis**) less common in middle mediastinum than lymphoma.
Imaging: cannot distinguish between inflammatory and neoplastic lymphadenopathy.

Neuroblastoma–Ganglioneuroblastoma–Ganglioneuroma Complex

See **Fig. 2.38**.
Pathology: embryonic tumor of sympathetic nervous system. **Neuroblastoma** is least differentiated = most malignant. Mature forms = **ganglioneuroblastoma, ganglioneuroma**. Paraspinal mass, sometimes with straddling and erosion of ribs, fo-

raminal enlargement. Intraspinal extension may occur (dumbbell tumors).
Imaging: MRI is modality of choice, especially for intraspinal extension.

Frequent irregular or granular calcifications (more common in older children with ganglioneuroma). Cervical-to-thoracic or thoracic-to-intraabdominal spread may occur.

> **!** Intraspinal extension must be detected preoperatively (risk of spinal cord injury at surgery).

Cystic Foregut Malformations

Pathology: bronchogenic cysts lined by respiratory epithelium, usually with subcarinal and right paratracheal location. **Duplication cysts of esophagus** lined by gastrointestinal mucosa, occur at paraspinal sites. Distinguished by histological examination.
Imaging: cysts are round or oval lesions with sharp margins and thin walls; they do not enhance after contrast administration. Contents of water density; protein-rich fluid after intracystic hemorrhage, also soft-tissue density. Air–fluid level signifies communication with bronchial system or GI tract.

Congenital Anomalies of the Vascular System

General: vascular rings (completely encircling of trachea and esophagus) and vascular loops (partially encircling) → respiratory distress in newborns, stridor and/or dysphagia in older children. Some vascular anomalies are clinically silent (incidental findings).
Imaging: initial detection and differentiation on chest radiographs (evaluation of aortic arch position!). Contrast imaging of esophagus in strictly AP and lateral projection for evaluation of vascular indentations.

Aortic Arch Anomalies

See also Sect. 2.5.
Pathology: hypothetical double aortic arch during embryonic development explains all aortic arch anomalies (**Fig. 2.39**). This double arch encircles esophagus and trachea, has a ductus arteriosus

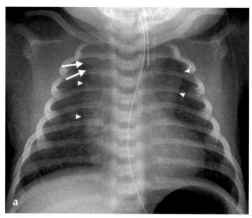

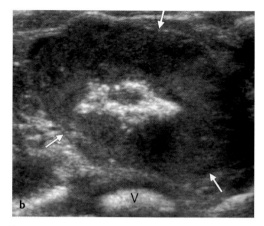

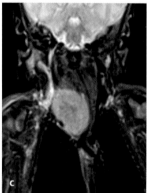

Fig. 2.38a–c   Neuroblastoma in 3-week-old newborn.
a AP chest radiograph. Mediastinal widening by thymus (arrowheads) accompanied by right-sided mediastinal mass appearing as dense apical opacity (arrows). Mass had displaced trachea (endotracheal tube) and esophagus (stomach tube) to left.
b Suprasternal transverse US scan shows hypoechoic mass (arrows) with dense central calcification and scattered punctate calcifications (V, vertebral body).
c MRI. Coronal TIRM sequence shows hyperintense mass with central hypointense calcification displacing trachea to left.

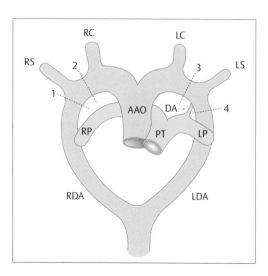

Fig. 2.39   Diagrammatic representation of Edwards' hypothetical double aortic arch. Sites of regression with:
1 normal left aortic arch,
2 left aortic arch with aberrant right subclavian artery (arteria lusoria),
3 right aortic arch with aberrant left subclavian artery,
4 right aortic arch with mirror-image vessel origins.
Ascending aorta (AAO), pulmonary trunk (PT), right pulmonary artery (RP), left pulmonary artery (LP), ductus arteriosus (DA), right subclavian artery (RS), left subclavian artery (LS), right common carotid artery (RC), left common carotid artery (LC), right descending aorta (RDA), left descending aorta (LDA). (Diagram: G. Schweigmann after R. M. Freedom.)

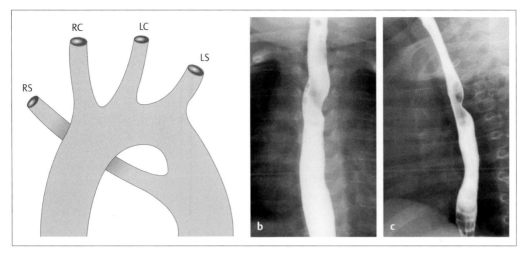

Fig. 2.40a–c **Left aortic arch with aberrant right subclavian artery in 2-month-old boy.**

a Diagrammatic representation (graphic: T. Geley). Right subclavian artery (RS), left subclavian artery (LS), right common carotid artery (RC), left common carotid artery (LC).

b, c Anteroposterior (**b**) and lateral (**c**) esophagrams show aberrant right subclavian artery indenting posterior wall of esophagus from lower left to upper right.

(DA) on each side, aorta descends in midline. Each arch gives rise to its own common carotid and subclavian artery (right common carotid artery [RC], left common carotid artery [LC]) and subclavian artery (right subclavian artery [RS], left subclavian artery [LS]).

Normal left-sided arch: interruption of right arch between subclavian artery and descending aorta = brachiocephalic trunk (1 in **Fig. 2.39**).

Absent or abnormal interruption of double aortic arch → aortic arch anomalies.

Left Aortic Arch with Aberrant Right Subclavian Artery

See **Fig. 2.40**.

Regression of right arch between RC and RS (2 in **Fig. 2.39**). RS = last branch of aortic arch, passes always behind esophagus to right arm. Most common aortic arch anomaly, no vascular ring, usually asymptomatic, rarely causes dysphagia by extrinsic compression.

Imaging: chest radiograph normal. AP esophagram—posterior oblique indentation of esophagus from lower left to upper right; lateral view: small posterior indentation of esophagus. US—first aortic arch branch shows absence of branching (no brachiocephalic trunk); small vessel in cross-section behind esophagus. CT/MRI—only in symptomatic patients.

Right Aortic Arch with Mirror-Image Origin of Cervical Vessels

Pathology: regression of left arch distal to LS. First vessel = left brachiocephalic trunk, then RC and RS (4 in **Fig. 2.39**).

Clinical features: no vascular ring, no stridor, no dysphagia. Often associated with cardiac anomalies.

Imaging: chest radiograph—trachea indented on right side, deviated to left side. Esophagram—esophagus indented on right side, no posterior indentation. US—aortic arch on right side of trachea and esophagus with mirror-image branching CT/MRI—only if necessary for evaluating associated cardiac anomalies.

Right Aortic Arch with Aberrant Left Subclavian Artery

See **Fig. 2.41**.

Pathology: interruption of left aortic arch between LC and LS. Aberrant LS arises as last branch from a usually large Kommerell diverticulum in descending aorta. DA or ligamentum arteriosum passes from diverticulum to left pulmonary artery (LP) = complete vascular ring (3 in **Fig. 2.39**).

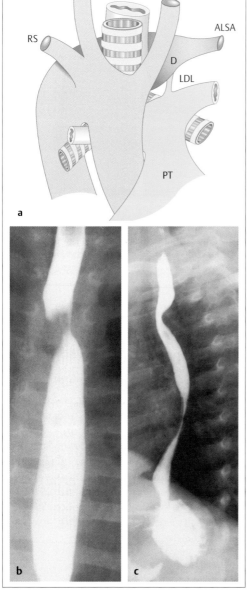

a

b   c

Fig. 2.41a–c Right aortic arch with aberrant left subclavian artery in 18-month-old boy.

a Diagrammatic representation (graphic: T. Geley). Pulmonary trunk (PT), left ductal ligament (LDL), right subclavian artery (RS), aberrant left subclavian artery (ALSA), right common carotid artery (RC), left common carotid artery (LC), Kommerell diverticulum (D).

b, c Anteroposterior (**b**) and lateral (**c**) esophagrams show indentation of esophagus from right side and marked posterior indentation (Kommerell diverticulum).

Clinical features: symptomatic vascular ring. Not associated with cardiac anomalies.

Imaging: chest radiograph—right aortic arch and frequent right descending aorta. Trachea indented on right side, deviated to left. Esophagram—indentation of esophagus on right and also large oblique posterior indentation (Kommerell diverticulum) from lower right to upper left; sometimes indentation on left with tight ductus or ligamentum arteriosum (mimicking double aortic arch). US—right aortic arch, first vessel arising from aorta does not branch (= LC), large "vessel cross-section" behind esophagus (= Kommerell diverticulum). CT/MRI—complete visualization of vascular anomaly.

Double Aortic Arch

See **Fig. 2.42.**

Pathology: both aortic arches persist. Each arch gives rise to only two main vessels (ipsilateral common carotid artery and subclavian artery). Right aortic arch is usually larger in diameter and higher in position than left arch. One segment may be atretic (usually left). Aorta descends on right or left side. This complete vascular ring encircles trachea and esophagus; symptomatic in newborns and infants. Usually no other anomalies associated.

Imaging: chest radiograph—trachea fixed in midline position between both arches, poorly delineated due to compression. Esophagram—bilateral indentation, higher on right than left, and with large posterior indentation. US—suprasternal parasagittal scans show one arch with only two vessels on right and left side of esophagus, respectively. Transsternal axial scan displays complete vascular ring. CT/MRI—to document size of both arches and to exclude coarctation.

Anomalies of the Pulmonary Arteries

Pulmonary (Artery) Sling (Aberrant Left Pulmonary Artery)

See **Fig. 2.43.**

Pathology: left PA arises extrapericardially from right PA, hooks around carina, and passes behind trachea and in front of esophagus to left lung. Forms sling around airways with extrinsic compression of distal trachea and right main bronchus → hyperinflation or atelectasis of right lung.

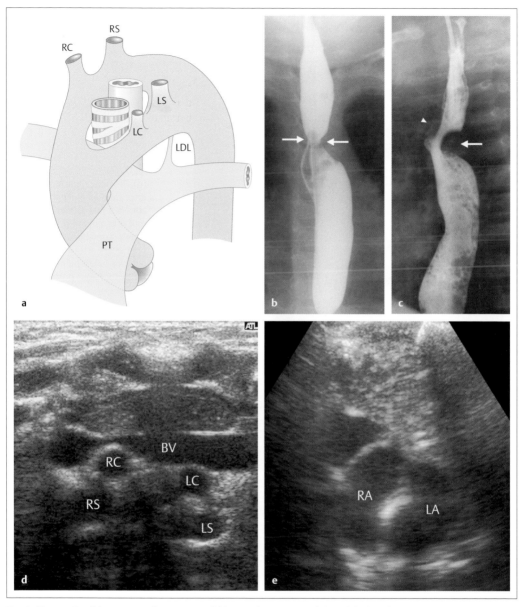

Fig. 2.42a–e   Double aortic arch in 1-year-old boy. Pulmonary trunk (PT), left ductal ligament (LDL), right subclavian artery (RS), left subclavian artery (LS), right common carotid artery (RC), left common carotid artery (LC), left brachiocephalic vein (BV), right aortic arch (RA), left aortic arch (LA).

a   Diagrammatic representation (graphic: T. Geley).
b, c   Anteroposterior and lateral esophagrams show bilateral indentation of esophagus (arrows). Lateral view (**c**) shows broad posterior indentation (arrow) accompanied by significant tracheal narrowing (arrowhead).

d   Transsternal axial US scan shows symmetrical origins of supra-aortic vessels.
e   Transsternal axial US scan displays complete vascular ring.

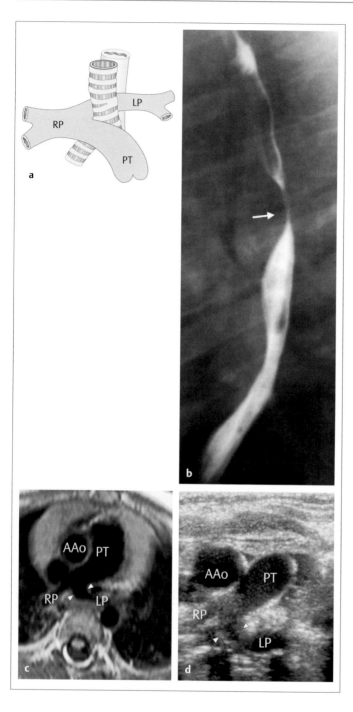

Fig. 2.43a–d Pulmonary sling in 1-year-old boy. Ascending aorta (AAo), pulmonary trunk (PT), right pulmonary artery (RP), left pulmonary artery (LP).

a Diagrammatic representation (T. Geley).

b Lateral esophagram shows aberrant left pulmonary artery indenting esophagus anteriorly (arrow).

c, d MRI, axial HASTE sequence (**c**), and transsternal axial US scan (**d**). Proximal right pulmonary artery and ascending aorta have almost equal diameters. Aberrant origin of left pulmonary artery (arrowheads) from right pulmonary artery. The trachea anterior to left pulmonary artery, esophagus posterior.

Classification: based on associated tracheobronchial anomalies:

- **Type I:** normal tracheobronchial tree, extrinsic compression by aberrant PA
- **Type II** (more common): associated tracheobronchial anomaly—long segmental tracheal stenosis with absence of membranous part and complete cartilage rings, anomalous bronchial branching pattern (middle and right lower lobe supplied by "bridging bronchus" arising from left main bronchus and crossing mediastinum)

Imaging: Chest radiograph—cross-section of aberrant PA in right tracheobronchial angle; in type II, long-segment tracheal stenosis and low-lying pseudocarina (inverted T pattern) due to bridging bronchus. Esophagram—lateral view: anterior pulsating indentation of esophagus at level of carina.

> Pulmonary sling = only vascular anomaly that causes anterior indentation of esophagus!

US—suprasternal scan in plane of aortic arch shows both right and aberrant left pulmonary artery in cross-section beneath aortic arch. Parasternal transverse scan shows absence of normal origin of left pulmonary artery and can display origin of left PA from right PA. CT/MRI—shows vascular anomaly, associated tracheobronchial stenosis, and abnormal bronchial pattern.

Proximal Interruption of Pulmonary Artery (Ductal Origin of Pulmonary Artery)

Pathology: congenital absence (atresia/interruption of proximal right/left PA)—intrapericardial segment of involved PA absent. Interrupted PA supplied by patent DA; after DA closure by acquired bronchial collateral circulation.

Imaging: Chest radiograph—interrupted PA, usually opposite side of aortic arch! Affected lung smaller with mediastinal shift toward affected side. Transpleural collaterals may cause pleural thickening. Enlarged hilar vascular structures on unaffected side. US—parasternal axial scan shows absence of PA bifurcation. Suprasternal parasagittal scan shows either large PA (absent left PA) or no PA (absent right PA) posterior to ascending aorta. CT/MRI—confirms diagnosis, shows small PA on affected side.

Anomalies of Systemic Veins

Persistent Left Superior Vena Cava

Pathology: usually opens into coronary sinus, rarely drains directly into left atrium. Left brachiocephalic vein absent or very small. Associated with congenital heart disease or isolated anomaly.

Imaging: Chest radiograph/US—central venous catheter (CVC) introduced from left side may enter left superior vena cava.

Azygos Continuation

Pathology: Absent hepatic segment of IVC. Hepatic veins drain directly into right atrium. IVC continues as azygos vein—more posteriorly located than normal IVC, anteriorly crossed by right renal artery (diagnostic clue in cross-sectional imaging). Association with heterotaxy syndrome (e.g., polysplenia syndrome).

Anomalies of Pulmonary Veins

See also Sect. 2.5.

Scimitar Syndrome

Pathology: hypoplasia of right lung with abnormal right pulmonary venous drainage, usually into inferior vena cava and anomalous systemic arterial supply to hypoplastic right lung.

> Look for scimitar vein in patients with unexplained right pulmonary hypoplasia.

Imaging: Chest radiograph—small right hemithorax, often with decreased lucency. Sharply defined, curved scimitar vein that widens as it descends (scimitar = Turkish sword). US—displays scimitar vein and abnormal systemic arterial vessel. CT(A)/MRI(A)—for complete visualization.

2

Situs Anomalies

Situs solitus and Situs inversus

Definition and classification: Bronchial division determines situs. In case of dextrocardia, thoracic situs can be determined from branching pattern of bronchi.

- **Situs solitus** (normal organ arrangement): right main bronchus more vertical than left and has epiarterial (high-origin) upper lobe bronchus. Left main bronchus less vertical with hypoarterial (low-origin) upper lobe bronchus
- **Situs inversus:** mirror image of normal organ arrangement

Situs ambiguous
(Asplenia and Polysplenia Syndrome)

Pathology: symmetrical arrangement of asymmetrically developed organs. A normally unilateral organ may be bilateral, overdeveloped, or absent.

Asplenia Syndrome

Pathology: bilateral right-sidedness or dextroisomerism. Spleen absent. Both lungs have three lobes with bilateral eparterial upper lobe bronchus. Left lobe of liver same size as right. Bowel malrotation usually coexists. Almost always associated with complex cyanotic heart disease.
Imaging: chest radiograph—both lungs have horizontal interlobar fissure (between upper and middle lobes), small symmetrical tracheobronchial angle, bilateral high origin of upper lobe bronchus.

Cardiac apex right or left. Liver symmetrical, occupies whole upper abdomen. US/CT/MRI—confirms absence of spleen. Liver symmetrical with hepatic veins and portal vein. IVC and aorta both to left or right of spinal column. IVC anterior to aorta. Cyanotic heart disease with bilateral morphologic right atrial appendages. Absent coronary sinus.

Polysplenia Syndrome

Pathology: bilateral left-sidedness or levoisomerism. Spleen consists of multiple small spleens (in right/left hypochondrium). Both lungs bilobed with bilateral hyparterial upper lobe bronchi. Frequent bowel malrotation and acyanotic heart disease. Dextrocardia in 50% of cases.
Imaging: chest radiograph—large symmetrical tracheobronchial angle with bilateral low origin of upper lobe bronchus. US/CT/MRI—multiple small spleens in right/left hypochondrium. Hepatic segment of IVC absent (azygos continuation). Hepatic veins open directly into right atrium.

Bibliography

1 Franco A, Mody NS, Meza MP. Imaging evaluation of pediatric mediastinal masses. Radiol Clin North Am 2005; 43(2): 325–355, 405–419
2 Lucaya J, Strife JL. Pediatric Chest Imaging. Heidelberg: Springer; 2002: 1–25, 187–208
3 Siegel MJ, Coley BD. The Core Curriculum: Pediatric Imaging. Philadelphia: Lippincott Williams & Wilkins; 2006: 33–64
4 Swischuk LE. Imaging of the Newborn, Infant and Young Child. 5th ed. Philadelphia: Lippincott Williams & Wilkins; 2004: 1–29, 151–163

2.3   Basic Principles of Thoracic Ultrasound in Children

Gisela Schweigmann, Ingmar Gassner

General

The pediatric mediastinum is accessible to US scanning through nonossified sternum and large thymus, especially in infants and newborns.

US detects masses in anterior mediastinum, can differentiate between pulmonary and pleural lesions, demonstrates pulmonary pathology (obscured by pleural effusion on chest films). US can characterize pleural effusions, detect aortic arch and pulmonary artery (PA) anomalies, and detect malposition and complications of central catheters. US can be used without sedation in incubators and at ICU.

Technique

- Always review recent images (including chest films) prior to US!
- Type of US probe depends on patient size and location of lesion to be evaluated. Use high-frequency linear/sector probes for preterms, newborns, and infants. Use probe with small contact area for suprasternal/supraclavicular scanning
- Reposition patient to improve visualization of position-dependent pathology. Fluid-filled stomach = good acoustic window

Mediastinum

- **Probe positions:** suprasternal and supraclavicular, transsternal (if sternum not yet ossified), parasternal, subxiphoidal, and subcostal. Aid supraclavicular/suprasternal scanning by raising shoulders (cushion, assistant's hand) or turning head to opposite side
- **Thymus** (**Fig. 2.36b**): bilobed, echogenicity < thyroid gland, equivalent to liver; linear and punctate connective-tissue echoes; scant vascularity; easily deformable (during respiration and crying) → does not compress adjacent vessels
- **Trachea:** hypoechoic tracheal cartilages, appearance of a necklace in longitudinal section
- **Esophagus:** hypoechoic muscle wall, hyperechoic mucosa and submucosa; movement of air and fluid clearly visible within lumen, especially during drinking

> Trachea and esophagus important in locating midline. Failure to identify trachea/esophagus may cause misinterpretation of aortic arch position (especially with midline shift due to pulmonary hypoplasia, etc.).

- **Aortic arch:** scanned from suprasternal, supraclavicular, or high parasternal transducer position. A plane from suprasternal notch directed toward right shoulder visualizes innominate artery and its bifurcation into right subclavian and carotid artery. (Right innominate artery implies left aortic arch and vice-versa!)
- **PA:** main trunk and bifurcation in axial transsternal and parasternal scans with slight anticlockwise rotation of transducer (left PA runs more cranially than the right!). Coronal suprasternal scan visualizes right PA just past origin of upper lobe artery. Oblique parasagittal scan in plane of aortic arch displays right PA in cross section beneath arch.

Pleura, Diaphragm, and Lung

- **Pleura:** most of pleura can be imaged from intercostal, subcostal, and subxiphoid sites. Liver and spleen = good acoustic windows
- **Lung:** aerated lung blocks sound penetration—linear, highly reflective interface with vertically directed comet-tail artifacts (subpleural interlobular septa) moves with respiration (gliding sign). This interface bordered by series of parallel echogenic lines (reverberation artifacts). Interface between aerated lung and diaphragm produces mirror-image artifacts from liver and spleen in longitudinal scans
- **Pleural effusion:** transudate = echo-free; exsudate = rarely echo-free, usually contains echogenic debris, mobile fibrin strands, septations. Dense fibrin septa → honeycomb appearance (**Fig. 2.44**)
- **Pneumothorax:** gliding sign and comet-tail artifacts replaced by static reverberations. Unless pneumothorax leads to total collapse of lung, junction of pneumothorax with normal lung appears as "lung point" that moves with respiratory excursions. Even very small pneumothorax detectable by US (intrapleural air always moves to highest level in chest!)
- **Pneumonia:** alveoli filled with fluid and inflammatory cells = good sound conduction (roughly isoechoic to liver). Air-filled bronchi with mobile gas bubbles converge toward pulmonary hilum (sonographic air bronchogram). Mucus- and secretion-filled bronchi = echo-free tubular structures (sonographic fluid bronchogram), distinguishable from pulmonary vessels on color duplex scans
- **Diaphragm:** scanned by intercostal, subcostal, or subxiphoidal approaches. Acoustic windows = liver, spleen, fluid-filled stomach. Both hemidiaphragms can be imaged simultaneously by tilting subxiphoidly positioned probe cranially (e.g., to evaluate diaphragmatic palsy). Muscular portion appears as hypoechoic bandlike struc-

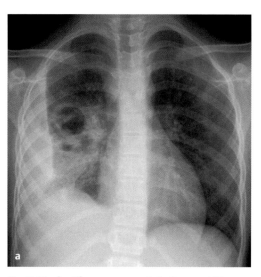

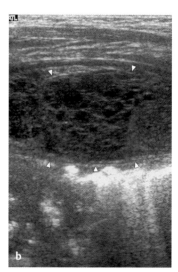

Fig. 2.44a, b   Pleuropneumonia in 8-year-old boy.

a PA chest radiograph shows right pleural effusion and infiltration of lung parenchyma with pneumatocele formation.

b Right intercostal oblique US scan. A broad effusion with multiple septa (arrowheads) borders on aerated lung and partially aerated, infiltrated lung.

ture. Detection of posterior (Bochdalek) and anterior (Morgagni) diaphragmatic hernia and eventration of diaphragm (congenital weakness of muscular portion).

Thoracic Ultrasound in Neonatal ICU

- Evaluation of central venous catheter (CVC) position

Detection of Catheter Complications

Sites and complications of common thoracic catheters and tubes (**Fig. 2.45a–e):**
- **Central venous catheter:** insertion from different sites (femoral, subclavian, external jugular, internal jugular, antecubital, saphenous vein) into thoracic cavity. Tip has to be in inferior or superior vena cava. Immediate complications: catheter malposition (in aorta, if catheter closer to midline than expected); pneumothorax and hematothorax secondary to insertion procedure; extraluminal placement with infusate extravasation. Late complications: infection, occlusion, thrombosis (inferior vena cava: may extend into renal veins with subsequent hema-

turia, hypertension, or renal failure; superior vena cava: lymphatic duct blockage with subsequent chylothorax), catheter tip migration (may lead to pericardial effusion, cardiac tamponade, or hydrothorax). **Caution:** curved catheter course in right atrium indicates contact of catheter tip with very thin atrial wall. This may lead to perforation or endothelial damage with subsequent increase in permeability (pericardial effusion!). Fibrin deposit around catheter frequently formed. Remaining fibrin sheath after catheter removal may mimic catheter fragment.
- **Pulmonary artery catheter:** tip in pulmonary artery, central or peripheral. Complications: coiling in right ventricle, dysrhythmia, damage to pulmonic valve, pulmonary artery erosion or infarction, balloon rupture, infection.
- **Umbilical vein catheter:** tip in right atrium (= ~ 1 cm above diaphragm). Complications: malposition in portal vein with possible liver necrosis (catecholamine application), perforation in liver parenchyma, thrombosis (may cause cavernous transformation of portal vein), hemorrhage.
- **Umbilical artery catheter:** tip in thoracal aorta at level of T6 to T10 or in abdominal aorta at level of L4 vertebral body. Complications: malposi-

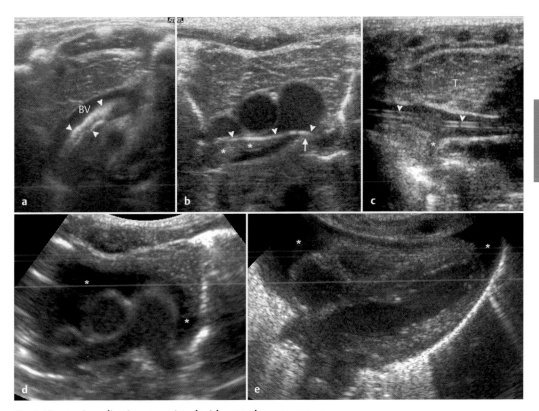

2

Fig. 2.45a–e   Complications associated with central venous access.

a Thrombus (arrowheads) in brachiocephalic vein (BV) around central venous catheter in 5-week-old girl. Transsternal axial scan.
b Embolization of broken catheter fragment into the pulmonary artery in 1-week-old boy. Transsternal axial scan. Fragment (arrowheads) with adherent thrombus (asterisks) overrides pulmonary artery bifurcation (arrow).

c Fibrin sheath of catheter left behind in superior vena cava after removal of central venous line in 10-day-old boy. Right parasternal longitudinal scan. Fibrin sheath (arrowheads), Azygos vein (asterisk), thymus (T).
d, e Pericardial effusion related to catheter tip in right atrium in 3-day-old girl. Transsternal high (**d**) and low (**e**) axial scans demonstrate significant amount of pericardial echo-free fluid (asterisks).

tion (i.e., left subclavian artery), retroperitoneal hemorrage after perforation, decreased femoral pulses, blanching of limbs and/or buttocks, aortic thrombi, infection with mycotic aortic aneurysm, renal artery thrombosis (hypertension!), embolization and infarction distal to tip.

- **Endotracheal tube:** tip should be in middle between vocal cords and carina at level of T2 vertebral body. Complications: tip in right main bronchus (atelectasis of right upper lobe), tip in esophagus (asphyxia, aspiration).
- **Enteral tube**: tip should be in stomach, duodenum or jejunum. Complications: malposition in airways (aspiration), perforation (pharyngeal

perforation may mimic esophageal atresia in newborns).

- **Chest tube drainage**: pneumothorax: puncture at 2nd/3rd intercostal space in medioclavicular line. Pleural effusion: puncture at 4th/5th intercostal space in anterior axillary line. Complications: subcutaneous position, posterior position in pneumothorax, perforation (lung, mediastinum, esophagus, pericardium, diaphragm, liver).
- **Pacemaker leads**: transvenous (tip in right atrium and right ventricular septum, apex or outflow tract) or epicardial. Complications: venous occlusion (transvenous), infection, perforation,

lead fracture, lead macro-dislocation, lead mi-cro-dislocation on X-ray not visible. Control of lead position: chest X-ray in two planes!

⚠ All venous catheters in patients with right to left shunt (i.e., cyanotic congenital heart disease) bear the risk of arterial infarction (brain, etc.).

Bibliography
1 Gassner I, Geley TE. Ultrasound of the neonatal thorax. In: Donoghue V, ed. Radiological Imaging of the Neonatal Chest. 2nd ed. Heidelberg: Springer; 2008: 197–225
2 Goya E, Xavier P. Chest ultrasound. In: Lucaya J, Strife JL, eds. Pediatric Chest Imaging. Heidelberg: Springer; 2002: 1–24
3 Riccabona M. Ultrasound of the chest in children (mediastinum excluded). Eur Radiol 2008; 18(2): 390–399

2.4   The Pediatric Breast

Gisela Schweigmann, Ingmar Gassner

General

Breast pathology is rare in children and adolescents.

⚠ Mammography generally contraindicated in children because of extremely low risk of breast cancer, increased risk of radiation-induced malignant changes in young glandular breast, and poor image quality due to dense fibroglandular breasts.

Primary imaging modality = US with high-frequency linear probe. Solid lesions can be evaluated by US-guided fine-needle aspiration—but biopsy and surgery should be avoided as they may cause deformity of developing breast.

Normal Breast Development

Normal breast development: **five stages** described by Tanner; correlate with characteristic US and histologic findings:

- **Tanner I:** prepubescent breast; only nipple visible; no palpable glands. US = hyperechoic retroareolar tissue with ill-defined borders
- **Tanner II:** glandular breast parenchyma and areola slightly raised to form breast bud. US = hyperechoic retroareolar nodule (= breast bud) with central stellate or linear hypoechoic region (represents simple branched ducts)
- **Tanner III:** breast parenchyma larger than areola. US = peripheral spread of echogenic glandular tissue from retroareolar region, continued presence of central hypoechoic spider-shaped center

- **Tanner IV:** gland in areolar region delineated from rest of breast. US = hyperechoic periareolar fibroglandular tissue; prominent hypoechoic central nodule; subcutaneous fat
- **Tanner V:** mature, rounded breast contour. US = hyperechoic breast parenchyma without central hypoechoic nodule as in stages II–IV, increased volume of anterior subcutaneous fat

Normal Variants and Abnormalities of Breast Development

Unilateral onset of breast development: one breast may develop up to 2 years before opposite breast; most common normal variant. US = normal breast tissue.

Premature thelarche: breast development begins before age 7½ years. May be isolated or associated with central precocious puberty, unilateral or bilateral. US = normal breast tissue (**Fig. 2.46**).

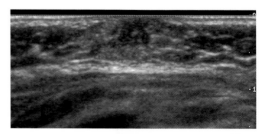

Fig. 2.46   Premature thelarche in 10-month-old girl. Axial US scan of right breast shows unilateral premature breast development. Breast parenchyma in this case has normal structure corresponding to Tanner stage II.

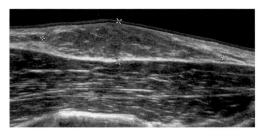

Fig. 2.47 Pubescent gynecomastia in 16-year-old boy. Sagittal US scan of left breast shows unilateral breast enlargement. Contralateral US examination did not show enlargement of the opposite right breast.

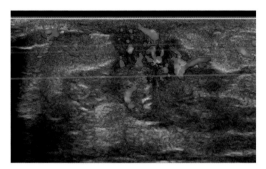

Fig. 2.48 Mastitis in 11-year-old girl. Axial color Doppler scan of left breast shows markedly increased retroareolar blood flow in hypoechoic inflammatory tissue with no abscess formation.

Congenital anomalies: polythelia (too many nipples), polymastia (too many breasts), congenital amastia (absence of mammary glands). Imaging usually unnecessary.

Gynecomastia: Physiologic gynecomastia (increased breast development in males) common, may be asymmetrical or unilateral. Breast development starts 1 year after onset of puberty approximately, regresses in 1 to 2 years. Gynecomastia may occur in setting of other diseases (Klinefelter syndrome, anorchia, etc.) or may be drug-induced. Isolated cases require mastectomy (**Fig. 2.47**). Rarely, US used for confirmation and size measurement of breast tissue. **Pseudogynecomastia** may occur in obesity (fat accumulation in breast). US diagnostic; can distinguish from other forms of breast enlargement.

Inflammatory Changes

Occur in newborns, children, and adolescents.

- **Abscesses:** may result from obstruction of glandular duct, infection of retroareolar cyst, irritation or desquamation of nipple, cellulitis of adjacent chest wall. US = round or oval mass with hypoechoic center (necrosis, liquefaction) and peripheral, vascularized abscess wall. Treatable by percutaneous aspiration under US guidance
- **Mastitis:** US also shows central blood flow, distinguishing it from peripheral vascularity of abscess (**Fig. 2.48**)

Benign Lesions

Benign Neoplastic Lesions

- **Fibroadenoma:** most common benign breast neoplasm in children and adolescents. US = hypoechoic round, oval, or lobulated mass with well-defined margins 1 to 20 cm in diameter. Multifocal in 10 to 15% of cases. 67% avascular by CDU, 33% have central vascularity
- **Hemangioma, papilloma, lymphangioma, lipoma**

Benign Non-Neoplastic Lesions

- **Breast cyst:** solitary or multiple, 1–5 cm in diameter, usually close to nipple/areola. US = well-defined, echo-free mass, occasionally with internal septa. When infected—multiple internal echoes, septations, sediment layer, increased peripheral blood flow
- Don't confuse with ductextasia (e.g., in female neonates)
- **Fibrocystic disease, galactocele, postoperative fibrosis, fat necrosis, hematoma, extramedullary hematopoesis**

Malignant Lesions

Primary Breast Malignancies

- **Cystosarcoma phylloides:** may develop from fibroadenoma or originate from breast tissue. Usually benign, 5% malignant. Very rare in adolescents, but most common malignant breast tumor in that age group. US = lobulated, round or

2

oval, hypoechoic with smooth margins, posterior acoustic enhancement; homogeneous or with cystic areas
- **Adenocarcinoma:** extremely rare in children, < 1% of breast tumors. May present as painless mass in first decade of life. US = variable, nonspecific; hypoechoic mass with irregular margins and inhomogeneous internal echoes
- **Lymphoma, rhabdomyosarcoma, angiomyosarcoma, ductal carcinoma in situ (DCIS)**

> Primary breast malignancies very rare in children and adolescents.

Secondary Breast Malignancies

- **Lymphoma, leukemia, rhabdomyosarcoma, neuroblastoma.** US = nonspecific. Look for primary tumor!

> Secondary breast malignancies in children more common than primary lesions!

Bibliography

1 García CJ, Espinoza A, Dinamarca V, et al. Breast US in children and adolescents. Radiographics 2000; 20(6): 1605–1612
2 Tea MK, Asseryanis E, Kroiss R, Kubista E, Wagner T. Surgical breast lesions in adolescent females. Pediatr Surg Int 2009; 25(1): 73–75
3 Weinstein SP, Conant EF, Orel SG, Zuckerman JA, Bellah R. Spectrum of US findings in pediatric and adolescent patients with palpable breast masses. Radiographics 2000; 20(6): 1613–1621
4 Welch ST, Babcock DS, Ballard ET. Sonography of pediatric male breast masses: gynecomastia and beyond. Pediatr Radiol 2004; 34(12): 952–957

2.5   Important Aspects of Cardiac Imaging in Newborns and Children

Erich Sorantin, Brigitte Povysil

Introduction

Incidence of congenital heart disease: 1% of all newborns.
Classification based on various factors:
- Anatomy: obstruction in left or right side of heart, septal and vascular malformations, complex cardiac anomalies, anomalous origins of great arteries (**Table 2.1**)
- Shunt characteristics: left-to-right, right-to-left, bidirectional, no shunt
- Clinical features: with/without cyanosis, lung perfusion decreased/normal/increased (**Table 2.2**)
- Degree of severity (**Table 2.3**)

Age distribution: rapid changes in recent decades—today more adults have congenital heart disease than children (increased life expectancy in this patient group, falling childhood incidence in western countries, fewer fetuses with cardiac anomalies carried to term) → problem not exclusive to pediatric radiology and pediatric cardiology.

Imaging: chest radiography and echocardiography—cornerstone for diagnosis and follow-up. CT, MRI, cardiac catheterization—specialized further testing.

Normal Findings on Chest Radiographs

Infants and small children (see also Sect. 2.1):
- cannot stand unaided → X-rayed in supine or sitting position
- cannot follow breath-hold commands—mostly expiratory views → normal cardiothoracic ratio up to 65%, higher than in adults
- have smaller pulmonary vessels for given imaging system resolution → normal vascular markings can be traced just into lateral half of lung (can be traced into lateral third of hemithorax in 95% of adults)
- Thymus dominant = pulmonary vessels just visible; even large vessels including PA main trunk (semitransparent structure) may be difficult to define (**Fig. 2.49**)
- Evaluating transverse diameter of central pulmonary arteries: compare right lower lobe ar-

Table 2.1   Classification of cardiac anomalies based on anatomical cause

Anatomical cause	Anomaly
Left heart obstruction	<ul><li>Valvular, sub-/supravalvular aortic stenosis (AS)</li><li>Coarctation of aorta (CoA), interrupted aortic arch</li><li>Hypoplastic left heart syndrome</li><li>Congenital mitral valve stenosis</li></ul>
Right heart obstruction	<ul><li>Valvular, sub-/supravalvular pulmonic stenosis (PS)</li><li>Pulmonary atresia (PA)</li><li>Tetralogy of Fallot (TOF)</li><li>Tricuspid atresia (TA)</li><li>Ebstein anomaly</li></ul>
Septal and vascular malformations	<ul><li>Atrial septal defect (ASD I, ASD II, ASD with partial anomalous pulmonary venous drainage)</li><li>Ventricular septal defect (VSD)</li><li>Total atrioventricular canal (AVC)</li><li>Patent ductus arteriosus (PDA)</li><li>Total anomalous pulmonary venous drainage (TAPVD)</li><li>Truncus arteriosus communis (TAC)</li></ul>
Complex congenital heart disease/ anomalous origins of great arteries	<ul><li>Complete transposition of great arteries (d-TGA)</li><li>Corrected transposition of great arteries (l-TGA)</li><li>Double-outlet right ventricle (DORV)</li><li>Univentricular heart (UVH), single ventricle (SV)</li></ul>

Table 2.2   Classification of cardiac anomalies based on cyanosis and lung perfusion

Without cyanosis Lung perfusion			With cyanosis Lung perfusion	
Increased	Decreased	Normal	Increased	Decreased
ASD	PS	AS	TGA	TOF
VSD	CoA		TAPVD	PA
PDA			DORV (without PS)	DORV and PS
			UVH	UVH without PS

Abbreviations: see **Table 2.1**.

Table 2.3   Degrees of severity of cardiac anomalies, in order of necessary treatment intensity

Degree of severity	Type
"Simple" anomalies	ASD, VSD, PDA
"Moderately severe" anomalies	AVC, valvular insufficiencies, CoA, ASD I, right ventricular outflow tract stenosis
"Severe" anomalies	Cyanotic heart defects, valvular atresias, TGA, UVH

Abbreviations: see **Table 2.1**.

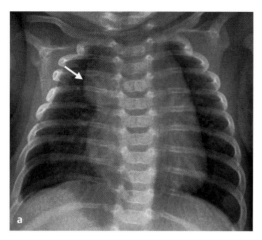 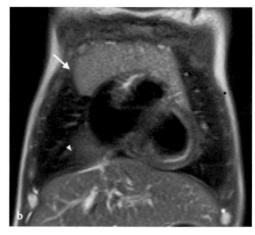

Fig. 2.49a, b Mediastinal widening referable to thymus. Chest radiograph (**a**) and T2-weighted MRI (**b**) show abnormal mediastinal and cardiac borders (arrows). Morgagni hernia (arrowhead) also present in **b**.

tery with trachea. In children with significant left-to-right shunt (> 2 : 1 = right ventricular stroke volume twice the left ventricular volume, as with atrial septal defect [ASD]), diameter of right lower lobe artery always greater than tracheal diameter

Basic Patterns of Findings on Chest Radiographs

Lung Perfusion

Increased lung perfusion: result of increased active or passive volume overload.

- **Actively increased lung perfusion:** always caused by shunting of blood from systemic circulation to low-pressure pulmonary circuit (ASD, ventricular septal defect [VSD], PDA, etc.). Volume overload → vessels elongated, traceable into periphery, sharp outlining
- **Passive overload:** usually results from left ventricular outflow tract obstruction (e.g., congenital critical aortic valve stenosis) or left ventricular failure → dilatation of pulmonary veins and fluid exudation into alveoli → indistinct vessel outlines, Kerley lines

Decreased lung perfusion: right ventricular outflow tract obstruction—e.g., tetralogy of Fallot (TOF), hypoplastic right heart syndrome, Ebstein anomaly.

Unequal lung perfusion intrinsic to certain heart diseases:

- TOF (usually less perfusion of left lung)
- Persistent truncus arteriosus (no side predominance)
- Congenital pulmonic stenosis (less perfusion of right lung)

Pulmonary Hila

Hila and central pulmonary arteries may be normal, dilated (widened), or narrowed.

Widened hila with laterally convex borders: left-to-right shunt, poststenotic dilatation due to pulmonary valve stenosis, pulmonary valve insufficiency (result of increased stroke volume due to diastolic regurgitation).

Narrowed hila: right ventricular outflow tract obstruction (e.g., TOF) or abnormal position (e.g., persistent truncus arteriosus), reactive due to unilateral pulmonary hypoplasia or airway obstruction (Euler–Liljestrand mechanism).

Aorta

Position of aorta: on left or right side, e.g., right descending aorta in 25% of patients with TOF.

Anomalies of shape: e.g., coarctation of aorta (CoA).

Small aortic knob: results from decreased aortic blood flow, e.g., ASD, VSD, hypoplastic left heart syndrome.

Aortic enlargement: ascending aorta, aortic knob, descending aorta. Enlarged ascending aorta → poststenotic dilatation (aortic valve stenosis), increased stroke volume (aortic insufficiency), central shunts (PDA, aortopulmonary window).

> **!** Older children—caution: Marfan syndrome.

Cardiac Chambers

Enlarged cardiac chambers: atrial dilatation develops relatively quickly, ventricular dilatation slowly. Two mechanisms:

- Increased inflow—receive more blood (left-to-right shunt, anomalous pulmonary venous drainage, etc.)
- Obstructed outflow (e.g., valvular stenosis—valvular/subvalvular/supravalvular)

Right atrium: widening of right cardiac silhouette, usually greatly enlarged in newborns = easy to diagnose.

Right ventricle: forms anteroinferior cardiac border; when enlarged → clockwise rotation of cardiac silhouette. If hypertrophy predominates → cardiac apex is rotated counterclockwise and points upward.

Left atrium: obliterated cardiac waist → left atrium forms right cardiac border. Elevation of left main bronchus, splaying of carina.

> **!** Caution: bronchomalacia of left main bronchus.

Left ventricle: counterclockwise rotation of cardiac silhouette, cardiac apex points downward.

Additional Findings

Rib notching: due to enlargement of intercostal neurovascular bundle (enlarged, tortuous intercostal arteries, increased pulsations → activation of osteoclasts).

Most frequent cause: CoA; 16 other possibilities (**Table 2.4**).

Musculoskeletal system: premature sternal fusion → thoracic deformity (pectus carinatum), rib mal-

Table 2.4   Causes of rib notching (after Felson 1973)

Organ system		Cause
Arterial	Obstruction of aorta	Coarctation of aorta
		Thrombosis of abdominal aorta
	Obstruction of subclavian artery	Blalock–Taussig operations
		Pulseless disease—Takayasu arteritis
		(Adults—atherosclerosis)
	Decreased pulmonary arterial flow	TOF
		Pseudotruncus
		Pulmonary valve stenosis
		Unilateral absence of a pulmonary artery
		Adults—pulmonary emphysema
Venous		Obstruction of superior vena cava
Shunts		Pulmonary AVF
		Intercostal AVF
		Intercostal to PA fistula
Neurogenic		Intercostal neurinoma
Osseous		Hyperparathyroidism
		Idiopathic—normal variant

Abbreviations: TOF, Tetralogy of Fallot; AVF, arteriovenous fistula; PA, pulmonary artery.

formations (bifid ribs, fused ribs—also acquired after cardiac surgery), postoperative widening of intercostal spaces (surgical approach), congenital scoliosis due to impaired vertebral body perfusion

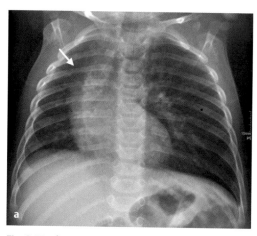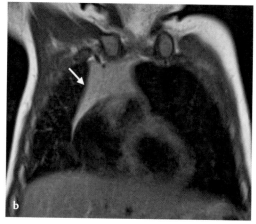

Fig. 2.50a, b   Dextroposition of the heart. Chest radiograph (**a**) and T2-weighted MRI (**b**) show heart displaced to right—aggravated by prominent thymus (white arrow).

or syndromic (see below), bone age retardation (generalized slow bone growth), widened medullary cavities and diminished trabecular pattern (spicules on flat bone—DD: Cooley anemia) = result of heart disease with cyanosis and secondary polyglobulia → medullary expansion.

Calcifications: intracardiac, vascular, valvular—e.g., calcified PDA remnant (incidental finding on chest radiograph), conduit calcifications after pulmonary valve replacement.

Aeration disorders: overaeration/atelectasis due to compression effects from abnormally positioned or enlarged vessels (possible bronchomalacia). Atelectasis most commonly affects left lower lobe (VSD, PDA, endocardial fibroelastosis). Generalized overaeration in anomalies associated with increased or decreased lung perfusion. Cause = increased respiratory excursions due to "air hunger."

Syndromes

Cardiac anomalies may also occur in syndromes. Common examples:

- VACTERL syndromes (**v**ertebral **a**nomalies, **c**ardiac malformations, **t**racheoesophageal fistula, **e**sophageal atresia, **r**enal dysplasia and **l**imb anomalies)
- "Heart–hand syndromes" (e.g., Holt–Oram syndrome = autosomal dominant genetic mutation with thumb, radius, and cardiac anomalies—frequent presence of ASD/VSD)

- Endocardial cushion defects (common in trisomy 21), increased incidence of CoA in girls with Turner syndrome (XO sex chromosomes).

Radiology of Selected Cardiac Anomalies

Malposition of the Heart

Dextroposition: heart in right hemithorax, no malrotation, no associated cardiac anomalies due to thoracic, mediastinal, pleural or other processes (e.g., funnel chest) (**Fig. 2.50**).

Differences: **dextrocardia**—heart on right side, atypical cardiac rotation. Most common form = mirror-image dextrocardia (apex points to right, complete inversion of otherwise normal heart).

Heterotaxy Syndromes (Ivemark Syndromes): Malposition with Asplenia or Polysplenia

Asplenia: trilobed left lung with accessory septum, cyanotic heart defect, flattened symmetrical bifurcation angle, malrotation.

Polysplenia: frequent acyanotic defect, dextrocardia present in 50% of cases, absence of coronary sinus, aplasia of intrahepatic IVC with azygos continuation.

Atrial Septal Defect

Classification:

- Primum type (ASD I—low position over atrioventricular valves, classified as atrioventricular defect)
- Secundum type (ASD II—most common, foramen ovale = patent foramen ovale [PFO])
- Sinus venosus defect (in upper part of interatrial septum/termination of superior vena cava [SVC], often associated with partial anomalous pulmonary venous drainage)

Hemodynamics: left-to-right shunt at atrial level → increased circulating blood volume in pulmonary circuit.

Radiology: findings depend on shunt volume—increased active lung perfusion, enlarged right atrium and ventricle and PA; small aortic knob.

Ventricular Septal Defect

Classification:

- Perimembranous type (in membranous part of septum, possible accompanying aneurysm)
- Muscular type (in muscular part of septum)
- Supraventricular type (supraventricular crest)

Hemodynamics: left-to-right shunt at ventricular level → increased circulating blood volume in pulmonary circuit, possible volume overload on left side. With large shunt volume—left ventricle "empties" into right ventricle = right volume overload → pressure elevation in pulmonary circuit, right ventricular hypertrophy, pressure reversal with right-to-left shunt (extreme case: Eisenmenger reaction; surgical correction no longer possible at that point).

Radiology: findings similar to ASD (depend on shunt volume and pulmonary vascular resistance, etc.)—prominent pulmonary segment, actively increased lung perfusion, dilated left atrium and ventricle, small aortic knob (**Fig. 2.51**).

Patent Ductus Arteriosus

Definition and etiology: connects left PA to descending aorta. After birth (spontaneous respiration), oxygen tension rises in blood → PDA contracts (normally remains functionally patent up to 48 hour postpartum). May calcify with regression.

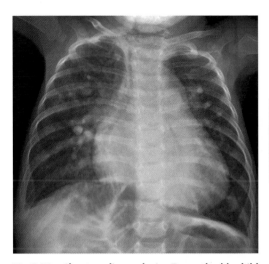

Fig. 2.51 Chest radiograph in 7-month-old child with membranous ventricular septal defect and cardiomegaly. Active pulmonary hyperperfusion. Left atrium forms almost all right cardiac border; bilateral pleural effusions. Right lower lobe artery same size as trachea—↑ due to shunt volume. Lower lobe dystelectasis in left lung, elevation of right hemidiaphragm.

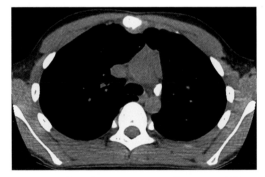

Fig. 2.52 Plain thoracic CT scan of 13-year-old boy, followed up for underlying oncologic disease. Calcification in aortopulmonary window has remained unchanged for years (calcified PDA remnant).

! Caution: do not confuse with calcified lymph nodes in aortopulmonary window (**Fig. 2.52**).

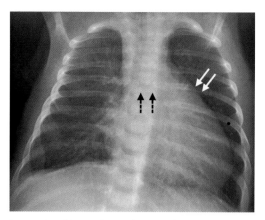

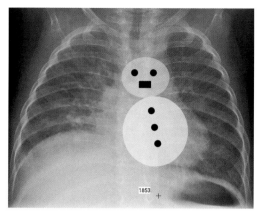

Fig. 2.53 Chest radiograph in newborn with patent ductus arteriosus. Left ventricle enlarged, left main bronchus elevated—expression of left atrial enlargement (broken black arrows). Cardiac waist effaced (solid white arrows); marked pulmonary hyperperfusion.

Fig. 2.54 Chest radiograph in infant with total anomalous pulmonary venous drainage. Cardiac vascular shadow shows typical "snowman" configuration with enlarged right heart and pulmonary hyperperfusion.

Hemodynamics: shunt depends on pulmonary vascular resistance (systolic and diastolic)—usually left-to-right shunt. With high pulmonary vascular resistance (e.g., persistent fetal circulation): right-to-left shunt (→ cyanosis).
Radiology: findings similar to VSD—active pulmonary hyperperfusion, enlarged left atrium and ventricle, prominent aortic arch (**Fig. 2.53**). "Ductus bump" sometimes present between aorta and PA.

Anomalous Pulmonary Venous Drainage

Classification: based on affected pulmonary veins. **Complete form** (= total anomalous pulmonary venous return [TAPVR]) and **incomplete form** (= partial anomalous pulmonary venous return [PAPVR])—abnormal draining pulmonary veins join to form collecting vessel → four types defined:
- **Type I** (50–55%): common supracardiac termination at persistent left superior vena cava, left brachiocephalic vein, SVC, or azygos vein
- **Type II** (30%): opens into right atrium or coronary sinus
- **Type III:** opens below diaphragm into IVC or portal vein, often associated with inflow obstruction
- **Type IV:** combination of types I–III

Scimitar syndrome: see Sect. 2.2.
Hemodynamics: complete form = complete bypass of left heart (left-to-right shunt). Blood from sys-

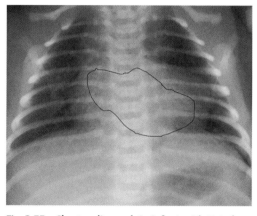

Fig. 2.55 Chest radiograph in infant with Tetralogy of Fallot. "Boot-shaped heart" outlined on film. Concomitant pulmonary hypoperfusion.

temic veins enters pulmonary circuit, returns to right heart via abnormal pulmonary veins. Lung perfused only through coexisting ASD/PFO. In type III, left-to-right shunt decreased due to venous obstruction, places rising pressure load on right heart.
Radiology: in types I and II, enlargement of right atrium and ventricle and active pulmonary hyperperfusion → "snowman" figure (**Fig. 2.54**). In type III, lung perfusion may be decreased, depending on venous obstruction.

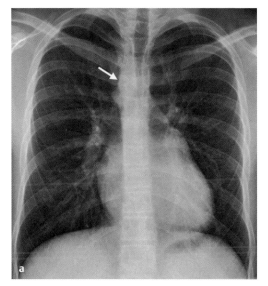
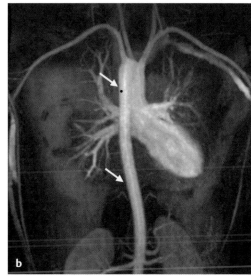

Fig. 2.56a, b   Tetralogy of Fallot and right descending aorta in 18-year-old male.

a Chest radiograph shows atypical aortic knob at right paravertebral location (white arrow).

b MRA demonstrates typical right aortic arch with left brachiocephalic trunk. Thoracal aorta descending to right.

Tetralogy of Fallot

Definition: cyanotic heart defect with pulmonary hypoperfusion. Consists of pulmonic stenosis, consequent right ventricular hypertrophy, high-sited VSD (aorta receives mixed blood from both ventricles—hence named "overriding aorta"); 50% of cases have pulmonary atresia instead of pulmonic stenosis. Pulmonary valve may be bicuspid. Possible associated anomalies/hypoplasia of pulmonary vessels—left PA most commonly affected. Aorta descends on right side in 25% of cases.

Primary correction of pulmonic stenosis and closure of VSD is almost always followed by pulmonary insufficiency (secondary right ventricular enlargement) and proximal stenosis of left and right PA → frequent secondary operations (pulmonary valve replacement, stent insertions).

Hemodynamics: right ventricular hypertrophy—cardiac apex directed upward due to hypertrophy ("boot-shaped" heart) and pulmonary hypoperfusion.

Radiology: boot-shaped heart, decreased pulmonary vascular markings, narrowed hila, possible asymmetric lung perfusion (usually on left side) due to concomitant hypoplasia/stenosis of PA (**Figs. 2.55** and **2.56**).

Transposition of Great Arteries (TGA)

Classification:

- **d-TGA** (dextro-TGA)—aorta arises from anatomic right ventricle, PA from anatomic left ventricle. Incompatible with life without shunts (PFO, ASD, VSD, PDA, systemic collaterals).
  Surgical treatment: early palliative Blalock–Taussig anastomosis. Later corrective surgery (Senning or Mustard operation) in which atrial septum is resected, newly created atrium assumes function of systemic venous atrium, atrial baffle routes SVC and IVC blood directly to mitral valve, and shunts are closed → restoration of normal blood flow.
  Current option, neonatal "switch operation": aorta and PA detached and connected to outflow tract of corresponding anatomic ventricle (PA to right ventricle, aorta to left ventricle); may include reimplantation of coronary arteries.
- **l-TGA** (levo-TGA)—additional inversion of ventricles → tricuspid valve supplies anatomic left ventricle, mitral valve supplies anatomic right

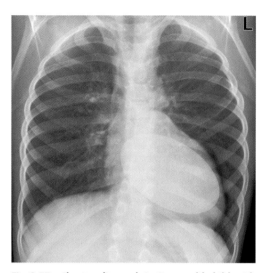

Fig. 2.57   Chest radiograph in 9-year-old child with transposition of great arteries shows narrow mediastinum and "egg-shaped" heart. Normal lung perfusion (after surgery).

ventricle. After Senning or Mustard operation or with l-TGA: anatomic right ventricle cannot permanently assume function of left ventricle → progressive ventricular dilatation in young adulthood, cardiac insufficiency, and cardiac arrhythmias = need for pacemaker implantation.

Hemodynamics:

- **d-TGA**—initially two completely separate circulations; survival relies on shunts (congenital/surgical). Atrial baffle after Senning/Mustard operation directs systemic venous blood through mitral valve to morphologic left ventricle (now functioning as subpulmonary ventricle), to PA, pulmonary venous blood flow is guided via newly created pulmonary venous atrium to anatomical right ventricle (now functioning as systemic ventricle), and finally to aorta.
- **l-TGA**—systemic venous return via right atrium and tricuspid valve to morphologic left ventricle and PA arising from it; systemic venous return via left atrium or mitral valve to morphologic right ventricle (= systemic ventricle) and aorta.

Radiology: rapid postpartum development of cardiomegaly due to shunts, active and passive hyperperfusion. Aorta and PA not side by side but one in front of the other in sagittal section ("double barrel shotgun" sign). Narrowed mediastinum, egg-shaped heart (**Fig. 2.57**).

Aortic Arch Anomalies

See also Sect. 2.2.

Aortic arch anomalies are rare (1% of all cardiac anomalies); 20% have genetic cause (chromosome 22q11 deletion).

Classification: double aortic arch—right aortic arch with mirror-image origins of supra-aortic vessels, right aortic arch with abnormal origins, left aortic arch with abnormal origins, cervical aortic arch (very rare), aberrant right subclavian artery. Abnormal origins and frequent bilateral PDA = complete vascular rings → frequent congenital stridor. Mirror-image right aortic arch present in TOF and truncus arteriosus.

Imaging: initial assessment by US/echocardiography. Give special attention to position of brachiocephalic trunk → include supra-aortic branches in all sectional imaging studies. MRI preferred, except for multiorgan imaging = CT (e.g., airway/lung investigations).

Coarctation of the Aorta

See also Sect. 2.2.

Definition: congenital constriction of aortic arch near DA ("juxtaductal"). Associated anomalies: bicuspid aortic valve, VSD; in girls—Turner syndrome.

In all symptomatic forms: blood pressure elevated in upper limbs, low in lower limbs. Palpable inguinal pulse often absent or diminished in infants.

Classification:

- Preductal (infantile) type: constriction proximal to DA → no intrauterine collateralization. Also hypoplasia of aortic arch = increased risk of aortic aneurysms in later life. Rapidly symptomatic after birth, at least by closure of DA
- Postductal (adult) type: intrauterine collateralization—clinical manifestations appear later than with infantile type

Hemodynamics: left ventricular hypertrophy due to hypertension.

Radiology: "figure 3" sign on chest radiograph (pre- and poststenotic dilatation) = dilated medial aortic border at pre- and postductal levels. Rib notches, left ventricular hypertrophy. Esophagram: mirror-image figure-3 sign = "E" sign. Later risk of spontaneous dissection and aortic dilatation → regular follow-ups with cross-sectional imaging.

Treatment: various surgical options (end-to-end anastomosis, subclavian flap procedure).

Cardiovascular Imaging in Congenital Heart Disease

Chest Radiograph

Displays abnormalities of organ shapes and position (situs evaluation), lung perfusion, associated pulmonary and skeletal changes.

Echocardiography and Mediastinal Ultrasound

For anatomical evaluation. Also permits visual assessment of cardiac contractility, functional assessment of regional and global cardiac function (ejection fraction—calculated, based on assumptions of ventricular geometry), gradients across valves and stenoses, and basic shunt evaluation.

> Reproducible quantification of right ventricular function is difficult. Geometric assumptions become less accurate with increasing cardiac size → greater deviation from measured values. Increasing age and postoperative changes/deformities make ultrasound more difficult/challenging.

Angiocardiography

"Gold standard," vessel mapping plus invasive pressure measurements (e.g., valvular gradients) and oximetry (determination of shunt volume). Ventricular volumes and derived indices (ejection fraction) can be calculated from biplanar views—based on assumption of given ventricular geometry (same problem as in echocardiography). Valvular insufficiency can be assessed visually and semiquantitatively (indicator dilution method = regurgitant fraction calculated from the dilution of a contrast bolus due to valvular insufficiency).

Treatment options: Rashkind procedure, balloon valvuloplasty, stent, valve insertions.

> Angiocardiography is burdened by high dosage, which depends, in part, on executing cardiologists.

Cardiac Magnetic Resonance Imaging

Noninvasive, yields morphologic information and much functional data. Sedation and β-blockers may be required.

Case Study 2.7

Clinical presentation: 11-year-old child with blood pressure differential between upper and lower limbs.

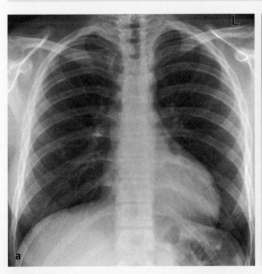
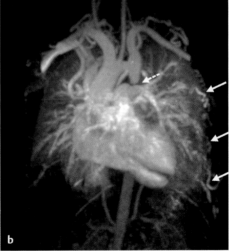

Fig. 2.58a, b

Findings: Fig. 2.58 a: Chest X-ray—discrete narrowing just below of aortic arch, rib notches. **Fig. 2.58b:** ce-MRA —subtotal narrowing with aortic isthmus (dashed arrow), collaterals are marked by white arrows.
Diagnosis: coarctation of aorta.

! Sedation and β-blockers should be used with caution in patients with right heart arrhythmias.

- Ventricular volumetry without need for geometric assumptions → global and regional cardiac function can be accurately assessed
- Flow measurements (velocity encoded imaging —VENC imaging) = valvular gradients and regurgitant fractions can be determined
- Contrast techniques: delayed enhancement (for diagnosing ischemia, DD of myocarditis), MRA
- MRA techniques: complex vascular malformations; with ECG and respiratory gating → can evaluate coronary vessels without contrast medium, even in spontaneously breathing children

Cardiac CT

Alternative when cardiac MRI contraindicated (e.g., pacemaker after TGA).
- Good anatomical imaging. CTA = accurate visualization of coronary vessels and great vessels.
- Volumetry: regional and global cardiac function can be assessed, valvular stenosis/insufficiency can be quantified (quantification of opening/closing area).

> Note: High radiation burden – Cardiac CT dose up to 25 mSv (or even higher). Heart rates > 60–90 bpm associated with higher exposures (rapid heart rate allows only parts of cardiac cycle to be acquired → prolonged scan time = greater exposure).

Cardiac Scintigraphy

Of minor importance in children.

Bibliography

1 Bailliard F, Hughes ML, Taylor AM. Introduction to cardiac imaging in infants and children: techniques, potential, and role in the imaging work-up of various cardiac malformations and other pediatric heart conditions. Eur J Radiol 2008; 68(2): 191–198
2 Felson B. The thoracic wall. In: Chest Roentgenology. Philadelphia: WB Saunders; 1973a: Ch 13, 450–463
3 Felson B. A review of over 30, 000 normal chest roentgenograms. In: Chest Roentgenology. Philadelphia: WB Saunders; 1973b: Ch 15, 494–501

4 Ferguson EC, Krishnamurthy R, Oldham SAA. Classic imaging signs of congenital cardiovascular abnormalities. Radiographics 2007; 27(5): 1323–1334
5 Kaemmerer H, Hess J. Adult patients with congenital heart abnormalities: present and future. [Article in German] Dtsch Med Wochenschr 2005; 130(3): 97–101
6 Rogel S, Schwartz A, Rakower J. The differentiation of dextroversion from dextroposition of the heart and their relation to pulmonary abnormalities. Dis Chest 1963; 44: 186–192
7 Schweigmann G, Gassner I, Maurer K. Imaging the neonatal heart—essentials for the radiologist. Eur J Radiol 2006; 60(2): 159–170
8 Swischuk LE. A scheme for roentgenographic interpretation. In: Plain Film Interpretation in Congenital Heart Disease. 2nd ed. Baltimore: Williams & Wilkins; 1979a: Ch II, 15–46
9 Swischuk LE. Cardiac malpositions, miscellaneous cardiac and vascular anomalies, and special problems in neonates and adults. In: Plain Film Interpretation in Congenital Heart Disease. 2nd ed. Baltimore: Williams & Wilkins; 1979b: Ch IV, 199–244
10 Taylor AM. Cardiac imaging: MR or CT? Which to use when. Pediatr Radiol 2008; 38(Suppl 3): S433–S438

Case Study 2.8

Clinical presentation: newborn with cyanosis and increased respiratory rate.

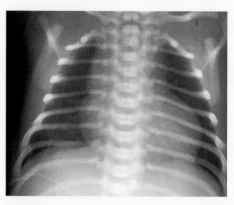

Fig. 2.59

Findings: First chest X-ray—cardiac silhouette widened and slightly boot-shaped, pulmonary circulation is diminished.
Diagnosis: Tetralogy of Fallot.

3 Imaging of the Pediatric Gastrointestinal Tract

Maria Sinzig

3.1 Imaging Modalities and Prerequisites

General

Quality assurance for radiographic imaging in children—two main principles: justification and optimization. Justification and patient selection for radiographic imaging are inseparable—if no alternative to X-rays (e.g., US vs. CT) → essential to optimize imaging procedure. Cornerstone of optimization = ALARA principle (see Chapter 1).

General rule: prerequisites for any imaging study = accurate history and clinical examination. Protect child from heat loss during examination. If possible, do not reposition child in neonatal ICU.

Methods

- **US:** first and only imaging study for many abdominal/GI investigations in children; various transducers required, especially high-frequency linear probes
- **Radiography:** plain abdominal radiograph, usually AP projection in supine position. Supine cross-table lateral or left-side-down decubitus views depend on indication and clinical status. Full-length thoracoabdominal radiograph ("babygram") may also be indicated. Immobilization (Babix holder, clear compression device made of radiolucent material, foam cushions, sandbags, manual immobilization by helper); accurate collimation (inadequate field size = common error in pediatric radiographs). Do not use scatter-reduction grid for infants < 1 year old.
- **FL:** pulsed FL systems; last-image-hold views preferred to reduce radiation exposure
- **Contrast media:** water-soluble, nonionic, iso-osmolar media (may be diluted with distilled water or physiologic saline solution)—safest option (but most costly)
- **CT:** adapt imaging protocol to clinical question and age; few indications (mainly trauma-related)
- **MRI:** no radiation exposure, therefore preferred over CT. Relative disadvantages = long examination time, sedation, (cost)

3.2 Congenital Anomalies of the Gastrointestinal Tract

Esophageal Atresia

General: esophagus and trachea develop from foregut, separate from each other in weeks 5 to 6 of embryonic development. Incomplete separation of esophagus from primitive trachea → esophageal atresia (EA) with/without tracheo-esophageal fistula (TEF). EA = most common congenital esophageal disorder (1 : 3,000 to 1 : 5,000 live births). Classified by Vogt types (**Fig. 3.1**). Most common type = proximal EA with distal fistula (Vogt type IIIb). 35% of babies with EA are premature. H-fistula = isolated TEF without EA.

Clinical features: inability of newborns to swallow saliva ("drooling"), choking, cyanosis, coughing on first attempt at feeding, tube cannot be passed into stomach.

H-fistula: coughing and choking during feeding, recurrent bronchopulmonary infections (diagnosis often delayed).

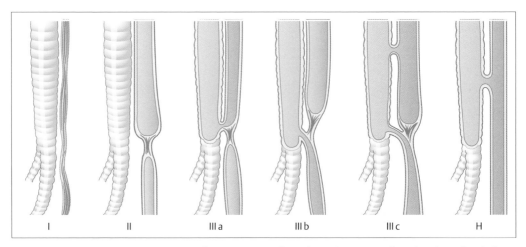

Fig. 3.1   Diagrammatic representation of various types of esophageal atresia with and without fistula (Vogt classification).

Imaging:

- **US:** EA detected prenatally in only about one-third of cases (stomach small/not visualized, polyhydramnios)

> With adequate communication between esophagus and trachea, amniotic fluid passage unimpaired; normal gastric filling, no polyhydramnios.

- **Radiography:** plain chest and abdominal radiographs—air-filled proximal esophageal pouch, gastric tube projected over thoracic inlet. Lower fistula: increased volume of intestinal gas (**Fig. 3.2**). No lower TEF: gasless abdomen; possible cardiac anomaly; aorta may descend on right or left side—decisive for surgeons, since thoracotomy on side opposite to aortic arch (if X-rays equivocal, define aortic arch with US). Possible malformations of spinal column (**Fig. 3.3**)
- **FL:** hardly necessary in types I to III. May be used in EA without distal fistula to define preoperative length of atretic segment: water-soluble contrast medium instilled into stomach via gastrostomy (lower pouch usually refluxive), or radiopaque tube advanced into lower esophageal blind pouch via gastrostomy while second radiopaque tube passed into upper pouch; distance between the two pouches assessed (**Fig. 3.4**).

H-fistula: imaged in lateral or prone position. Fistula passes forward and upward to trachea from anterior esophageal wall (**Fig. 3.5**).

> Some H-fistulas only intermittently patent → important to sufficiently opacify esophagus (have patient swallow water-soluble contrast or instill via tube with tip placed in upper third of esophagus; use 5 or 8 Fr feeding tube in newborns, may use double balloon technique if necessary).

> **!** Do not mistake aspirated contrast medium for contrast medium from nonvisualized fistula! Document contrast transit as far as duodenojejunal flexure to detect or exclude associated malrotation.

- Postoperative esophagram (leak, other complications): water-soluble contrast medium swallowed or instilled by tube.

DD: traumatic pharyngeal perforation by orogastric tube placement (differentiate gas-filled proximal esophageal pouch from pneumomediastinum). H-fistula with chronic or recurrent bronchopulmonary infections: GER, FB aspiration, immunodeficiency, CF.

Associated anomalies: VACTERL association (45%) (**Fig. 3.3**), intestinal atresias (**Fig. 3.3**), biliary atresia, esophageal stenosis (**Fig. 3.6**).

Treatment: atresia with distal fistula—usually primary anastomosis with fistula repair. Atresia without distal fistula—initial gastrostomy (primary repair rarely possible, usually long atretic segment), then repeated bougienage (to lengthen ends of esophagus for end-to-end anastomosis). If not possible, gastric pull-up operation or colon interposition.

Prognosis: depends on associated anomalies.

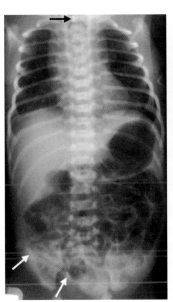

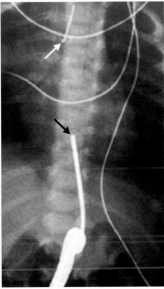

Fig. 3.2

Fig. 3.4

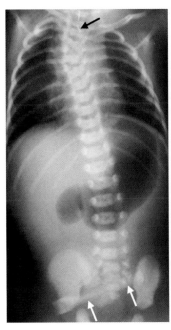

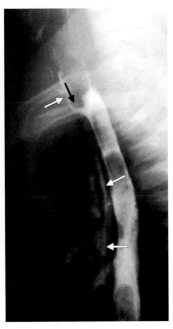

Fig. 3.3

Fig. 3.5

3

Fig. 3.2 Thoracoabdominal radiograph in male term infant on first day of life, type III b esophageal atresia. Gastric tube in proximal esophageal pouch (black arrow). Increased intestinal gas content suggests lower tracheo-esophageal fistula. Umbilical clamp (white arrows).

Fig. 3.4 Fluoroscopy in type II esophageal atresia. Radiopaque tube placed in distal end of esophagus via gastrostomy, second tube placed in proximal esophagus (arrows). Long gap between the two esophageal blind pouches.

Fig. 3.3 Thoracoabdominal radiograph in newborn girl with type III b esophageal atresia (EA) plus duodenal atresia and VATER association (vertebral defects, anal atresia, tracheo-esophageal fistula with EA, and radial dysplasia). Gastric tube in proximal end of esophagus (black arrow), gaseous distention of stomach and proximal duodenum ("double bubble" sign), rest of abdomen gasless. Upper thoracic vertebral anomalies. Umbilical clamp (white arrows).

Fig. 3.5 Esophagram with water-soluble contrast medium in lateral projection, H-fistula (black arrow). Contrast medium in bronchial system and trachea (white arrows).

Esophageal Stenosis

General: congenital stenosis very rare (1 : 25,000 to 1 : 50,000 live births). Three types: circumscribed fibromuscular hypertrophy, tracheobronchial rests in esophageal wall, or esophageal membrane with small central perforation. **Acquired stenosis** may result from epidermolysis, GER, surgery, or esophageal injury (caustic ingestion, etc.).

Clinical features: difficulty or inability to swallow solid foods/large bites, food gets stuck.

Imaging:

- **FL:** water-soluble contrast. Fibromuscular stenosis—smooth margins, typically at T8–T10 level (**Fig. 3.6**). Stenosis due to tracheobronchial rests—smooth margins, very tight, usually at T10–T11 level. Stenosis by membrane—thin web with regular contours, usually at T4 level.

DD: stricture caused by reflux esophagitis—mucosal abnormalities (mucosa appears endoscopically normal with fibromuscular stenosis or tracheobronchial rests; consider level of narrowness).

Treatment: Fibromuscular stenosis easily dilated. Stenosis due to tracheobronchial rests rigid—requires resection. Acquired stenosis often difficult to treat (repeated bougienage, stent insertion, esophageal replacement, etc.).

Gastroesophageal Reflux

General: GER = normal intermittent physiologic phenomenon, usually after eating, common in infants and small children.

Gastroestophageal reflux disease (GERD) = symptomatic GER = "disease."

Clinical features: vomiting, irritability, failure to thrive, bronchopulmonary infections, cough, abdominal pain, chest pain, dysphagia.

Imaging:

- **US:** retrograde flow of gastric contents into esophagus in infants and small children after fluid ingestion (US best done immediately after bottle feeding)
- **FL:** visualization of esophagus in upper gastrointestinal (UGI) series: fasted child, water-soluble contrast medium ingested or instilled by tube, esophagus imaged in AP and lateral views. Evaluate for anatomic abnormalities (e.g., aberrant right subclavian artery) and motility disorders; finally have child ingest tea (= water siphon test—improves GER detection rate). Follow contrast transit to duodenojejunal flexure (malrotation?)

> X-ray swallowing study indicated only in GERD (relatively high radiation exposure = ca. 2.6 mSv = about 130 chest radiographs) to exclude associated anatomic abnormalities (hiatal hernia, gastric outlet obstruction, malrotation).

DD: HPS, duodenal stenosis, achalasia, esophagitis due to different cause.

Treatment: GER usually resolves at 1 to 2 years; only about 1% require surgery (fundoplication).

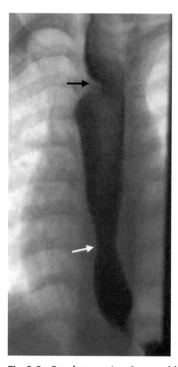

Fig. 3.6   Esophagram in a 3-year-old boy after end-to-end anastomosis for type III b esophageal atresia, congenital esophageal stenosis (white arrow). Circumscribed semicircular esophageal constriction at level of anastomosis (black arrow).

Duodenal Obstruction

General: two main groups (**Table 3.1**); intrinsic and extrinsic obstruction often coexist.

Duodenal Atresia and Stenosis

General: most common high intestinal obstruction in newborns (~ 1 : 3,400).
Clinical features: bile-stained vomiting (obstruction usually distal to Vater ampulla); nonbilious vomiting less common (obstruction proximal to Vater ampulla).
Imaging:

- **US:** about 50% fetal polyhydramnios; double-bubble sign from fluid-filled stomach and duodenum on pre- and postnatal scans. Possible annular pancreas, preduodenal portal vein, biliary anomalies. Obstruction by Ladd bands—vigorous peristalsis in obstructed duodenum.
- **Radiographs:** double-bubble sign (gas-filled stomach + gas-filled proximal duodenum), rest of abdomen gasless (duodenal atresia, **Fig. 3.3**); little intestinal gas distal to duodenum (duodenal stenosis, **Fig. 3.7**). Possible gas in bile ducts due to incompetent Oddi sphincter
- **FL:** UGI series (water-soluble contrast medium administered by tube); may be useful with incomplete obstruction (plain radiographs usually diagnostic)

> Y-shaped termination of pancreatic duct oral and aboral to atresia → gas entering aboral intestine → images show gas distal to atresia.

DD: differentiation extrinsic/intrinsic in most cases not definable preoperativly; malrotation with volvulus, duplication cyst.
Associated anomalies: annular pancreas, trisomy 21, cardiac anomalies, EA.

Table 3.1 Duodenal obstruction

Intrinsic	Extrinsic
- Duodenal atresia	- Ladd bands in malrotation
- Duodenal stenosis	- Midgut volvulus
- Duodenal web	- Annular pancreas
	- Preduodenal portal vein
	- Intestinal duplication

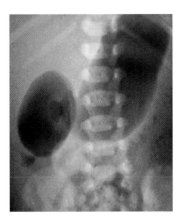

Fig. 3.7 Abdominal radiograph in 2-day-old girl with Down syndrome and duodenal stenosis. Double-bubble sign, scant intestinal gas distal to dilated proximal duodenum.

3

Treatment: surgery (urgent but not emergent); emergent for partial duodenal obstruction if volvulus cannot be excluded.

Malrotation

General: synonym for incomplete/absent bowel rotation (broad spectrum of abnormal intestinal rotation and fixation—classification schemes of little help). In weeks 6–11 of embryonic development, midgut makes three 90° counterclockwise rotations around long axis of superior mesenteric artery (SMA) → after total 270° rotation, duodenojejunal flexure in upper left quadrant of abdomen, cecum in lower right quadrant → taut fixation of small bowel mesentery (from upper left to lower right quadrant). Malrotation leads to short mesenteric root and lax fixation of small bowel with risk of midgut rotation around long axis of SMA (= volvulus).
Clinical features: Malrotation in itself is asymptomatic. Vomiting (bilious) results from associated peritoneal fixation (Ladd bands—from cecum to porta hepatis via second part of duodenum → duodenal obstruction, **Fig. 3.8**).
Imaging:

- **US:** relative positions of SMA and superior mesenteric vein (SMV); latter normally anterior and to right of SMA (**Fig. 3.9**).

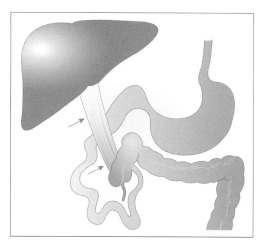

Fig. 3.8   Diagrammatic representation of intestinal malrotation, Ladd bands (arrows).

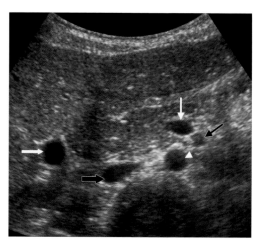

Fig. 3.9   Transverse ultrasound scan through mid-upper abdomen demonstrates normal relationship of superior mesenteric artery (black arrow) to superior mesenteric vein (white arrow). Aorta (arrowhead), inferior vena cava (thick black arrow), gallbladder (thick white arrow).

! A normal relationship of these vessels does not exclude malrotation.

If SMV to left of SMA, malrotation likely (**Fig. 3.10**).
- **FL:** UGI series—with normal bowel rotation—duodenojejunal flexure just to left of spinal column at level of duodenal bulb (**Fig. 3.11**). All other positions = malrotation (**Fig. 3.12**)

> Initial passage of contrast medium from duodenum gives nonsuperimposed view of flexure. Contrast enema not reliable for detecting/excluding malrotation (cecum may be mobile despite normal bowel rotation).

Associated anomalies: duodenal stenosis/atresia, Meckel diverticulum (MD), omphalocele, gastroschisis, situs ambiguus, polysplenia, asplenia, diaphragmatic hernia.

Volvulus

General: Midgut volvulus = abnormal rotation of small bowel around long axis of SMA, usually during neonatal period. Midgut volvulus = potential complication of abnormal intestinal rotation and represents life-threatening emergency—requires immediate surgery due to rapid onset of intestinal ischemia and necrosis.
Clinical features: bilious vomiting, (acute) abdominal pain.

Imaging:
- **Radiographs:** plain abdominal radiograph may be normal or show paucity of intra-abdominal gas (**Fig. 3.13**). Duodenum not significantly dilated despite obstruction (due to rapid progression of disease)
- **US:** whirlpool sign—highly specific for volvulus, occurs when small bowel, mesentery, and SMV wrap around SMA (**Figs. 3.14** and **3.15**). Bowel distal to obstruction collapsed or fluid-filled, has thickened walls (edema). Free intraperitoneal fluid (intestinal vascular compromise)
- **FL:** if radiographs and US do not exclude volvulus → UGI series with water-soluble contrast medium administered by gastric tube—beak-shaped termination or corkscrewlike configuration of duodenum (**Fig. 3.16**)

> Despite duodenal obstruction, double-bubble sign absent due to rapid development of bowel ischemia—not enough time to cause dilation.

DD: GER (vomiting not bilious), duodenal atresia/stenosis, annular pancreas, duodenal web (dilated proximal duodenum usually means long-standing obstruction).
Treatment: surgical emergency!

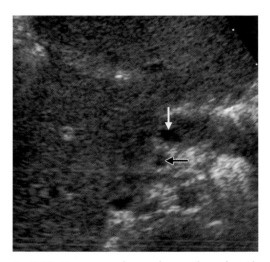

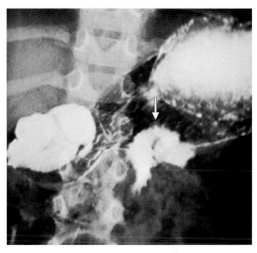

Fig. 3.10 Transverse ultrsound scan through mid-upper abdomen in malrotation. Superior mesenteric vein (white arrow) located at 1 o'clock position relative to superior mesenteric artery (black arrow).

Fig. 3.11 UGI series documents normal position of duodenojejunal flexure (arrow).

3

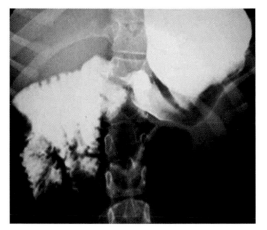

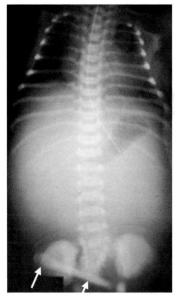

Fig. 3.12 UGI series in malrotation (nonrotation). Duodenojejunal flexure and proximal small bowel to right of spinal column.

Fig. 3.13 Thoracoabdominal radiograph in male infant several hours old with bilious vomiting, abdominal distention, volvulus. Gas in stomach, rest of abdomen gasless; duodenum not defined. Umbilical clamp (arrows).

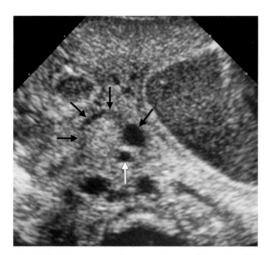

Fig. 3.14 Transverse ultrasound scan through mid-upper abdomen in newborn with bilious vomiting and volvulus. Whirlpool sign caused by superior mesenteric vein (black arrows) wrapped around superior mesenteric artery (white arrow).

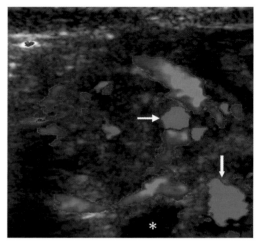

Fig. 3.15 Color Doppler scan through mid-upper abdomen in 10-day-old newborn with bilious vomiting and volvulus. Whirlpool sign caused by superior mesenteric vein wrapped around superior mesenteric artery (thinner white arrow). Aorta (thicker white arrow); inferior vena cava (*).

Jejunal/Ileal Atresia/Stenosis

General: jejunal atresia/stenosis = most common congenital small bowel obstruction (1 : 750 live births). Early vascular insult may be causative. Four types:

- Type I: single intraluminal web
- Type II: solid cord, connects both intestinal blind pouches
- Type III: intestinal blind pouches are completely separated, associated mesenteric defect
- Type IV: familial form with multiple atresias ("apple peel")

Clinical features: proximal atresia → bilious vomiting. More distal obstruction causes abdominal distention with absent/delayed meconium passage.

Imaging:

- **Radiographs:** number of dilated bowel loops reflects level of obstruction—many dilated bowel loops = distal obstruction (small and large bowel radiographically indistinguishable in newborns —haustrations not yet present). Few dilated loops = jejunal/proximal ileal obstruction (**Fig. 3.17**). High jejunal obstruction may also present with single, grossly dilated bowel loop —diagnosis should be recognized from that sign (**Fig. 3.18**)

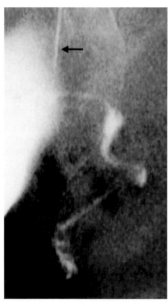

Fig. 3.16 UGI series with water-soluble contrast medium in 3-day-old boy with bilious vomiting and volvulus. Right lateral decubitus view. Note corkscrewlike appearance of opacified duodenum. Gastric tube (arrow).

- **US:** sometimes shows meconium pseudocyst or meconium peritonitis (following intrauterine perforation), bowel dilated oral to obstruction
- **FL:** contrast enema with water-soluble medium in distal intestinal obstruction—microcolon ("unused colon"). The more distal the small bowel obstruction, the smaller the colon lumen (with high obstruction, adequate fluid and shed intestinal mucosal cells = "intestinal juice," so colon often has normal caliber)

> Microcolon absent with distal small bowel obstruction developing shortly before birth (colon had time to reach normal diameter). Microcolon diagnostic for long-standing distal small bowel obstruction, but normal colon caliber does not exclude that entity.

DD: meconium ileus, meconium plug syndrome (small left colon syndrome), Hirschsprung disease.
Treatment: surgical resection.

Colonic Atresia/Stenosis

General: Rare (~1:40,000 live births); probable cause = vascular insult. Proximal atresia more common than distal atresia. Classification based on anatomical features (as in small bowel).
Clinical features: abdominal distention, absent/delayed meconium passage (>24–48 hours), bilious vomiting.
Imaging:
- **Radiographs:** multiple dilated bowel loops (nonspecific)
- **FL:** contrast enema with water-soluble medium: small-caliber colon distal to atresia, "wind sock" sign in type I (intraluminal web with central perforation, **Fig. 3.19**)

DD: Hirschsprung disease, ileal atresia, meconium ileus, meconium plug syndrome.
Treatment: surgical.

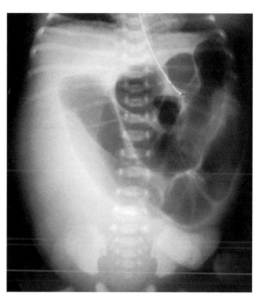

Fig. 3.17 Abdominal radiograph in female term infant, first day of life, jejunal atresia. Intestine distal to gas-distended small bowel loops devoid of gas.

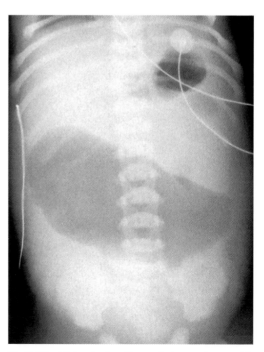

Fig. 3.18 Abdominal radiograph in newborn with high jejunal atresia shows single, grossly dilated bowel loop in midabdomen.

3

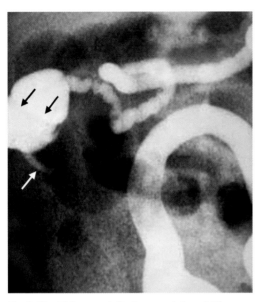

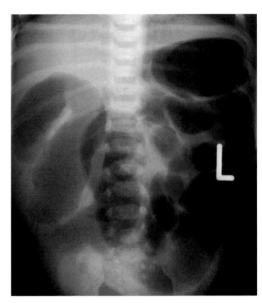

Fig. 3.19 Male term infant, second day of life; contrast enema shows "wind sock" sign in type I colonic atresia (intraluminal web—black arrows). Appendix (white arrow). Relatively small colon lumen.

Fig. 3.20 Abdominal radiograph in male newborn with meconium ileus, second day of life. Multiple dilated bowel loops, "soap bubble" pattern in right hemiabdomen caused by mixture of gas and viscous meconium.

Meconium Ileus/Peritonitis

General: distal ileal obstruction by abnormally viscous meconium; usually associated with CF (but only 10–20% of patients with CF have meconium ileus; see Chapter 2). (Intrauterine) perforation → meconium peritonitis.

Clinical features: absence of meconium passage, abdominal distention, bilious vomiting.

Imaging:

- **Radiographs:** signs of low intestinal obstruction —multiple dilated bowel loops, bubbly–granular pattern in lower right quadrant (soap-bubble effect caused by gas–meconium mixture, **Fig. 3.20**). Usually no air–fluid levels (abnormal secretion from mucinous glands), but air–fluid levels do not exclude meconium ileus. Peritoneal calcifications in meconium peritonitis (**Fig. 3.21**). Also scrotal calcifications in children with patent vaginal process. Some cases show meconium pseudocyst formation with peripheral calcification (leakage of meconium)
- **US:** dilated bowel loops with hyperechoic contents. Peritoneal calcifications in meconium

peritonitis. Circumscribed inhomogeneous mass, possibly with calcified echogenic wall (meconium pseudocyst)

- **FL:** contrast enema with water-soluble (iso-osmolar) medium—microcolon, multiple filling defects in terminal ileum (meconium pellets)

> Soap-bubble effect on radiographs is common but not pathognomonic for meconium ileus (also seen in ileal atresia, meconium plug syndrome, colonic atresia, Hirschsprung disease, etc.) → therefore contrast enema often necessary in children with signs of low intestinal obstruction. Any obstruction with perforation may lead to meconium peritonitis. Undiluted Gastrografin (sodium amidotrizoate and meglumine amidotrizoate, hyperosmolar) contraindicated since iso-osmolar contrast medium equally effective and safer.

DD: ileal atresia, total aganglionosis of colon, meconium plug syndrome.

Treatment: clearing of meconium ileus by repeated contrast enemas with 15–20% solution of N-acetylcysteine and water-soluble iso-osmolar contrast medium (~33% success rate). Otherwise, or in case of perforation → surgical treatment.

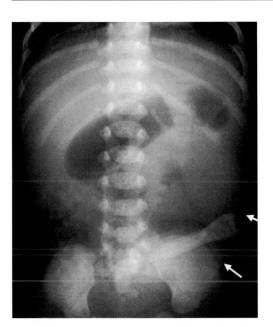

Fig. 3.21   Meconium peritonitis with pseudocyst in male newborn with bilious vomiting, first day of life. Radiograph shows calcified wall of large pseudocyst (arrows) and multiple flecks of peritoneal calcification, most prominent in right midabdomen.

Meckel Diverticulum

General: remnant of omphalomesenteric duct (connects yolk sac to midgut). MD found in 2–4% of autopsies = most common congenital GI tract anomaly, always on antimesenteric side, up to 100 cm oral from ileocecal valve. Wall layers identical to small bowel (true diverticulum); contains ectopic gastric mucosa (in 15%) or ectopic pancreatic tissue (in 5%) → predisposes to ulcers and bleeding. Rare cases with giant MD (diameter ≥ 5 cm)

Clinical features: usually asymptomatic. Small children with symptomatic diverticulum: usually painless rectal bleeding (may be profuse). Intestinal obstruction (forms lead point for ileocolic intussusception). Meckel diverticulitis presents with fever, vomiting, and abdominal pain.

Imaging:
- **Radiographs:** giant MD appears as large, gas-filled mass, sometimes with intraluminal enteroliths

- **US:** modality of choice in intussusception with (inverted) MD as lead point; inflammatory change in bowel wall structure (similar to appendicitis) in MD.
- **Scintigraphy:** ^{99m}Tc-pertechnetate scans most reliable (when gastric mucosa present). Sensitivity in children 85%, specificity 95%

> Symptomatic MD = imaging challenge. MD that becomes symptomatic in children is often associated with ectopic gastric mucosa.

DD: appendicitis, intestinal duplication, bowel wall hemangioma.
Treatment: surgical.

Gastrointestinal Duplication Cysts

General: three characteristics—wall composed of smooth muscle, lined with epithelium from specific portion of GI tract, current/prior communication with GI tract. Cysts contain ectopic gastric mucosa in 2% of cases (colon) to 43% (esophagus). Sites of occurrence: 75% abdominal (usually ileum), 20% thoracic, 5% thoracoabdominal. Often associated with (intra)spinal anomalies (neuroenteric cysts).
Clinical features: children usually present in first year of life with abdominal pain, vomiting, intestinal obstruction/intussusception. Presence of gastric mucosa → peptic ulceration with intestinal bleeding (melena). Sometimes detected incidentally at US.
Imaging:
- **US:** high-frequency linear probe; pathognomonic layered wall structure (= "gut signature"): high-level entry echo (at mucosal interface), hypoechoic lamina propria, hyperechoic submucosa, hypoechoic lamina muscularis, hyperechoic serosal interface. Echo-free lumen, sometimes with septations or echogenic debris.
- **Radiographs:** contribute little to diagnosis
- **FL:** contrast examination—displacement/obstruction of adjacent bowel loops; duplication cyst opacified in rare cases
- **Scintigraphy:** ^{99m}Tc-pertechnetate scan (when gastric mucosa present—more common in upper GI tract)
- **CT/MRI:** used mainly for intrathoracic duplication cysts

3

DD: MD, ovarian cyst/teratoma, ovarian torsion, mesenteric cyst, mesenteric lymphangioma, meconium pseudocyst, urachal cyst, hydrometrocolpos, exophytic liver cyst, choledochal cyst, pancreatic pseudocyst.
Treatment: surgical.

Hirschsprung Disease

General: congenital megacolon (1:4,500 live births), most common in term infants. Disturbance of craniocaudal neuroblast migration in embryonic/fetal period → absence of ganglion cells in myenteric and submucous plexus. Normally, ganglion cells descend along GI tract—reach distal colon by week 12 of embryonic development. If migration arrested, bowel distal to that level is aganglionic. Most common sites are rectum and sigmoid colon (~80%, preponderance of males); total aganglionosis of colon in 5 to 10% (no sex predilection). Aganglionosis starting from duodenum and ultrashort segment (= transition zone at anorectal junction) very rare. Absence of ganglion cells → absent/deficient relaxation of affected bowel segment = functional obstruction. Skip lesions questionable (inconsistent with concept of ganglion cell migration)—probably areas with absent ganglion cells due to intrauterine ischemic bowel insult.
Clinical features: absent/delayed meconium passage, abdominal distention, bilious vomiting, constipation problems starting at birth, enterocolitis.
Imaging:
- **Radiographs:** numerous dilated, gas-filled bowel loops (in newborns, **Fig. 3.22**). Increased stool proximal to aganglionic segment (in older children); (almost) no gas in rectum
- **FL:** contrast enema with water-soluble medium in unprepared patients (no bowel lavage or rectal examination at least 2 days prior); rectal diameter smaller than sigmoid colon (rectosigmoid index < 1, normally ≥ 1, **Fig. 3.23**). Transition zone = bowel segment forming junction between "normal-caliber" aganglionic segment and more proximal, dilated bowel with normal ganglion cells (**Fig. 3.24**). Irregular, uncoordinated contractions in aganglionic segment (~20%). Delayed contrast excretion on late images. Total colonic aganglionosis—less specific signs → imaging diagnosis difficult or

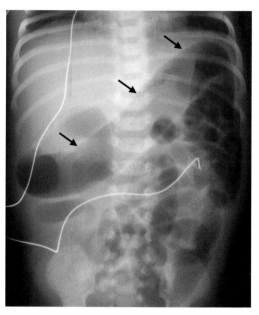

Fig. 3.22 Abdominal radiograph in male term infant, 6 days old, with delayed meconium passage in Hirschsprung disease. Numerous distended bowel loops suggest low intestinal obstruction. Transverse colon identified by its location; haustrations physiologically still absent (arrows).

impossible (sometimes colon slightly shorter, flexures rounded)

> Classic narrow aganglionic segment may not yet be visible in first 10 to 14 days of life. Absence of transition zone/narrow segment does not exclude Hirschsprung disease. Clinical signs of distal intestinal obstruction with no apparent cause on contrast enema → further investigation.

Other tests: manometry, diagnostic accuracy = 75%; rectal (suction) biopsy—can exclude Hirschsprung disease in 100% of cases (presence of ganglion cells).
Serious complication: with high mortality rate = enterocolitis/toxic megacolon (owing to delayed diagnosis and treatment).
DD: meconium plug syndrome, meconium ileus, ileal atresia, immature colon in preterm infant, neuronal intestinal dysplasia, colonic atresia.
Associated anomalies: chromosome abnormalities (trisomy 21).

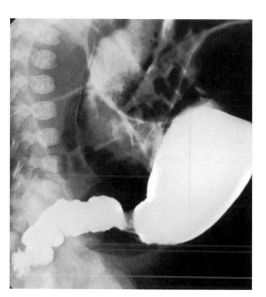

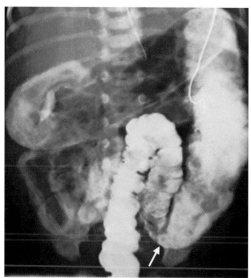

Fig. 3.23 Contrast enema, left lateral decubitus, in 5-week-old boy constipated since birth reveals Hirschsprung disease. Note abrupt transition from aganglionic rectum to more proximal colon, which already shows marked dilatation.

Fig. 3.24 Contrast enema in Hirschsprung disease (same child as in Fig. 3.22) clearly displays transition zone at junction of descending colon with sigmoid colon (arrow). Irregular contractions in aganglionic sigma/rectum. Colon oral to that segment dilated.

Treatment: (sub)total resection of aganglionic segment, pull-through of normally innervated bowel.
Postoperative complications: constipation, encopresis, diarrhea, enuresis.

Omphalocele

General: herniation of abdominal organs (usually small bowel and liver) into umbilical cord. Associated with chromosome abnormalities in 50% of cases.
Clinical features: marked enlargement of umbilical cord at birth.
Imaging:
- **US:** intestine normally has returned to abdominal cavity by week 11 of embryonic development—allows for early intrauterine diagnosis. Postpartum: GER, malrotation
- **FL:** UGI series—malrotation.

  Omphalocele covered by amniotic epithelium.

DD: umbilical hernia (covered by skin).
Treatment: surgical.

Gastroschisis

General: paraumbilical defect in anterior abdominal wall—usually on right side—with herniation of small bowel; rarely includes colon (**Fig. 3.25**) and stomach. Bowel loops exposed to amniotic fluid in utero—damage to bowel wall (sterile inflammation with bowel wall edema and fibrogelatinous coating) → frequent cause of life-long bowel motility problems (hypoperistalsis syndrome).
Clinical features: abdominal wall defect with herniated, exposed intestine.
Imaging:
- **US:** intrauterine—herniated bowel, polyhydramnios—suggests associated intestinal atresia
- **FL:** UGI series—malrotation, intestinal hypomotility with prolonged transit time, intestinal obstruction by adhesions, GER
DD: ruptured omphalocele.
Treatment: surgical.

3

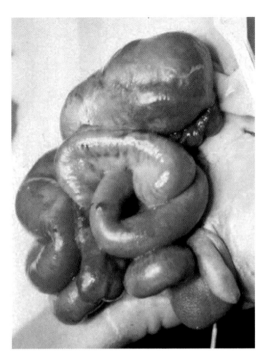

Fig. 3.25   Gastroschisis in newborn. Herniated small and large bowel. Fibrin coatings visible on bowel walls.

Congenital Diaphragmatic Hernia

General: herniation of abdominal organs into chest. Bochdalek hernia = posterior hernia (most common, incidence = 1 : 2,200, more common on left side). Morgagni hernia = anterior hernia (3%, more common on right side).

Clinical features: respiratory distress immediately after birth, flat abdomen; occasional late presentation (late onset of diaphragmatic hernia).

Imaging:

- **US:** prenatal—intrathoracic abdominal contents, mediastinal shift, possible abnormal position of gastric bubble. Postnatal—intrathoracic bowel loops; possible herniation of stomach, liver, spleen; malrotation

- **Radiographs:** immediate postnatal films show dense opacity in corresponding hemithorax; later films (after air has entered GI tract) show "cystic" mass, contralateral mediastinal shift, and few or no intra-abdominal gas-filled bowel loops (**Fig. 3.26**). Right-sided hernia often contains liver (dense intrathoracic mass, **Fig. 3.27**). Hypoplasia of ipsilateral lung and possibly of contralateral lung, possible abnormal gastric tube position above diaphragm (intrathoracic stomach). Contralateral deviation of intrathoracic course of gastric tube, atypical course of umbilical vein catheter (with intrathoracic liver, **Fig. 3.27**).

- **CT:** not indicated.

- **MRI:** almost only in fetal period; multiple hyperintense structures (T2-weighted images) in chest (bowel loops), mediastinal shift, decreased lung volumes, few intra-abdominal bowel loops, possible herniated liver (hypointense). Important prognostic parameters: lung volumes, position of liver.

Main complication = pulmonary hypoplasia with persistent fetal circulation. Early herniation is associated with more pronounced hypoplasia. Immediate postpartum placement of gastric tube prevents severe gaseous bowel distention, reduces mass effect (less respiratory distress). Malrotation is usually present.

DD: congenital pulmonary airway malformation (CPAM), congenital lobar emphysema, pneumatoceles in pneumonia (streptococci, staphylococci), eventration of diaphragm.

Treatment: extracorporeal membrane oxygenation (ECMO) may be necessary for stabilizing patient. Definitive treatment = surgery.

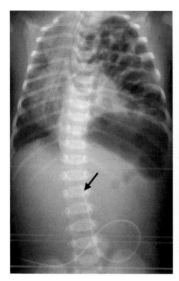

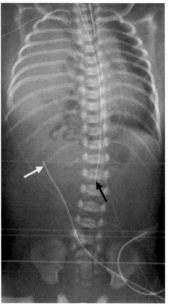

Fig. 3.26

Fig. 3.27

Fig. 3.26 Thoracoabdominal radiograph several hours after birth of child with respiratory distress syndrome and left diaphragmatic hernia. Film shows multiple radiolucencies due to gas-filled bowel loops in left hemithorax with contralateral shift of heart and mediastinum. Stomach intra-abdominal, rest of abdomen almost gasless. Position of umbilical vein catheter too low (arrow).

Fig. 3.27 Thoracoabdominal radiograph several hours after birth of child with respiratory distress syndrome and right diaphragmatic hernia. Almost entire intestine and portion of liver intra-thoracic (atypical course of umbilical vein catheter—white arrow). Stomach intra-abdominal, gastric tube in place (black arrow).

3

3.3 Neonatal Gastrointestinal Problems and Complications

Vomiting in Newborns

General: Vomiting is common in neonates. Bilious vomiting = danger sign.

! Caution: volvulus.

Full-term newborns pass meconium within 24 to 48 hours. Absent/delayed meconium passage → increasing abdominal distention (cause: obstruction, pneumoperitoneum, mass, free fluid, necrotizing enterocolitis [NEC], intestinal paralysis)—often associated with vomiting.

Imaging:

- **Radiographs:** basic workup for neonatal GI problems includes evaluation of
  - bowel gas distribution (gas normally in distal ileum 5 to 11 hours after birth, in rectum by 24 hours); paucity of intra-abdominal gas usually more alarming that multiple distended bowel loops—DD: volvulus (see **Fig. 3.13**)
  - width of bowel loops (colon and small bowel indistinguishable in newborns)
  - possible pneumatosis, abnormal calcifications, free air, separation of bowel loops (thickened bowel walls, free fluid), mass (e.g., meconium pseudocyst); supine or left lateral decubitus (LLD) cross-table view may be necessary (free air)
- **US:** detection or exclusion of volvulus; possible free fluid, (free air), pneumatosis, gas in portal venous system, peritoneal calcifications, meconium pseudocyst, intestinal paralysis
- **UGI series:** water-soluble, nonionic contrast medium via gastric tube (with "high" obstructions plain radiographs usually diagnostic)

! Volvulus—always obtain UGI series if radiographs and US inconclusive.

- **Contrast enema:** for "low" obstructions (distal small bowel, colon); use 8-Fr feeding tube and water-soluble, nonionic contrast medium (**Figs. 3.19, 3.23, 3.24**).

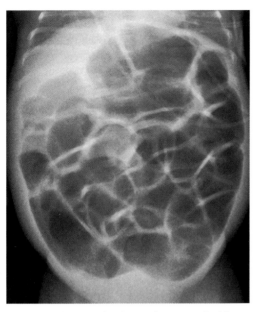

Fig. 3.28   Abdominal radiograph in 2-week-old pre-term infant with CPAP belly shows multiple distended bowel loops. Gaseous bowel distention resolved spontaneously in a few days, progression to normal feeding tolerated without problems.

Table 3.2   Causes of free intraperitoneal air in newborns

With perforation of GI tract	Necrotizing enterocolitis
	Gastric perforation, spontaneous or iatrogenic
	Isolated perforation of small bowel/colon (without associated anomaly)
	Perforated Meckel diverticulum (ectopic gastric mucosa with ulceration)
	Colon perforation (usually iatrogenic by rectal thermometer, intestinal lavage catheter, enema)
	Perforation due to intestinal obstruction (atresia, meconium ileus, Hirschsprung disease)
	Anastomotic leak after GI surgery
Without perforation of GI tract	Pulmonary air leak (pneumomediastinum, pneumothorax)

DD: GER (immaturity of lower esophageal sphincter), malrotation and volvulus, intestinal obstruction, sepsis, gastroenteritis (GE), hiatal hernia, incarcerated inguinal hernia, CPAP belly syndrome (small bowel and colon distention in preterms due to aerophagia and decreased peristalsis during nasal CPAP, **Fig. 3.28**; CPAP = continuous positive airway pressure).
Treatment: based on cause.

Pneumoperitoneum

General: free intraperitoneal air, most commonly due to gastrointestinal perforation (**Table 3.2**). NEC = leading cause in neonatal ICU. Spontaneous gastric perforation—not unusual in full-term infants; rectal perforation usually iatrogenic. With pneumomediastinum or pneumothorax, gas may enter abdomen through normal openings in diaphragm.
Clinical features: usually difficult to assess. Abdominal distention, sepsis, vomiting.

Imaging:
- **Radiographs:** signs often subtle in AP projection: increased lucency of upper abdomen (**Fig. 3.29**); football sign (increased central abdominal lucency with visualization of falciform ligament); Rigler sign (outlining of inner and outer borders of bowel walls, **Fig. 3.29**). "Triangles" of gas between bowel loops, scrotal gas. Supine or LLD cross-table view may resolve doubts.

> PIE/pneumothorax suggests extraintestinal cause (to resolve preoperative doubts by administer nonionic, water-soluble contrast medium via gastric tube). "Pseudo-Rigler sign" after oral contrast administration!

- **US:** in experienced hands, very sensitive for free air—use high-resolution linear probe with light pressure
Treatment: surgical for GI perforation. Exception: extreme prematurity—drainage may be alternative to surgery.

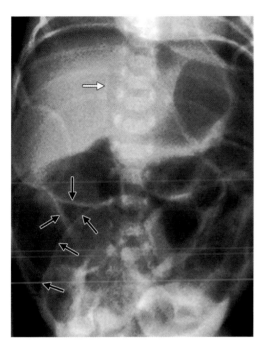

Fig. 3.29 Abdominal radiograph in preterm infant with necrotizing enterocolitis and free intraperitoneal air due to intestinal perforation. Note increased lucency below both diaphragm leaflets with Rigler sign (black arrows) and football sign (white arrow).

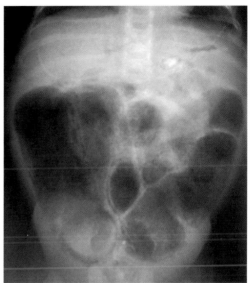

Fig. 3.30 Abdominal radiograph in preterm infant with severe necrotizing enterocolitis. Intramural gas appears as cystic and bandlike lucencies along numerous segments of bowel. Portal venous gas in liver. Unlike gas in intrahepatic bile ducts, portal venous gas extends to periphery of liver (gas in bile ducts—extremely rare in children, may result from biliary tract surgery or massive high obstruction).

Necrotizing Enterocolitis

General: severe disease mainly affecting preterm infants (1–3 : 1,000 live births). Most common in first 2 weeks of life. Cause not fully understood—multifactorial etiology such as ischemia, hyperosmolar feeding, intestinal hypomotility, immature immune response → damage to intestinal mucosa, bacterial invasion of bowel wall. Terminal ileum and proximal colon most commonly affected. Main risk factor = prematurity; occurs rarely in stressed term infants. Forms range from mild to rapidly progressive (transmural necrosis, perforation, peritonitis); possible fatal outcome.

Clinical features: bile retention, bilious vomiting, abdominal distention, bloody stools, lethargy, tachycardia, tachypnea, sepsis.

Imaging:

- **Radiographs:** films in early stage show nonspecific bowel distention (diffuse/localized), may show dilated bowel loop that remains constant over time ("persistent loop sign") = indicator of advanced disease. Individual bowel loops appear separated owing to bowel wall edema and/or free fluid. Intestinal pneumatosis—linear and/or cystic—caused by submucous/subserous air (gas results from bacterial metabolism), portal venous gas in liver (**Fig. 3.30**). Possible free intraperitoneal air (may be demonstrable by supine or LLD cross-table view)

- **US:** high-frequency linear probe; fluid-filled bowel loops with thickened walls, absence of peristalsis, free fluid, possible high-level echoes in bowel wall (pneumatosis), air echoes in portal vein and intrahepatic portal vein branches, (free air)

- **Doppler ultrasound:** spikes (artifacts due to tiny gas bubbles) in portal vein (**Fig. 3.31**)

- **FL:** after surgery with stoma construction; prior to reversal use FL to define efferent limb and exclude significant strictures

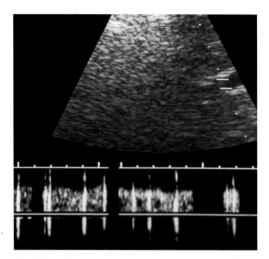

Fig. 3.31   Doppler spectrum from portal vein of preterm infant with necrotizing enterocolitis displays typical spikes (artifacts caused by small gas bubbles).

Pneumatosis intestinalis may occur in all diseases of intestines with impaired circulation, in case of severe bowel obstruction, idiopathic.

On plain abdominal radiographs, differentiation between small intraluminal gas bubbles and pneumatosis can be difficult—in doubtful cases, safer to overdiagnose. Pneumatosis in NEC in about 66%; nevertheless, diffuse pneumatosis usually marker for advanced disease. However, even in severe NEC, pneumatosis may never develop.
US (high resolution linear transducer) may demonstrate intramural gas bubbles and intraportally travelling gas (Doppler "blibbs" on spectral analysis).

DD: intestinal obstruction, immature colon in preterm infant, gaseous distension, idiopathic pneumatosis.
Treatment: gastric tube, parenteral hydration and nutrition, antibiotics. Pneumoperitoneum = solely commonly accepted indication for surgery.
Complications: perforation, lethality (about 25%), intestinal strictures/stenosis (singular or multiple), small bowel syndrome.

3.4   Acquired Gastrointestinal Changes after the Neonatal Period

Hypertrophic Pyloric Stenosis

General: idiopathic thickening of pylorus muscle (most frequent cause of gastric outlet stenosis), incidence = 1 : 500 live births. Typical age of onset 3 to 6 weeks, with preponderance of males (4–5 : 1). Rare in preterm infants (but may be congenital).
Clinical features: increasing not bile-stained vomiting, finally projectile, with weight loss, dehydration, and palpable "olive" (hypertrophic pylorus) in epigastrium.
Imaging: US: classic sonographic diagnosis. Define gallbladder with linear probe (at least 6 MHz); pylorus typically located just medial to it. Image pylorus in transverse and longitudinal scans. Transverse = hypoechoic hypertrophic muscular ring with central echogenic mucosa ("donut" sign). Longitudinal = central echogenic mucosa bilateral bounded by hypertrophic, hypoechoic pylorus muscle (**Fig. 3.32**). Measure muscle thickness, length of pyloric canal, pyloric diameter—reference values: muscle thickness > 3 mm, pyloric canal length > 16 mm, pyloric diameter > 15 mm.

Reference dimensions do not apply in cases with very early onset of manifestations—evaluate function.

DD: GER, malrotation with volvulus (bilious vomiting), duodenal stenosis, atrial web or polyp.
Complications: dehydration, metabolic dysfunction.
Treatment: surgical (pylorotomy).

Intussusception

General: invagination of one bowel segment (intussusceptum) into aboral segment (intussuscipiens). Peristalsis propels invaginated segment distally. Affects various combinations of bowel segments: jejunojejunal, ileoileal, ileocolic, ileo-ileocolic, colocolic. Terminal ileum most commonly affected—ileocolic intussusception = most common abdominal emergency in infants and small children (3–24 months). Incidence = 2–4 : 1000. Cause: idiopathic in > 90%. Lymph nodes and abnormal peristalsis may have causal significance (increased incidence during/after viral infection). Outside typical age group, usually arises from "lead point": MD, appendix, intestinal polyp (Peutz–Jeghers syndrome), non-Hodgkin lymphoma, duplication cyst (jejunojenunal), hemangioma, bowel wall hematoma in Schoenlein–Henoch purpura.

Mesentery of affected bowel segment with its feeding and draining vessels trapped between intussusceptum and intussuscipiens → decreased venous return → bowel wall edema and bleeding into bowel lumen due to venous congestion → restricted arterial inflow → bowel wall ischemia, necrosis, perforation.

Clinical features: classic presentation—sudden abdominal pain, intermittent, recurrent episodes of crying, initially separated by intervals in which child feels well. Untreated cases show deterioration, vomiting, bloody stool (raspberry jelly-like), lethargy, shock. Approximately 50% of children have palpable intra-abdominal cylindrical mass.

Imaging:

- **US:** imaging modality of choice for detecting **and** excluding intussusception; linear probe (> 6 MHz). Usually located in right midabdomen/upper abdomen or at inferior hepatic border. Transverse scan: persistent rounded structure about 2.5–4 cm in diameter with some concentric rings = target sign. With edematous swelling due to venous congestion, rings widened ("donut sign"): hyperechoic center (intussusceptum mucosa) surrounded by hypoechoic ring (intussusceptum wall), hyperechoic outer ring (intussuscipiens mucosa), hypoechoic outer zone (intussuscipiens muscle; **Fig. 3.33**). Longitudinal scan: thickened bowel wall with widened, hyperechoic center ("pseudokidney sign"); usually shows dilated prestenotic fluid-filled bowel loops, often shows some free intra-abdominal fluid. Mesenteric lymph nodes inside (and outside) intussusception figure. Color duplex scan: may show absence of flow signals in intussusceptum (bowel wall necrosis)

- **Radiographs:** mass of soft-tissue density, little gas in lower right quadrant— uncertain, however; radiography of little value in establishing diagnosis; helpful to assess perforation (pneumoperitoneum?) prior to image-guided reduction (perforation = contraindication to image-guided reduction)

DD: post-intussusception target sign = markedly swollen ileocecal valve (note diameter = 1.5–2.4 cm —smaller than ileocolic intussusception!). Ileoileal intussusception (mobility of small bowel loops → usually resolves spontaneously, diameter usually < 2 cm).

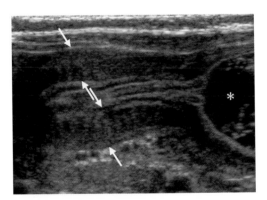

Fig. 3.32 Hypertrophic pyloric stenosis in 5-week-old male term infant with projectile vomiting. Longitudinal ultrasound scan through elongated pylorus shows thickened pyloric muscle (arrows) and fluid-filled stomach (*).

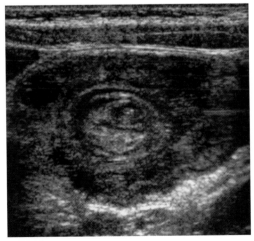

Fig. 3.33 Transverse ultrasound scan through ileocolic intussusception. Intussusceptum forms double-target pattern ("donut sign") within thickened hypoechoic wall of ascending colon.

Treatment:

1. Hydrostatic reduction under US/FL control in sedated child; IV line and continuous infusion; large-bore enema tube—instill physiologic saline solution (US) or water-soluble contrast medium (FL) from enema bag (drip height 80–100 cm), watch for reduction of intussusceptum leading edge (**Fig. 3.34**). Criteria for successful reduction: intussusceptum leading edge moves past ileocecal valve, intussusception figure disappears, clear ileocecal valve is defined (**Fig. 3.35**); visible reflux of fluid/contrast medium into terminal ileum, fluid-/contrast-filled loops of terminal ileum.

2. Pneumatic reduction under FL (rarely US) guidance: gas (air) administered by enema tube (maximum pressure 120 mmHg), usually via manual balloon pump.

3. Surgery if conservative treatment unsuccessful or contraindicated (peritonitis, intestinal perforation, hemodynamically unstable child—hypovolemia shock), or attempted conservative treatment has caused iatrogenic perforation.

> Prolonged history and bowel obstruction do not contraindicate image-guided reduction attempt.

Complications: perforation (spontaneous/during reduction in ~ 0.5–3%), bowel wall necrosis, bowel obstruction.

Chronic Inflammatory Bowel Diseases

Crohn Disease
(Terminal Ileitis, Regional Enteritis)

General: chronic recurring, segmental, granulomatous inflammatory bowel disease mainly affecting young adults (4% younger than 10 years, very few younger than 6 years). Ileocolic region most commonly involved; affects all layers of bowel wall.

Clinical features: recurring gastrointestinal complaints—abdominal pain, (bloody) diarrhea, anorectal fistula (often first sign—perianal changes in children strongly suspicious for Crohn disease in ~ 40%), pseudo appendicitis, fever of unknown ori-

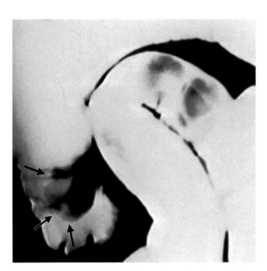

Fig. 3.34 Incomplete hydrostatic reduction of ileocolic intussusception with water-soluble contrast medium under fluoroscopic control. Filling defect (residual intussusceptum) appears at level of ileocecal valve (arrows). Terminal ileum not opacified.

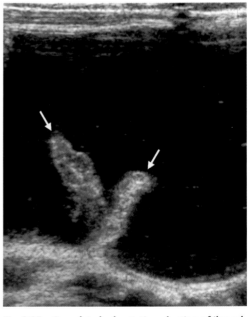

Fig. 3.35 Complete hydrostatic reduction of ileocolic intussusception with physiologic saline solution under US guidance. Ileocecal valve (arrows) clear and surrounded by fluid.

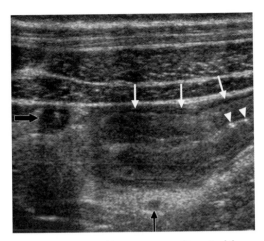

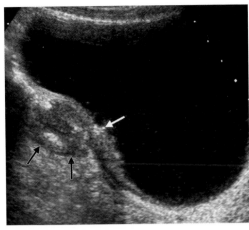

3

Fig. 3.36 Sonographic appearance of terminal ileum (longitudinal scan, white arrows) in Crohn disease. All layers of bowel wall thickened and hypoechoic. Bowel lumen greatly narrowed (arrowheads). Posterior fat shows inflammatory changes with small lymph node (thin black arrow). Note concomitant involvement of thickened appendix wall (thick black arrow).

Fig. 3.37 Longitudinal ultrasound scan through bladder of 14-year-old boy with Crohn disease. Terminal ileum shows asymmetric wall thickening (black arrows) and fistulous connection with bladder. Small air bubbles entering bladder lumen (white arrow). Posterior bladder wall thickened.

gin, associated joint pains, failure to thrive, anorexia nervosa–like symptoms, erythema nodosum.

Imaging:

- **US:** high-frequency linear probe shows thickened bowel wall. Transmural involvement → loss of typical wall stratification (**Fig. 3.36**). Ulcers, increased perfusion (color Doppler), narrowed bowel lumen, dilated bowel loops oral to change, hypoechoic hypertrophic and inflamed perifocal mesenteric fat, mesenteric lymph nodes, possible fistulas (**Fig. 3.37**), (intramural) abscesses
- **Radiographs:** bowel wall thickening (thumbprinting) in colitis, displacement of bowel loops by inflammatory mass (chiefly in right lower quadrant), signs of intestinal obstruction, gas in urogenital tract with abscess/fistula (**Fig. 3.37**)
- **FL:** enteroclysis via duodenal tube ("small bowel double-contrast study," Sellink)—largely superseded by MRI
- **MRI/MR enteroclysis:** rarely via duodenal tube, usually by oral ingestion (avoids FL-guided tube insertion) of hyperosmolar solutions (e.g., Mucofalk, mannitol, ethylene glycol suspension). Sequences: T2-weighted True FISP (fast imaging with steady-state precession), balanced FFE/SSFP (fast field echo, steady-state free preces-

sion), T2-weighted TSE SPIR (turbo-spin echo, spectral presaturation with inversion recovery), fat-suppressed T1-weighted SE before/after IV Gd-DTPA (gadolinium diethylenetriamine pentaacetic acid), more recent diffusion weighted sequences for active inflammation, and cine acquisitions (thick slab SSFP) for peristalsis (before administering Buscopan): contrast enhancement of affected bowel segment in active phase, bowel wall thickening, "comb sign" (mesenteric vessels of affected bowel segment arranged like teeth of comb due to inflammatory hypervascularity), proliferation of mesenteric fat ("creeping fat"), mesenteric lymph nodes, fistulas, abscesses (**Fig. 3.38**), obstruction with lack of bowel motility at stenotic site and prestenotic hyperperistalsis

- **CT:** MRI preferred! CT may be useful for detecting abscesses and directing drainage (if MRI unavailable, US guidance not possible)

DD: infectious enteritis (*Eschericia coli*, salmonella, *Shigella*, *Yersinia*, Tb), ulcerative colitis, appendicitis, mesenteric lymphadenitis, intestinal lymphoma.

Complications: perforation, peritonitis, fistula (to adjacent bowel loops, bladder, abdominal wall, perineum), cellulitis, abscess, bowel obstruction, GI

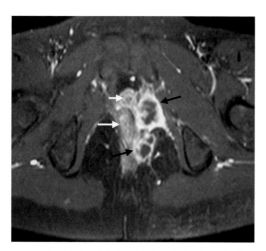

Fig. 3.38   Axial pelvic MRI (T1-weighted SPIR after contrast administration) in 10-year-old girl with Crohn disease. Perianal abscesses (black arrows), anal canal (long white arrow), urethra (short white arrow).

changes in adjacent fat; ulcerations potentially only seen after NaCl-enema ("US-hydrocolon")
- **Radiographs:** diffuse dilatation of colon with thickened haustra, absence of haustrations
- **FL:** usually colonoscopy and biopsy; double contrast enema rarely used
- **CT:** not indicated owing to radiation issues
- **MRI:** similar technique as with MR enteroclysis in Crohn disease, but after rectal enema

DD: Crohn disease, pseudomembranous colitis, infectious colitis, typhlitis.

Complications: intestinal bleeding, toxic megacolon, obstruction (postoperative), risk of malignant transformation, growth retardation (rarer than in Crohn disease).

Extraintestinal manifestations: pyoderma gangrenosum, sclerosing cholangitis, chronic active hepatitis, arthritis, ankylosing spondylitis, iritis.

Treatment: treatment of choice = colectomy.

bleeding, iliofemoral venous thrombosis, growth retardation.

Extraintestinal manifestations: sclerosing cholangitis, cholecystolithiasis, kidney stones, arthritis.

Treatment: conservative = corticosteroids, 5-aminosalicylic acid, azathioprine, infliximab, 9-mercaptopurine, metronidazole; iron, folic acid, vitamins B12, A, D, E, and K replacement; diet. Absolute indications for surgery: perforation, intra-abdominal and perianal abscess, bowel obstruction.

Ulcerative Colitis

General: idiopathic inflammatory disease affecting colonic mucosa and submucosa (DD: Crohn disease). Almost always begins in rectum, then spreads proximally by contiguous spread (no skip lesions—DD from Crohn disease). Rectosigmoid affected in 95% of cases. Backwash ileitis in 10–40%. Age distribution: mainly adolescents and young adults; infantile form may take fulminating fatal course.

Clinical features: bloody diarrhea, cramping abdominal pain, fever, weight loss, anemia, hypoalbuminemia, leukocytosis.

Imaging:
- **US:** thickened mucosa and submucosa, normal muscularis propria, no/less inflammatory

Appendicitis

General: inflammation of vermiform appendix. Most frequent cause of acute abdomen/abdominal surgery in pediatric age group (however, 11–32% of appendectomized children had normal appendix).

Clinical features: abdominal pain, vomiting, fever, local tenderness, rebound pain, leukocytosis, elevated CRP. The younger the child, the more difficult to localize pain, and the less specific the symptoms.

Imaging:
- **US:** modality of choice; shows aperistaltic, usually hypervascular, noncompressible structure ending in blind pouch. Possible intraluminal appendicolith. Transverse scan = target sign > 6 mm in diameter, often surrounded by hyperechoic inflamed fat and mesentery (**Fig. 3.39**). Possible mesenteric lymphadenopathy, free fluid

> Wall vascularization not increased/missing in necrotizing/gangrenous appendicitis. If only part of appendix seen, "normal" appendicitis not to be ruled out!

Perforated appendix often not visualized (appendix diameter may decrease again), inhomogeneous "mass," possible perityphlitic abscess, extraluminal appendicolith. Surrounding bowel loops fluid-

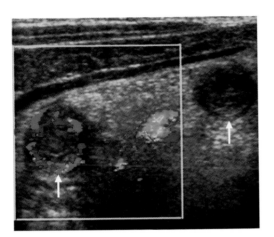

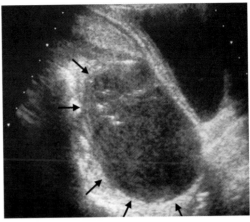

Fig. 3.39 Sonographic appearance of acute appendicitis. Appendix cut twice (arrows) by transverse scan. Color Doppler image shows increased wall vascularity and hyperechoic perifocal fat.

Fig. 3.40 Longitudinal ultrasound scan through lower midabdomen shows extensive abscess formation posterior to bladder (cul-de-sac abscess) due to perforated appendicitis (arrows).

filled, dilated, aperistaltic (paralytic ileus), mesenteric reaction, free fluid, lymph nodes

- **Radiographs:** rarely necessary (exclusion of free air); left convex lumbar scoliosis, obliterated ipsilateral psoas shadow, appendicolith, signs of bowel obstruction
- **CT:** rarely necessary (e.g., obese patients and clinically equivocal, with unclear US)
- **MRI:** can diagnose appendicitis, rarely used for cost and availability reasons

> Prominent lymphatic tissue in children sometimes responsible for enlarged, uninflamed appendix (in this case, no increased wall perfusion or hyperechoic perifocal fat). Mesenteric lymphadenitis does not exclude appendicitis. "Sonopalpation" very helpful. Appendicitis accompanying other bowel diseases. "Pseudoappendictis" in patients with cystic fibrosis.

DD: mesenteric lymphadenitis, MD, ovarian pathology, Crohn disease, omental infarction, torsion of appendages; in some cases urinary tract infection or urolithiasis.

Complications: perforation, perityphlitic or cul-de-sac abscess (**Fig. 3.40**), diffuse peritonitis, paralytic ileus.

Treatment: usually surgical at present.

Gastroenteritis

General: common childhood disease, often fatal in underdeveloped countries. Causative organisms: bacteria (salmonella, shigella, *E. coli, Yersinia,* campylobacter), viruses (rotavirus, norovirus, adenovirus), parasites (worms, especially *Ascaris lumbricoides*).

Clinical features: vomiting, diarrhea, abdominal pain, dehydration.

Imaging:

- **US:** usually not indicated; fluid-filled small bowel loops, sometimes with thickened walls, and parasite in bowel lumen (**Fig. 3.41**). Increased peristalsis, enlarged mesenteric lymph nodes, free intraperitoneal fluid, may show intermittent ileo-ileal intussusception (diameter < 2 cm, resolves spontaneously)
- **Radiographs:** usually not indicated; dilated bowel loops with air–fluid level(s)

DD: appendicitis, ileocolic intussusception.

Treatment: fluid administration, progressive bland diet; anthelmintic therapy as needed.

Ascariasis

General: most common human worm infection (= 1 billion infected persons worldwide). Causative organism: *Ascaris lumbricoides,* roundworm (nema-

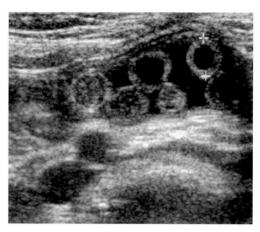

Fig. 3.41   Ultrasound demonstrates multiple round-worms in transverse diameter occupying fluid-filled small bowel loop in left lower quadrant.

tode) up to 35 cm long inhabiting human small intestine. Ingested larvae penetrate bowel wall, travel in bloodstream to lung, are coughed up and reswallowed, and develop to mature worms in bowel. Eggs transmitted by dust, raw fruit/vegetables, hand to mouth. Risk factor: poor hygiene and sanitation.

Clinical features: cough, respiratory distress, fever, malaise, eosinophilia (during larval migration to lung); abdominal pain, vomiting, worms in stool. Massive infection → malabsorption, intestinal obstruction or ileus, perforation, peritonitis. Diagnosis = detection of eggs in stool.

Imaging:

- **Radiographs:** chest radiograph shows areas of lung consolidation during migration phase (often with eosinophilia). Plain abdominal radiograph may show individual worms in air-filled bowel loops or aggregates of worms (medusa head)
- **US:** worms occasionally visible in bowel lumen (in common bile duct, in gallbladder) (**Fig. 3.41**)

DD: appendicitis, amebiasis, other nematode infections.

Complications: spread to biliary tract → acute cholangitis, liver abscess, pancreatitis.

Treatment: mebendazole, albendazole (single dose). All family members should be treated concurrently.

Filariasis

General: infection with filarial nematodes in tropical countries—complicated life cycle, humans definitive host.

Lymphatic filariasis (lymphedema) and onchocerciasis ("river blindness") most common prevalent diseases (120 million and 17 million people infected, respectively).

Diagnosis: identifying microfilariae on Giemsa-stained blood film smears, antigen/antibody assays, US (may show filaria moving = "dancing" in some fluid-filled structure, potentially Doppler ultrasound), lymphoscintigraphy, X-ray (calcified adult worms in lymphatics).

Treatment: global program to eliminate lymphatic filariasis (GPELF)—based on mass drug administration (MDA): combination of albendazole and ivermectin.

Swallowed Foreign Bodies, Bezoars

General: swallowing FBs—common in children. Most FBs pass through GI tract without problems. Retained FBs most often located in esophagus (thoracic inlet), less commonly at level of left main bronchus, rarely above lower esophageal sphincter. Indigestible material may accumulate in stomach = bezoars. Swallowed hairs = trichobezoar, fruit/vegetable fibers = phytobezoar, curdled milk = lactobezoar (in preterm infants).

Clinical features: dysphagia, stridor, respiratory distress, choking, vomiting, anorexia, bloated feeling.

Imaging:

- **Radiographs:** chest, abdomen, lateral trachea: may show radiopaque FB (coin in esophagus always oriented with flat side facing front or back, coin in trachea with flat side facing right or left)
- **US:** bezoar—filled stomach in fasted child; proximal echogenic band with posterior acoustic shadow (trichobezoar)
- **FL:** rarely esophagram or UGI series with barium (due to perforation risk with water-soluble contrast medium) for nonradiopaque FB → filling defect, inhomogeneous mass on delayed images caused by retained barium (trichobezoar, **Fig. 3.42**)

Complications: ulcer, perforation, bleeding, mediastinitis, peritonitis.

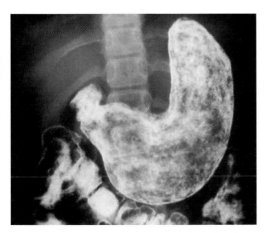

Fig. 3.42 Abdominal radiograph 4 hours after barium UGI series in 10-year-old girl with bloated feeling and palpable upper abdominal mass: trichobezoar. Mass of hairs mixed with retained barium completely fills stomach.

> FBs that reach stomach are usually excreted without problems → no radiologic follow-up in asymptomatic children. Always problematic: ingestion of more than one magnet!

Treatment: usually none. Endoscopic/surgical retrieval: batteries from esophagus and stomach; all FBs lodged in esophagus; multiple magnetic objects (single magnetic FB does not cause problems) anywhere in GI tract (mutual attraction of magnets in various bowel segments may quickly lead to ulceration, perforation, fistulation); refractory bezoars.

Chronic Constipation

General: change in frequency, volume, and consistency of stool, change in painless defecation. Frequency variable, age-dependent (declines from infant to older child). Chronic constipation—affects up to 8% of children and adolescents, may lead to encopresis (fecal incontinence in toilet-trained children over 4 years of age).

Causes: functional (90–95%), neurogenic (Hirschsprung disease, neuronal intestinal dysplasia), chronic intestinal pseudo-obstruction (most severe form = megacystis–microcolon–hypoperistalsis syndrome), cerebral palsy, spinal column/

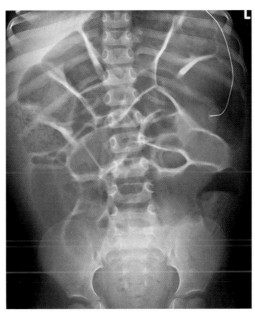

Fig. 3.43 Abdominal radiograph in 3½-year-old boy with megacystis–microcolon–intestinal hypoperistalsis syndrome (= most severe form of chronic intestinal pseudo-obstruction). Massive intestinal dilatation. Distended bladder completely occupies the small pelvis.

cord anomalies (e.g., myelomeningocele, anal fissure/stricture).

Clinical features: decreased stool frequency, painful defecation, encopresis, abdominal pain, gaseous distention, anorexia, vomiting.

Imaging:

- **Radiographs:** abdomen plain film not routinely indicated; dilated bowel loops filled with stool/gas (**Fig. 3.43**), sometimes with air–fluid levels, absence of gas in rectum/sigmoid colon (may signify Hirschsprung disease). With therapeutic implications in severe forms, determine transit time
- **US:** enlarged transverse diameter of stool-filled rectum, gaseous distention
- **FL:** contrast enema in newborns with delayed meconium passage (see Sect. 3.2). Defecography (after 4 years of age): contrast enema instilled to left colic flexure—with absence of aganglionic segment or transition zone, fluoroscopy table placed upright and child placed on small commode—lateral images acquired at rest, during defecation, and straining. Defecation normally associated with relaxation of puborectalis mus-

3

cle and flattening of anorectal angle (ARA = angle between longitudinal axis of anal canal and line along posterior rectal wall, usually about 90 degrees during rest, widening during straining, i.e., angle becomes obtuse). Impaired relaxation/paradoxical contraction of puborectalis with unchanged or decreased ARA seen with functional constipation, Hirschsprung disease. Internal sphincter normally relaxes in filling phase (due to rectal distention) and start of defecation (when external anal sphincter still contracted). Anterior bulge of proximal anal canal—

absent in Hirschsprung disease but always present in functional constipation. Megarectum usually present in functional constipation
Further tests: anorectal manometry, rectal (suction) biopsy.
Treatment: modification of diet, physical exercise, adequate fluid intake, pelvic floor exercises; Laevolac may be considered for functional constipation. Symptomatic treatment advised for chronic intestinal pseudo-obstruction. Hirschsprung disease, see Sect. 3.2.

3.5   Congenital and Acquired Abnormalities of the Liver, Bile Ducts, and Pancreas

Choledochal Cyst

General: spectrum of malformations affecting intra-/extrahepatic bile ducts, especially common in Japan. Theory on pathogenesis: abnormal communication ("common channel") between common bile duct (ductus hepatocholedochus [DHC]) and pancreatic duct (PD) with reflux of pancreatic secretions and digestion of wall by pancreatic enzymes. Todani classification:

- Type I: dilatation of DHC over variable length (80–90%)
- Type II: one or more diverticula in DHC
- Type III: choledochocele (dilated intraduodenal DHC segment, into which PD also opens)
- Type IV A: type I plus intrahepatic cysts
- Type IV B: multiple extrahepatic cysts
- Type V: **Caroli disease** = segmental, nonobstructive dilatation and cysts of intrahepatic bile ducts

Clinical features: jaundice, acholic stools, hepatomegaly, palpable mass, abdominal pain.

Imaging:
- **US:** dilated intra-/extrahepatic bile ducts (DHC dilatation > 10 mm in children almost always associated with biliary tract malformation), variable cyst size and shape (up to 15 cm)—see Todani classification, "second" gallbladder appearance, intraluminal sludge/calculi
- **CT:** superseded by MRI
- **MRI/MRCP:** accurate preoperative evaluation of ductal anatomy (**Fig. 3.44**); may be difficult to

assess "common duct" phenomenon, does not always resolve undilated ducts in very small infants and neonates (resolution restrictions)
DD: obstructive choledocholithiasis, chronic cholangitis, pancreatic pseudocyst, echinococcal cyst, duplication of duodenum, mesenteric cyst, liver cyst, biloma.
Complications: lithiasis, cholangitis, cirrhosis, spontaneous cyst rupture (bilious peritonitis), pancreatitis, bile duct carcinoma (20-fold increase in risk), intrahepatic abscess (Caroli).

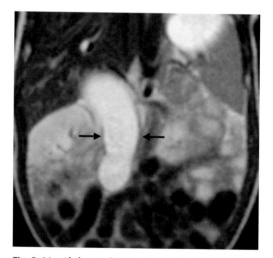

Fig. 3.44   Abdominal MRI, T2-weighted coronal image in 2-year-old girl with type I choledochal cyst (arrows).

Associated malformations: hepatic fibrosis, medullary sponge kidney, infantile polycystic kidneys, nephronophthisis.

Treatment: cyst excision, biliary-enteric anastomosis (choledocho-, hepatojejunal anastomosis with Roux-en-Y technique); if Caroli limited to one hepatic lobe (usually left) → lobectomy; involvement of both lobes with liver failure → liver transplantation.

Biliary Atresia

General: BA and neonatal hepatitis are probably different stages of same pathophysiologic process (fetal inflammatory cholangiopathy). Portions of bile ducts (focal, intra-/extrahepatic) become completely obliterated (DD: neonatal hepatitis—bile ducts patent).

Clinical features: protracted jaundice (> age 4 weeks, up to 90% associated with BA/neonatal hepatitis), acholic stools.

Imaging:
- **US:** BA and neonatal hepatitis = hepatomegaly, echo texture of liver altered or normal, gallbladder absent or small (longitudinal diameter < 20 mm; longitudinal diameter > 30 mm in fasted newborn excludes BA). Intrahepatic bile ducts not dilated; "triangular cord sign"—triangular echogenic area anterior to portal vein bifurcation (fibrotic remnant of DHC)—relatively specific for BA (sensitivity 84%, specificity 98%). Postprandial shrinkage of gallbladder usually absent in BA.
- **MRI/MRCP:** for imaging biliary malformation and possible periportal fibrosis
- **Scintigraphy:** hepatobiliary scintigraphy (premedicate with phenobarbital to optimize hepatic excretion) normal liver enhancement, no activity in GI tract (delayed scans up to 24 hours)

> Radiopharmaceutical detection in GI tract does exclude BA; absence of enhancement inconclusive—severe neonatal hepatitis may impair liver function so severely that small amounts of excreted radiotracer are not detectable.

- **Percutaneous cholecystocholangiography:** at some centers, demonstration of DHC to exclude BA in equivocal cases

- **Exploratory laparotomy and intraoperative cholangiography:** to define intra- and extrahepatic bile ducts (liver biopsy not always diagnostic)

DD: neonatal hepatitis, choledochal cyst, Alagille syndrome (arteriohepatic dysplasia).

Associated syndromes: in about 10% polysplenia, left isomerism of lungs, preduodenal portal vein, azygos continuation, anomalies of hepatic arteries.

Complications: cholangitis, cirrhosis, portal hypertension.

Treatment: portoenterostomy (Kasai operation)—up to 50% success rate when done by third month of life → early diagnosis is critical. Liver transplantation undertaken in patients with complications. Neonatal hepatitis treated medically.

Cholecystolithiasis, Choledocholithiasis

General: cholecystolithiasis much rarer in children than adults. Causes:
- In newborns/small children: parenteral nutrition and intensive care, diuretics, dehydration, infection, hemolytic anemia, short bowel syndrome, congenital biliary tract anomalies, medication/antibiotics
- In older children: idiopathic, sickle-cell anemia, pancreatic diseases, inflammatory bowel diseases, CF, short bowel syndrome, hemolytic anemia, antibiotics, parenteral nutrition and intensive care

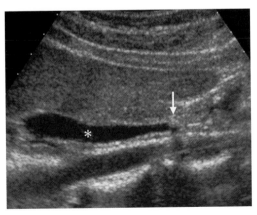

Fig. 3.45   Upper abdominal ultrasound scan in a 14-year-old girl with right upper quadrant pain shows choledocholithiasis (arrow), dilated common bile duct (*).

3

Gallstones sometimes detectable prenatally—usually resolve spontaneously during first year of life.
Clinical features: asymptomatic in most infants and small children. Symptoms in older children usually similar to adults—colicky pains in right upper quadrant, nausea, vomiting, especially in choledocholithiasis.
Imaging:
- **US:** hyperechoic objects in gallbladder, may cause acoustic shadow depending on stone size/composition, move with position changes. DHC dilated in choledocholithiasis (those stones can usually be detected by US, **Fig. 3.45**)
- **CT:** hardly ever necessary
- **MRCP:** clearly defines bile ducts in patients with equivocal US findings. Gallstones usually hypointense on T2-weighted MRI
- **Endoscopic retrograde cholangiopancreaticography (ERCP):** gallstones appear as filling defects; stone extraction during same procedure possible

DD: gallbladder polyp, sludge.
Complications: choledocholithiasis, cholecystitis, cystic duct/infundibular stone with gallbladder hydrops, cholangitis, biliary pancreatitis. Acalculous cholecystitis unusual (hypotheses: gallbladder ischemia, atypical bile composition, high ampullary pressure).
Treatment: none in asymptomatic patients, cholecystectomy in patients with complaints. Medical treatment tried in some cases (Ursofalk, etc.).

Cholangitis

General: ascending cholangitis associated with biliary obstruction (congenital/acquired), potentially life-threatening → rapid diagnosis and treatment.

Primary sclerosing cholangitis: inflammatory fibrosing process (probably autoimmune) in chronic inflammatory bowel diseases (ulcerative colitis), Langerhans cell histiocytosis (LCH), cystic fibrosis, idiopathic—predominantly affects intrahepatic bile ducts.
Clinical features: abdominal pain, jaundice, diarrhea, fever.
Imaging:
- **US:** hepatomegaly, dilated intrahepatic (and extrahepatic) bile ducts with irregularly thickened walls, thickened gallbladder wall, possible cholecystolithiasis. With cirrhosis: liver surface irregularities, signs of portal hypertension

- **MRCP/ERCP:** irregular bile ducts with proximal strictures and dilatation

Treatment: ascending cholangitis—eliminate cause to establish biliary drainage and prevent liver damage. Sclerosing cholangitis—no specific treatment, prognosis usually poor; liver transplantation for liver failure.

Hemangioma, Hemangioendothelioma

General: mesenchymal vascular tumors (~50% of benign liver tumors). Nomenclature confusing: the term infantile hemangioendothelioma, generally preferred in pathologic literature; infantile hepatic hemangioma = the name adopted by International Society for the Study of Vascular Anomalies. Nearly 90% diagnosed within first 6 months of life.
Clinical, pathological features, and outcome: usually asymptomatic; possible abdominal pain, hepatomegaly, vomiting (pressure on nearby structures). Life-threatening complications from large hemangioendotheliomas due to consumption coagulopathy (Kasabach–Merritt syndrome), heart failure (arteriovenous shunts), rupture with hemorrhage. Multifocal: small with no central necrosis, proliferation followed by involution. Focal: large with central necrosis, hemorrhage or fibrosis, involute by age 12–14 months—considered as the hepatic counterpart of cutaneous rapidly involuting congenital hemangioma (RICH). Diffuse: liver enlarged and replaced by masses, complicated clinical course.
Imaging:
- **US:**
  - Multifocal: usually hypoechoic with sharp margins (typical hyperechoic appearance of adult hemangioma = uncommon in infantile hemangio-endothelioma)
  - Focal: often heterogeneous with central hemorrhage, necrosis, fibrosis, rich blood supply, usually large (up to 20 cm). Frequent abrupt decrease in aortic diameter below celiac trunk (= large intrahepatic arteriovenous shunt volume)
  - Contrast-enhanced US may help DD in equivocal cases (lesion characterization as in adults or on dynamic MRI)
  - Color/spectral Doppler—variety of flow patterns

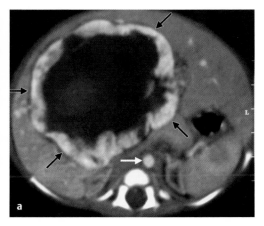
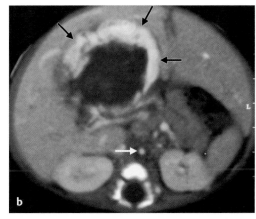

Fig. 3.46a, b   Upper abdominal CT immediately after bolus contrast injection in 14-day-old girl with cardiac decompensation and large hepatic hemangioendothelioma. Note intense peripheral contrast enhancement (black arrows) and hypodense center.

a Aortic diameter larger above origin of celiac trunk (white arrow).

b Aortic diameter smaller below origin of celiac trunk (white arrow).

- **CT:**
  - Precontrast scans: well-circumscribed hypodense mass, may be calcified.
  - Postcontrast scans: nodular peripheral enhancement spreading to center of mass (**Fig. 3.46**); later periphery isodense to liver parenchyma—central hypodensity may persist in large lesions (fibrosis, thrombosis). Note: diameter of abdominal aorta above and below origin of celiac trunk (**Fig. 3.46**)
- **MRI:**
  - Low signal intensity in T1 (hyperintense foci—hemorrhage), high signal intensity in T2, larger focal lesions often heterogeneous (thrombosis, necrosis, fibrosis); nodular contrast enhancement spreads from periphery to center

DD: hepatoblastoma, metastatic neuroblastoma, mesenchymal hamartoma, hepatocellular carcinoma (HCC).

Treatment: depends on severity—steroids, interferon, embolization, surgical resection.

Echinococcosis

General: in humans echinococcus granulosus most common; dog = definitive final host; sheep, cattle, pigs = intermediate hosts. Humans become intermediate host when infected by direct contact with final host or contaminated water, vegetables, etc.

Eggs develop into larvae in human bowel, penetrate bowel wall, and travel to liver via portal vein circulation—75% of echinococcal (hydatid) cysts (contain brood capsules with scolices) in liver, 15% in lung. Systemic dissemination may occur (10%).

Clinical features: depend on organ involvement. Echinococcosis of liver = right upper quadrant pain, jaundice (compression); sometimes asymptomatic.

Classification of cystic echinococcosis (CE)/stage (based on US appearance):

- Cystic lesion (CL): simple cyst, cyst wall not visible, may be due to different etiologies (parasitic, congenital, biliary, neoplasms) → further diagnostic tests necessary; if CE – active stage
- Type CE 1: unilocular, simple cyst, may contain fine echos – hydatide sand ("snow flake" sign—brood capsules), cyst wall visible; active stage; pathognomonic signs include visible cyst wall and snowflake sign
- Type CE 2: multiseptated cyst, daughter cysts may completely fill unilocular mother cyst; active stage; US features pathognomonic
- Type CE 3: anechoic content with detachment of laminated membrane from cyst wall ("water-lily" sign) or unilocular cyst containing unechoic daughter cysts and echoic areas; transitional stage (starting to degenerate); US features pathognomonic
- Type CE 4: heterogeneous contents, no daughter cysts; "ball of wool" sign; mostly not fertile. US

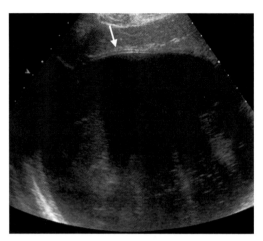

Fig. 3.47 Upper abdominal ultrasound scan in 10-year-old boy with right upper quadrant pain, large echinococcal cyst in right lobe of liver. Note three-layered structure of capsule (arrow) and fine internal echoes.

features not pathognomonic → further tests required to confirm diagnosis

- Type CE 5: cysts with thick calcified wall; majority not fertile. Diagnosis uncertain (features not pathognomonic but highly suggestive)

Imaging:

- **US:** cystic lesion with three-layered wall (pericyst, ectocyst, endocyst, **Fig. 3.47**), possible mural calcification, echogenic debris (hydatid sand), intralesional septa (classification and image appearance—see above)
- **CT:** rarely necessary. May show cyst wall calcification better than US
- **MRI:** low T1 signal intensity, high T2 signal intensity

Complications: cyst rupture, dissemination of parasites.

Treatment: surgical or interventional ablation (instillation of hypertonic saline solution/95% alcohol with image guidance).

Pancreas Divisum, Annular Pancreas, Pancreatitis, Pancreatic Changes in Cystic Fibrosis

General:

- **Pancreas divisum**—most common congenital pancreatic anomaly, found in about 8% of patients examined by ERCP. Caused by incomplete fusion of dorsal (accessory pancreatic duct, duc-

tus Santorini) and ventral (duct of Wirsung) pancreatic ducts. Both ducts open into duodenum via separate papillae (minor and major duodenal papillae)

- **Annular pancreas** = rare anomaly; ventral bifid pancreatic rudiment encircles descending part of duodenum and narrows its lumen. Ring-shaped portion of pancreas often has separate excretory duct that opens into duodenum on opposite side of Vater papilla.
- **Pancreatitis** rare in children. Causes: sepsis, shock, trauma, hemolytic uremic syndrome, viral infection, congenital anomaly, metabolic disease, familiar chronic recurrent pancreatitis (with secondary changes such as ductectasia, varying size, stenoses)
- **Cystic fibrosis (CF)**—common multisystem recessive genetic disease, dysfunction of exocrine glands

Clinical features: pancreas divisum—often asymptomatic. Annular pancreas—often presents shortly after birth with (bilious) vomiting (duodenal obstruction). Pancreatitis—nausea, vomiting, fever, abdominal pain.

Imaging:

- **US:** annular pancreas—see Sect. 3.2; pancreatitis—possible enlargement of pancreas, dilated pancreatic duct, echogenicity usually normal, varies with duration; CF—depends on stage/severity, usually echogenic and smaller than normal unless acutely active; may develop cysts and ductectasia
- **Radiographs:** annular pancreas—see Sect. 3.2; CF—rarely visible calcification
- **CT:** annular pancreas—pancreatic tissue encircles descending part of duodenum; pancreatitis—pancreas normal-sized (up to 70%) or enlarged, irregular outlines, diffuse or focal hypodensity (edema/necrosis), ductectasia, peripancreatic inflammatory changes and fluid collections; contrast enhancement may be normal, increased, or (focally) decreased; CF—focal or diffuse decreased (fatty replacement)/increased attenuation (fibrotic replacement), calcification; MRI preferred
- **MRI/MRCP:** more sensitive to congenital pancreatic (duct) changes than CT. Pancreatitis—high T2 signal intensity, associated changes/necrosis as in CT (**Fig. 3.48**); CF—diffuse hyperintense pancreas (lipomatous replacement)
- **ERCP** (if necessary): direct demonstration of ducts

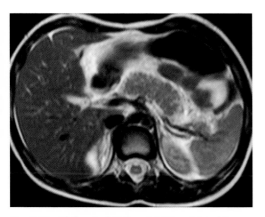

Fig. 3.48 Abdominal MRI, axial T2-weighted image in 3-year-old girl with abdominal pain and fever, acute pancreatitis. Note edematous enlargement of pancreas, thin peripancreatic fluid collections, and free intraperitoneal fluid.

! Caution: ERCP may exacerbate inflammation.

In case of chronic (recurrent) pancreatitis, nondiagnostic MRCP, treatment of stone-induced pancreatitis.

Complications: pancreatitis in pancreas divisum and annular pancreas, pancreatic necrosis, abscess, pancreatic pseudocyst.

Associated malformations: annular pancreas—duodenal stenosis/atresia, trisomy 21, malrotation, esophageal malformations, anal atresia, cardiac anomalies.

Treatment: annular pancreas with duodenal obstruction—surgical; pancreatitis—parenteral nutrition, gastric tube, pain management, causal treatment.

3

3.6 Important Disorders of the Spleen

General: spleen = largest lymphatic organ. Accessory spleen(s) = most common congenital anomaly. Wandering spleen—inadequate fixation allows spleen to occupy atypical site, usually in lower left quadrant → risk of torsion.

- Asplenia = right isomerism (absent spleen, liver has two right lobes, two trilobed lungs, frequent cardiac anomalies, malrotation, stomach on right or left side)
- Polysplenia = left isomerism (multiple small spleens, liver on midline, two bilobed lungs, complex cardiac anomalies, azygos continuation, frequent preduodenal portal vein)
- Splenunculus: often seen, normal variant or associated with splenomegaly, may torse and cause acute complaints. Differentiate from lymph nodes and pancreatic tail.
- Splenomegaly: in children due to infectious/inflammatory processes (e.g., mononucleosis), reticuloendothelial hyperplasia (e.g., hemolytic anemia), vascular congestion (hepatic cirrhosis, portal vein thrombosis), infiltrative process (e.g., Gaucher disease, Niemann–Pick disease, LCH, leukemia, lymphoma).

- Focal splenic lesions—rare, usually cystic, mostly benign: epidermoid, dermoid, mesothelial cyst (true cysts), posttraumatic (false cyst, no wall structure), parasitic (e.g., echinococcosis).
- Other benign tumors—also rare: hemangioma, lymphangioma, hamartoma.
- Malignant lesions most common in leukemia (splenomegaly with diffuse splenic involvement) or lymphoma (splenomegaly with diffuse involvement or focal lesions).
- Trauma to spleen, see Chapter 6.

Imaging:
- **US:** spleen size determined in relation to age—rule of thumb: inferior border of spleen should not be lower than inferior renal pole (in normal-sized kidney). Spleen size—frequent question to US, seldom rewarding (size changes may persist for months after disease, large inter-/intraindividual variations in measured values).
- **CT:** normal spleen has unenhanced density of 40 to 60 HU, shows typical heterogeneous enhancement in (early) arterial phase after contrast administration
- **MRI:** normal spleen has lower T1 signal intensity than liver, higher signal intensity than muscle; T2 signal intensity higher than in liver

Case Study 3.1

History: 9-year-old boy constipated since birth.

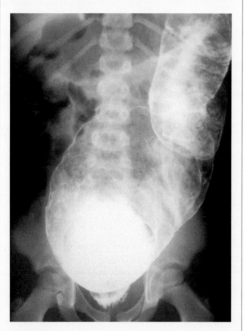

Fig. 3.49

Imaging: irrigoscopy, AP projection.
Findings: greatly dilated colon proximal to normal-caliber rectum.
Diagnosis: Hirschsprung disease.

Case Study 3.2

History: polyhydramnios on fetal US.

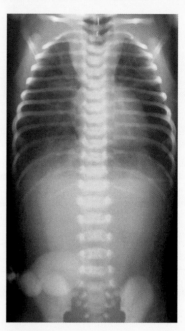

Fig. 3.50

Imaging: thoracoabdominal radiograph immediately after birth.
Findings: gastric tube terminates in dilated, air-filled upper esophagus. Abdomen devoid of gas.
Diagnosis: EA without lower tracheo-esophageal fistula (type II).

Case Study 3.3

History: complex cardiac anomaly known from fetal US.

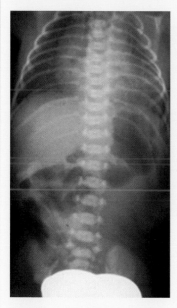

Fig. 3.51

Imaging: thoracoabdominal radiograph shortly after birth.
Findings: gas-filled oral small bowel loops to right of spinal column. Intestinal gas did not yet reach distal small bowel and rectum.
Diagnosis: malrotation (nonrotation).

Case Study 3.4

History: newborn with clinically abnormal abdomen.

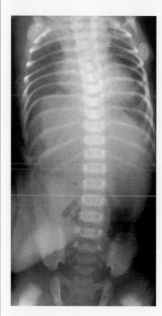

Fig. 3.52

Imaging: thoracoabdominal radiograph immediately after birth.
Findings: indrawn abdomen, "mass" of soft-tissue density extends outside right half of abdomen.
Diagnosis: omphalocele.

3

███ **Case Study 3.5** ███

History: 10-year-old girl with anorexia, bloated feeling, upper abdominal pain.

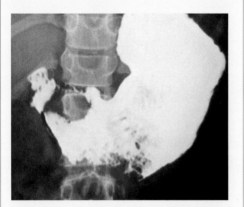

Fig. 3.53

Imaging: barium UGI series in fasted state.
Findings: opacified stomach with filling defect in gastric body, deep contrast pool on lesser curve.
Diagnosis: (Tricho)bezoar with gastric ulcer (complication).

███ **Case Study 3.6** ███

History: Peutz–Jeghers syndrome, status post-intussusception and ileal resection, anemia, abdominal pain.

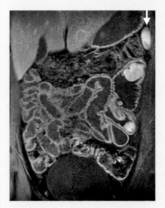

Fig. 3.54

Imaging: MRI after oral Metamucil, coronal T1 after contrast administration.
Findings: three enhancing lesions of different size projecting into small bowel lumen. The hyperintense mass in upper left quadrant (arrow) part of spleen cut by image plane.
Diagnosis: three small bowel polyps in left hemi-abdomen, Peutz–Jeghers syndrome.

Quiz Case 3.1

History: 6-week-old girl with constipation and abdominal distention.

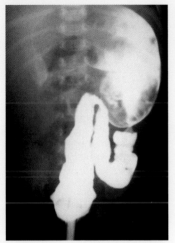

Questions	Correct answers
What primary and subsequent studies are available?	US, abdominal radiograph, contrast enema
What changes does the contrast enema show?	Circumferential narrowing of descending colon with significant dilatation of more proximal colon
Diagnosis?	Colonic stenosis
DD?	Hirschsprung disease
Is further imaging necessary?	No
How is the diagnosis confirmed?	Rectal (suction) biopsy (to exclude Hirschsprung disease)
Treatment?	Resection of stenosis

Fig. 3.55

3

Quiz Case 3.2

History: 17-year-old girl with abdominal pain, chronic diarrhea, weight loss, suspicion of Crohn disease.

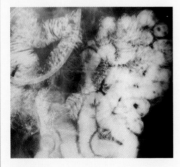

Questions	Correct answers
What primary and subsequent studies are available?	US, enteroclysis (conventional or MRI)
What changes are shown by conventional enteroclysis?	Mixed pattern of round and tubular filling defects in multiple small bowel loops
Diagnosis?	Ascariasis
DD?	Other intestinal parasites
Is further imaging necessary?	No
How is the diagnosis confirmed?	Stool examination for helminth eggs
Treatment?	Medical (mebendazole, albendazole)

Fig. 3.56

History: 14-month-old girl with sudden onset of dysphagia.

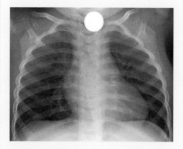

Fig. 3.57

Questions	Correct answers
What primary and subsequent studies are available?	Lateral radiograph of cervical soft tissues, chest radiograph; possible X-ray swallowing study with water-soluble contrast
What changes does the chest radiograph show?	Circular opacity at level of suprasternal notch, flat side facing AP
Diagnosis?	Swallowed radiopaque coin (2-cent piece) lodged in upper esophagus
DD?	Aspiration
Is further imaging necessary?	No
Treatment?	Endoscopic FB retrieval

History: female term infant, 6th day of life, with bilious vomiting and equivocal US findings.

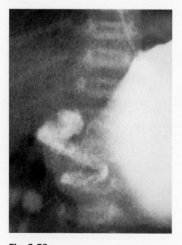

Fig. 3.58

Questions	Correct answers
What primary and subsequent studies are available?	Abdominal radiograph, US, possible contrast study of stomach and proximal small bowel (UGI series)
What changes does the UGI series show?	Corkscrewlike configuration of duodenum
Diagnosis?	Small bowel volvulus
DD?	None
What study is definitive for excluding small bowel volvulus?	UGI series
Treatment?	Surgical emergency

Quiz Case 3.5

History: 14-month-old boy with abdominal pain, no US abnormalities.

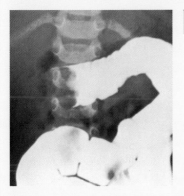

Fig. 3.59

Questions	Correct answers
What primary and subsequent studies are available?	US, possible abdominal radiograph (to exclude free air); contrast enema may be done if findings equivocal
What diagnostic-therapeutic options are available?	Contrast enema for hydrostatic reduction of ileocolic intussusception
What changes does the contrast enema show?	Cutoff of contrast column in transverse colon
Diagnosis?	Ileocolic intussusception
DD?	None
Is further imaging necessary?	No
Interventional procedure?	Hydrostatic reduction under US/FL guidance or pneumatic reduction under FL guidance; surgery if needed
When is hydrostatic/pneumatic reduction contraindicated?	Hemodynamically unstable child, free air/signs of peritonitis

3

Bibliography

1 Andronikou S, Welman CJ, Kader E. Classic and unusual appearances of hydatid disease in children. Pediatr Radiol 2002; 32(11): 817–828

2 Chung EM, Cube R, Lewis RB, Conran RM. From the archives of the AFIP: Pediatric liver masses: radiologic-pathologic correlation part 1. Benign tumors. Radiographics 2010; 30(3): 801–826

3 Delaney L, Applegate KE, Karmazyn B, Akisik MF, Jennings SG. MR cholangiopancreatography in children: feasibility, safety, and initial experience. Pediatr Radiol 2008; 38(1): 64–75

4 Dufour D, Delaet MH, Dassonville M, Cadranel S, Perlmutter N. Midgut malrotation, the reliability of sonographic diagnosis. Pediatr Radiol 1992; 22(1): 21–23

5 Fitoz S, Erden A, Boruban S. Magnetic resonance cholangiopancreatography of biliary system abnormalities in children. Clin Imaging 2007; 31(2): 93–101

6 Fotter R. Imaging of constipation in infants and children. Eur Radiol 1998; 8(2): 248–258

7 Goske MJ, Applegate KE, Boylan J, et al. The Image Gently campaign: working together to change practice. AJR Am J Roentgenol 2008; 190(2): 273–274

8 Hernanz-Schulman M. Imaging of neonatal gastrointestinal obstruction. Radiol Clin North Am 1999; 37 (6): 1163–1186, vi–vii

9 Hörmann MN. MR imaging of the gastro-intestinal tract in children. Eur J Radiol 2008; 68(2): 271–277

10 Kuhn JP, Slovis TL, Haller JO. Caffey's Pediatric Diagnostic Imaging. 10th ed. Philadelphia: Mosby; 2004: 1455–1459

11 Mann EH. Inflammatory bowel disease: imaging of the pediatric patient. Semin Roentgenol 2008; 43(1): 29–38

12 Nijs E, Callahan MJ, Taylor GA. Disorders of the pediatric pancreas: imaging features. Pediatr Radiol 2005; 35 (4): 358–373, quiz 457

Quiz Case 3.6

History: 2-year-old girl with fever, nausea, abdominal pain.

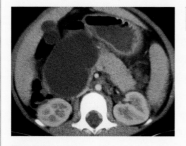

Fig. 3.60

Questions	Correct answers
What primary and subsequent studies are available?	US, MRI (MRCP), CT (with contrast, if MRI unavailable), very rarely ERCP (common channel)
What changes does CT show?	Large, well-circumscribed, hypodense lesion in region of pancreatic head; does not enhance after contrast administration
Diagnosis?	Choledochal cyst (Todani type I)
DD?	Pancreatic pseudocyst, echinococcal cyst, mesenteric cyst, duodenal duplication cyst, possible choledocholithiasis with obstruction
Is further imaging necessary?	MRCP/ERCP may be done preoperatively to define anatomic details
Treatment?	Surgical (cyst resection, cholecystectomy, hepaticojejunostomy)

13 Riccabona M, Avni FE. MR imaging of paediatric abdomen. In: Gourtsonyiannis N, ed. Clinical MRI of the Abdomen. Why, How, When. Heidelberg: Springer; 2011: 639–676

14 Pracros JP, Sann L, Genin G, et al. Ultrasound diagnosis of midgut volvulus: the "whirlpool" sign. Pediatr Radiol 1992; 22(1): 18–20

15 Sinzig M, Nickl S, Kraschl R, Fasching G, Hausegger KA. Giant Meckel's diverticulum associated with oesophageal atresia, tracheo-oesophageal fistula and cleft lip and palate. Pediatr Radiol 2005; 35(2): 216–217

16 Stringer DA, Babyn PS. Pediatric Gastrointestinal Imaging and Intervention. 2nd ed. Hamilton, London: B.C. Decker; 2000: 731–786

17 WHO Informal Working Group. International classification of ultrasound images in cystic echinococcosis for application in clinical and field epidemiological settings. Acta Trop 2003; 85(2): 253–261

4 Imaging of the Pediatric Central Nervous System and Spine

4.1 Radiography, Computed Tomography, and Magnetic Resonance Imaging in Pediatric Neuroradiology

Maria Sinzig, Ianina Scheer

Imaging Modalities and Indications

Computed Tomography

General principles, indications: CT = relatively high radiation exposure: **check indication**—use MRI/US if available, which may yield same or more diagnostic information!

- Example A: CT ordered for child with acute neurologic abnormalities. MRI = modality of choice. If MRI contraindicated/unavailable for other reasons → use high-quality CT to answer as many questions as possible and avoid repeat examinations.
- Example B: trauma raises question: fracture, pneumocephalus, or mass hemorrhage? Goal = rapid examination, prompt diagnosis for acute therapeutic implications, not highest quality → CT (low radiation dose!). If indicated, follow-up with MRI when child is stable.
- Example C: shunt assessment—do not use high-dose CT; use US/MRI whenever possible.

Technique: axial scans parallel to canthomeatal line, age-adjusted protocol. **Older children:** same scan parameters as for adults (basic rule: scan parameters depend on indication). **Children < 7 years:** usually scanned with sedation, slice thickness > 2.5 mm. Neonatal brain has high water content—use proper window setting (see also Chapter 1).

Magnetic Resonance Imaging

General principles, indications: MRI = modality of choice (cerebral and spinal imaging). Disadvantages: time-consuming, requires immobilization. Young/uncooperative children require sedation/general anesthesia (difficult to wait for "natural sleep").

Technique: standard protocol is T1- and T2-weighted sequences in all three planes, one FLAIR (fluid-attenuated inversion recovery) sequence in children > 1 year, one axial diffusion-weighted sequence. Axial images parallel to AC–PC line (anterior commissure, posterior commissure). Sequence parameters appropriate for child's age and indication—have age-appropriate protocols stored in system memory.

- Example for neonatal head: slice thickness/spacing 2.5 mm/0.2 mm, T2-weighted images in three planes, axial T1-weighted imaging (to assess myelination), diffusion-weighted imaging (perinatal hypoxia? acute focal ischemia?), consider inversion recovery (IR) and FLAIR sequences, proton spectroscopy in basal ganglia and white matter (perinatal hypoxia: presence of lactate peak → information on severity of hypoxia and prognosis). Abnormal peaks may suggest metabolic disorders.

Arterial/venous infarctions—add MRA/MRV. If necessary, supplement with T2*/susceptibility-weighted sequences (visualization of blood and blood breakdown products).

Depending on clinical question, slice thickness may be reduced to 1 mm, or to 0.8 to 0.6 mm for high-resolution T2-weighted imaging (inner ear), potentially 3D isotropic volume acquisition.

Radiography

General: immobilize patient! Collimation: inadequate field size = most common error in pediatric radiography—no more than a maximum of 1 cm should be added to the necessary field of view in newborns, no more than 2 cm after neonatal period.

Indications: suspected child abuse (part of skeletal status), syndromic evaluation, craniosynostosis, clinical abnormality ("bump") without neurologic symptoms, FBs.

> Mild head trauma in child without neurologic abnormalities = not an indication for cranial radiographs.

Technique: use extra filtering (Al, Cu). Do not use scatter-reduction grid for infants and small children < 6 months, use grid in older children. Film–focus distance 110 cm, 60 to 70 kV.

Normal Findings

Development of Central Nervous System

The embryonic neural plate folds to form the neural tube. Cranial part develops into brain, caudal part into spinal cord. Corpus callosum and commissures begin to develop in gestational week 7. Brain is initially smooth. First sulcus = sylvian fissure (brain resembles figure "8"), gyral development approximately starts in week 22, not complete until term. Neurons begin to form in subependymal lateral ventricle (LV) wall layers around week 7 (germinal matrix zone); they start migrating to definitive cortical sites around week 8. In cortex: neurons become organized, arranged in cell layers (= cortical organization). Myelination of white matter starts

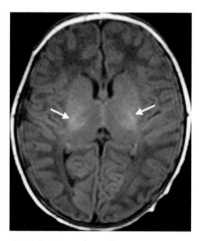

Fig. 4.1   Normal myelination in term newborn.
T1-weighted axial MRI without contrast medium.
Myelinated posterior limb of internal capsule
appears hyperintense (arrows).

in week 20. The medulla oblongata, dorsal midbrain, superior and inferior cerebellar peduncles, and posterior limb of internal capsule become myelinated by birth (**Fig. 4.1**). Further myelination after birth follows established timetable (see specialized textbooks). Subcortical white matter matures last, beginning in occipital lobes and spreading to frontal and temporal lobes. Myelination equals adult pattern by 18 to 24 months of age.

Imaging: MRI—unmyelinated white matter T2 hyperintense, T1 hypointense (Note: T2-weighted appearance of neonatal brain similar to T1-weighted appearance of adult brain).

Closure of Cranial Sutures

Head consists of three parts: neurocranium, facial skeleton (viscerocranium), and skull base. Bones of neurocranium form by membranous ossification (bone develops directly from embryonic connective tissue = mesenchyme). Calvarial bone divided by sutures and fontanelles—six constant fontanelles located at four corners of parietal bone (two in midline = anterior and posterior fontanelles, two on each side = anterolateral and posterolateral fontanelles). Fontanelles and sutures become smaller and narrower with age. Posterior fontanelle closes between birth and several months of age; anterior fontanelle closes later. Large sutures have fused by approximately the middle of third decade. Metopic suture closes during third year of life, mendosal suture during second year. Most cranial growth occurs during first 2 years of life; skull reaches definitive size by about 20 years old.

Pneumatization of Paranasal Sinuses

Maxillary sinuses develop first (rudimentary medial to orbits at birth, reach hard palate by ~ 9 years). Frontal sinuses develop last (by end of puberty). Timetables for sinus pneumatization, see specialized textbooks. Degree of pneumatization highly variable: aplasia, hypoplasia (uni-/bilateral), prominent intrasinusoidal septa = normal variants.

Congenital Malformations of the Brain, Spinal Cord and Spinal Column, and Metabolic Disorders

Anomalies of the Corpus Callosum

General: agenesis of corpus callosum = complete absence of corpus callosum. Partial absence (usually posterior) = hypogenesis. Absence of anterior portions of corpus callosum with intact posterior portions = usually due to secondary damage. Structure develops from anterior to posterior between gestational weeks 7 and 20. Complete corpus callosum: rostrum, genu, body, isthmus, splenium.

Clinical features: isolated agenesis of corpus callosum—may be asymptomatic or associated with macrocephaly, developmental delay, epilepsy, hypothalamic dysfunction.

Imaging:
- **CT:** parallel LVs spaced well apart, occipital horns often dilated (colpocephaly); may be associated with midline cysts or corpus callosum lipoma
- **MRI:** eversion/absence of cingulate gyrus; radial arrangement of gyri and sulci, directed toward third ventricle (sagittal image). Third ventricle communicates with interhemispheric fissure (**Fig. 4.2**). Probst bundles indent LV from medial side → characteristic steer-horn configuration of anterior horns (coronal image). Elongated foramen of Monro, meandering course of anterior cerebral artery (ACA). Frequent heterotopia and cortical dysplasia

DD: secondary change due to trauma, infarction, or hypoxic-ischemic encephalopathy (HIE). Corpus callosum may be thinned in hydrocephalus.

Associated intracranial malformations: corpus callosum lipoma, interhemispheric cyst, heterotopia, holoprosencephaly (HPE), lissencephaly (LIS), schizencephaly.

Associated syndromes: Aicardi syndrome, Apert syndrome, morning glory syndrome, Chiari II malformation, Dandy–Walker malformation. Agenesis of corpus callosum = most common cerebral malformation in fetal alcohol syndrome.

Schizencephaly

General: full-length cleft in brain, lined by gray matter—creates communication between outer cortical brain surface and LV ependyma. Types: closed-lip and open-lip schizencephaly (depending on cleft width). Malformation may be unilateral (60%) or bilateral (40%), may have genetic or acquired cause.

Clinical features: epilepsy, hemiparesis (mainly in open-lip type), developmental delay.

Imaging:
- **CT:** cleft lined by gray matter; large atypical veins in proximity
- **MRI:** cleft often lined by dysplastic gray matter, usually pre-/postcentral (**Fig. 4.3**). Deformed LVs (sometimes just convex lateral LV wall). Septum pellucidum often absent. Calvarium may show focal bulging in open-lip schizencephaly (CSF pulsations). Closed-lip schizencephaly is sometimes difficult to diagnose.

DD: porencephaly, hydrancephaly, HPE.

(Classic) Lissencephaly

General: LIS = agyria–pachygyria complex (impaired neuronal migration). LIS = "smooth brain" (physiologic stage of embryonic development, gyral development starts in week 22). **Agyria** = complete absence of gyri, thickened cortex. **Pachygyria** = small number of broad, flat gyri, thickened cortex. Classic LIS has high association with chromosome abnormalities.

Clinical features: developmental delay, epilepsy, facial dysplasia.

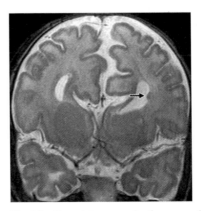

Fig. 4.2 Complete agenesis of corpus callosum in a 4-month-old girl. T2-weighted coronal MRI displays steer-horn configuration of anterior horns and communication of third ventricle with interhemispheric fissure. Small focus of subependymal heterotopia (arrow) visible on left side.

4

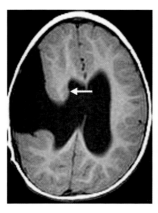

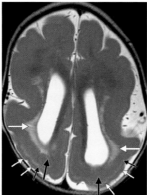

Fig. 4.3   **Fig. 4.4**

Fig. 4.3 Right-sided open-lip schizencephaly in 2-year-old girl. T1-weighted axial MRI shows direct communication between inner and outer CSF spaces and partial dysplasia of cleft lined with gray matter (arrow).

Fig. 4.4 Partial lissencephaly in 8-month-old girl. T2-weighted axial MRI shows isolated shallow gyri and sulci and thickened cortical band. Narrow T2-hyperintense parenchymal band (short black arrows) visible between thin outer cortex (short white arrows) and thick layer of neurons arrested in their migration (longer black arrows). Note dilated Virchow–Robin spaces (longer white arrows).

Imaging: CT/MRI in complete classic LIS = figure-of-8 brain configuration ("figure 8 LIS"—smooth brain, shallow sylvian fissure). Incomplete LIS (**Fig. 4.4**) more common—zones with agyria and pachygyria (cortex thickened, shallow sulci, broad gyri), may be associated with hypo- or agenesis of corpus callosum, cerebellar hypoplasia.

DD: polymicrogyria, cobblestone LIS, bilateral diffuse bandlike heterotopia.

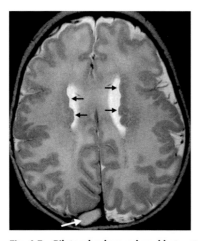

Fig. 4.5 Bilateral subependymal heterotopia in 3-week-old girl. T2-weighted axial MRI demonstrates subependymal heterotopia (black arrows) associated with bilateral parietal polymicrogyria and subdural hemorrhage residues (white arrow).

Heterotopia

General: heterotopia = focal collection of nerve cells outside cortex and basal ganglia. Neurons often "stall" on their way from subependymal germinal matrix to cortex = neuronal migration disorder. Bandlike heterotopias often have chromosomal cause (X-chromosome). Classified by location: subependymal, focal subcortical, bandlike.

Clinical feature: epilepsy.

Imaging: MRI—subependymal heterotopia = rounded/oval nodules bordering on ventricle wall, isointense to gray matter (**Fig. 4.5**). Focal subcortical heterotopia = nests of gray matter cells in white matter —single/multiple, rounded/oblongated; bandlike heterotopia = homogeneous band of gray matter between LV and cortex, separated from both by white matter ("double cortex").

DD: tuberous sclerosis (TS) (subependymal nodules have variable MRI signal intensity, often calcified). Focal subcortical heterotopia may be mistaken for tumor.

> Affected cortex in heterotopia usually thin and dysplastic. Heterotopia never associated with perifocal edema!

Holoprosencephaly

General: HPE = defect in differentiation and splitting of prosencephalon or abnormal formation of separate hemispheres from the telencephalon. HPE is highly associated with maternal diabetes. Septooptic dysplasia = mild form of HPE.

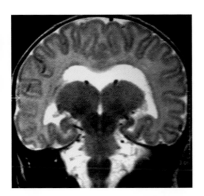

Fig. 4.6 Semilobar holoprosencephaly in 5-day-old boy. T2-weighted coronal MRI. Hemispheres fused anteriorly. Anterior portions of corpus callosum and septum pellucidum absent.

Clinical features: mental retardation, epilepsy, microcephaly, midline facial anomalies (ranging to cyclopia), hypothalamic–pituitary dysfunction.

Imaging:

- **CT:** alobar = lack of hemispheric differentiation (no interhemispheric fissure, no falx cerebri), monoventricle in continuity with large posterior cyst; semilobar = hemispheres are fused anteriorly, separate posteriorly. Septum pellucidum is absent, posterior horns are rudimentary, temporal horns also rudimentary in most cases; lobar = septum pellucidum absent, anterior horns usually deformed.
- **MRI:** alobar = absence of corpus callosum (T1, sagittal); semilobar (**Fig. 4.6**); lobar = posterior corpus callosum present, anterior portions absent (= only exception to rule that absence of anterior portions equals secondary lesion)

DD: hydrocephalus, open-lip schizencephaly, agenesis of corpus callosum with interhemispheric cyst, hydrancephaly.

Associated syndromes: Edward syndrome (trisomy 18), Patau syndrome (trisomy 13).

Chiari Malformations

Chiari Malformation Type I

General: downward herniation of cerebellar tonsils through foramen magnum due to malformation of posterior cranial fossa (PCF), craniovertebral junction anomalies, basilar invagination. Type I may also occur without associated anomalies.

Clinical features: headache, nystagmus, lower cranial nerve palsies, scoliosis.

Imaging:

- **CT:** completely filled foramen magnum; absence of CSF around upper cervical cord.
- **MRI:** position of cerebellar tonsils best appreciated in sagittal images. Low cerebellar tonsils sometimes hyperintense in T2-weighted images, do not enhance after contrast administration (DD: dura thickened in low-CSF-pressure syndrome, enhances after contrast administration)

> Always look for syringomyelia in children with Chiari malformation type I—image entire cord.

Treatment: surgical decompression of PCF.

DD: tonsillar herniation due to increased intracranial pressure, Chiari malformation type II, achondroplasia, low-CSF-pressure syndrome due to CSF leak.

> Displacement of cerebellar tonsils < 6 mm below line between basion and opisthion—physiologic in asymptomatic children. Greater displacement/clinical manifestations, diagnostic of Chiari malformation type I.

Chiari Malformation Type II

General: complex malformation—nearly always present in children with myelomeningocele (MMC). Small PCF, low attachment of tentorium, downward displacement of cerebellar and brainstem structures. Often associated with supratentorial anomalies; 80% of children develop hydrocephalus after MMC closure (often requiring shunt).

Clinical features: MMC; with brainstem compression at level of foramen magnum or C1→ stridor, apnea, swallowing difficulties, arm weakness.

Imaging:

- **CT:** small PCF, fourth ventricle narrow or obliterated, hypoplastic falx cerebri, interdigitations (gyri herniate through falx defect to opposite side, create interdigitating pattern), hydrocephalus, *lückenschädel* (lacunar skull) due to calvarial ossification defects
- **MRI:** small PCF, herniation of portions of vermis and possibly of cerebellar tonsils through foramen magnum into spinal canal, cerebellar hemispheres encircle medulla oblongata, kink at junction of medulla oblongata and cervical cord, fourth ventricle shallow and elongated

4

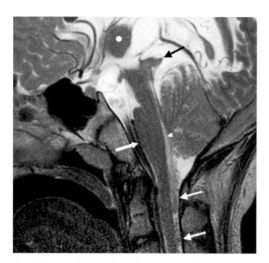

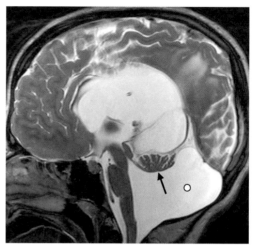

Fig. 4.7   Lumbosacral myelomeningocele in 10-year-old boy with history of Chiari II malformation with corpus callosum hypogenesis and shunted hydrocephalus. T2-weighted sagittal MRI. Posterior cranial fossa too small, vermis has herniated downward (white arrows). Pons and fourth ventricle markedly flattened (thick white arrow, arrowhead). Beaked appearance of quadrigeminal plate (black arrow), thickened interthalamic adhesion (white dot).

downward ("normal" fourth ventricle signifies impaired CSF circulation), quadrigeminal plate displaced downward and posteriorly ("tectal beaking," sagittal images), hypo- or agenesis of corpus callosum, prominent massa intermedia (**Fig. 4.7**), dilated LV

DD: Chiari malformation types I, III, IV (Chiari III = herniation of cerebellum through a posterior spina bifida at C1 to C2 level; Chiari IV = severe cerebellar hypoplasia, small brainstem, large posterior fossa CSF spaces).

Dandy–Walker Complex

General: Dandy–Walker complex is subdivided into three groups:

- **Dandy–Walker malformation** (DWM) = enlarged PCF, high attachment of tentorium, cerebellar vermis hypoplastic and rotated superiorly, cystic dilatation of fourth ventricle. Often associated with hydrocephalus and corpus callosum anomaly, less commonly with heterotopia, occipital encephalocele, or syringohydromyelia
- **Dandy–Walker variant** = not consistently defined—term no longer used

Fig. 4.8   Dandy–Walker malformation in 8-year-old girl. T2-weighted sagittal MRI shows hypoplastic cerebellar vermis that is rotated upward (arrow), also cystic dilatation of fourth ventricle (black circle), corpus callosum anomaly, and hydrocephalus.

- **Megacisterna magna** = large PCF due to enlargement of cisterna magna with normal vermis and fourth ventricle

Clinical features: developmental delay, epilepsy, hearing loss, vision problems.

Imaging:

- **CT:** large cyst (in PCF) communicating with fourth ventricle. Hydrocephalus present in 90% of cases at diagnosis; anterolateral displacement of cerebellar hemispheres
- **MRI:** fourth ventricle opens posteriorly into large cyst, vermis hypoplastic and rotated superiorly (**Fig. 4.8**). Brainstem pressed against clivus. Variable cerebellar hypoplasia/dysplasia (vermis normal in megacisterna magna). Possible corpus callosum anomalies, syringohydromyelia.

DD: retrocerebellar arachnoid cyst, Walker–Warburg syndrome, Chiari IV, Joubert syndrome, cerebellar hypoplasia.

Phacomatoses

Phacomatoses = congenital malformations mainly affecting structures composed of ectoderm (nervous system, skin, eyes). Visceral organs much less commonly affected.

Neurofibromatosis Type I

General: von Recklinghausen disease; autosomal dominant mode of inheritance.

Clinical features: café-au-lait spots, axillary freckles, cutaneous neurofibromas (usually at onset of puberty), Lisch nodules (iris hamartomas), learning disability, macrocephaly, short stature, scoliosis.

Imaging:

- **Radiographs:** scoliosis with vertebral body dysplasia, sphenoid dysplasia, widened superior orbital fissure
- **CT:** widened superior orbital fissure (sphenoid dysplasia), enlarged skull base foramina (depending on growth of plexiform neurofibromas), lambdoid suture defect
- **MRI:** various findings and manifestations:
  - Optic gliomas—usually pilocytic astrocytomas, rare high-grade malignancies; gliomas of any WHO grade. Hyperintense in T2-weighted and STIR sequences, usually enhance markedly after contrast administration. Multiple T2- and FLAIR-hyperintense lesions in brainstem, cerebellar white matter, globus pallidus, corpus callosum—no mass effect, no vasogenic edema, nonenhancing. Develop after 2 years of age, increase in size and number until puberty, decline thereafter
  - Plexiform neurofibromas (poorly organized aggregation of Schwann cells, neuromas, and connective tissue)—spread diffusely along nerves, locally aggressive, create mass effect. Intra-/extraspinal neurofibromas
  - Vascular malformations, vascular stenoses, aneurysms

DD: neurofibromatosis (NF) II, tuberous cerebral sclerosis, demyelination (e.g., acute disseminated encephalomyelitis [ADEM]), cerebral gliomatosis.

Neurofibromatosis Type II

General: NF II with bilateral acoustic neuromas (schwannomas); autosomal dominant mode of inheritance; less common than NF I.

Clinical features: affected children are often asymptomatic. Rare: epilepsy (cerebral meningiomas), café-au-lait spots, cranial nerve palsy (schwannomas), cutaneous schwannomas, cataracts.

Imaging:

- **Radiographs:** scoliosis, enlarged neuroforamina (nerve sheath tumors)

- **CT:** uni-/bilateral iso-/hypodense mass in cerebellopontine angle, enlarged internal auditory canal (acoustic schwannomas); hyperdense intra-axial calcifications, mass abutting dura (meningioma)
- **MRI:** cranial nerve schwannomas usually T2-hyperintense and T1-hypointense. Meningiomas hypointense on T1- and T2-weighted images. Both show diffuse contrast enhancement. Paraspinal nerve sheath tumors (schwannomas, neurofibromas), intraspinal meningiomas, intramedullary tumors (mostly ependymomas).

> Schwannomas and meningiomas = unusual tumors in patients < 30 years of age—always suspicious for NF II in young patients.

DD: schwannomatosis, cerebellopontine angle tumors (epidermoid), multiple meningiomas, Tb.

Tuberous (Cerebral) Sclerosis

General: Bourneville–Pringle disease; autosomal dominant inheritance.

Clinical features: depigmented nevi, sebaceous adenoma (after 1 year of age), epilepsy, mental retardation (~50%), microphthalmos, and leukocoria due to retinal hamartomas (DD: retinoblastoma).

Imaging:

- **Radiographs:** foci of osteosclerosis, cysts in metacarpals and phalanges
- **CT:** (calcified) subependymal nodules (hamartomas), cerebral hamartomas (tubers), cortical and in white matter—hypodense (unless calcified); possible hydrocephalus
- **MRI:** tubers in cortex and white matter/subependymal nodules along ventricle wall—hyperintense in T2 and FLAIR sequences, T1-isointense to myelinated white matter (DD: heterotopia—isointense to gray matter!). In newborns, hyperintense to unmyelinated white matter in T1-weighted images, calcify with age (**Fig. 4.9**). May show contrast enhancement, rarely undergo malignant transformation
  Giant cell astrocytomas = enhancing subependymal masses that tend to enlarge, usually close to foramen of Monro (follow-up!). Hydrocephalus due to ipsilateral CSF obstruction

DD: cortical dysplasia, congenital infections (TORCH), Taylor dysplasia, tumors (dysembryo-

4

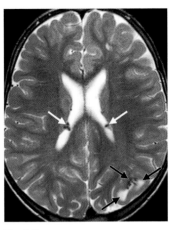

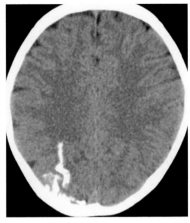

Fig. 4.9   **Fig. 4.10**

Fig. 4.9   Tuberous sclerosis in 5-year-old boy. T2-weighted axial MRI. Subependymal calcified nodules have very low T2 signal intensity (white arrows). Partially calcified subcortical tuber (black arrows).

Fig. 4.10   Sturge–Weber syndrome in 5-year-old girl. Unenhanced axial CT shows calcifications distributed along cortical gyri in right occipital lobe. Adjacent calvarium thickened.

plastic neuroectodermal tumors, subependymoma, central neurocytoma).

Extracerebral manifestations: renal AML (angiomyolipoma), pulmonary lymphangioleiomyomatosis, cardiac rhabdomyomas.

Von Hippel–Lindau Disease

General: CNS angiomatosis—autosomal dominant inheritance.

Clinical features: visual disturbances (retinal angiomas), cerebellar symptoms (hemangioblastomas), hearing loss (endolymphatic sac tumors).

Imaging: CT/MRI—hemangioblastoma (usually cerebellar): fluid-filled cyst with small, hypervascular mural nodule; one-third of hemangioblastomas solid (contrast administration!). Spinal hemangioblastomas: easily missed without contrast administration (indirect sign = syrinx). Papillary cystadenomas of endolymphatic sac (CT: surrounding bone destruction with calcium stipples; MRI: marked, heterogeneous contrast enhancement).

DD: solitary hemangioblastoma (without gene alterations), pilocytic astrocytoma, small arteriovenous malformation (AVM), vascular metastases (e.g., renal cell carcinoma).

Manifestations outside CNS: renal cell carcinoma, pheochromocytoma, papillary cystadenoma (epididymis), angiomas (liver, kidneys).

Sturge–Weber Syndrome

General: encephalotrigeminal (meningofacial) angiomatosis, usually with sporadic occurrence.

Clinical features: facial port-wine stain (trigeminal nerve distribution), epilepsy, hemiparesis, hemianopsia (angiomatosis of choroid), mental retardation.

Imaging:

- **Radiographs:** tortuous "tram-track" calcifications
- **CT:** calcifications follow cortical gyri (**Fig. 4.10**). Calvarium thickened over angiomas
- **MRI:** early—intense pial contrast enhancement (angioma), accelerated myelination (transient hyperperfusion); late—"burnout" = absence of pial enhancement (thrombosed angioma), decreased T2-weighted cortical signal intensity (calcifications), atrophy, thickened choroid plexus

DD: blue rubber bleb nevus syndrome, Wyburn-Mason syndrome, Klippel–Trenaunay–Weber syndrome, meningoangiomatosis, meningitis (leptomeningeal contrast enhancement), leptomeningeal tumors, metastases.

Vascular Malformations

Vein of Galen Malformations

General: Classification—**vein of Galen aneurysmal malformation** (VGAM—dilated vein = embryonic vein of Galen precursor, corresponding to median prosencephalic vein). **Vein of Galen aneurysmal dilatation** (VGAD—usually in older child, less common than VGAM). **Dural AV shunts with aneurysmal vein of Galen dilatation** (most common in adults). **Vein of Galen varix** (vein of Galen dilatation, no AV shunts).

Clinical features: depend strongly on type of malformation and age at which it becomes symptomatic—neonatal heart failure, macrocephaly, and mild cardiac symptoms. Small children—hydrocephalus and seizures. Older children/adults—headache/subarachnoid hemorrhage (SAH).

Imaging:

- **Radiographs** (chest): cardiomegaly with heart failure (large shunt volume), present neonatally in VGAM
- **CT:** aneurysmal venous dilatation—slightly hyperdense, hydrocephalus (pressure on aqueduct), hypodense lesions (acute ischemia), subcortical calcifications (chronic venous ischemia). Imaging workup may include preinterventional CTA
- **MRI:** arterial feeders appear as flow voids; dilated median vein—T1-hypointense, inhomogeneous (turbulent flow); T2-hypointense, homogeneous (**Fig. 4.11**). Herniation of cerebellar tonsils, tectum compression, enlarged sulci (increased venous pressure, decreased CSF reabsorption), impaired diffusion in areas of acute/subacute ischemia. MRA and MRV!
- **Angiography**: digital subtractive angiography (DSA) is essential for neurointerventional planning

DD: dural AVF, giant aneurysm (not associated with venous anomalies), complex developmental venous anomaly (DVA).

Treatment: only treatment option = neurointerventional embolization in VGAM.

Encephaloceles

General: encephalocele (cephalocele) = congenital herniation of intracranial structures through defect in skull (rare). **Atretic cephalocele** = contains meninges, connective tissue. **Meningocele** = sac contains meninges, CSF. **Meningoencephalocele** = contains meninges, brain tissue, CSF. **Meningoencephalocystocele** = encephalocele that includes ventricular elements. **Gliocele** = CSF-filled cyst lined with glial cells.

Sites of occurrence: occipitocervical, occipital, parietal, frontal, temporal, frontoethmoidal, sphenomaxillary, spheno-orbital, nasopharyngeal, lateral.

Clinical features: occipital encephalocele usually visible at birth. Frontoethmoidal sac—nasal airway obstruction, facial dysmorphias.

Imaging:

- **Radiographs:** calvarial midline defects of variable size
- **CT:** cranial defect filled with intracranial structures. Displacement/distortion of brain morphology; microcephaly
- **MRI:** Thin-slice T2-weighted imaging = best sequence in newborns, clearly distinguishes among nerve tissue, CSF, vessels (sagittal images or isotropic 3D sequence; **Fig. 4.12**). MRA and MRV (vascular anatomy) if needed.

4

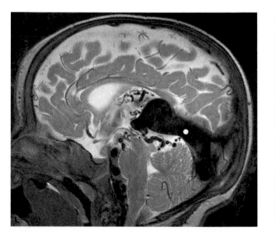

Fig. 4.11 Vein of Galen aneurysmal malformation in 5-month-old girl in T2-weighted sagittal MRI. Median vein of prosencephalon shows marked aneurysmal dilatation (white dot). Multiple arterial feeders visible.

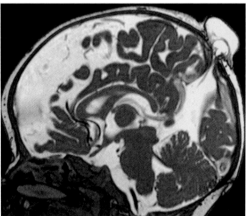

Fig. 4.12 Interparietal cephalocele. T2-weighted sagittal MRI displays cephalocele, absence of straight sinus, and upward deviation of cerebellar tentorium.

DD: nasal polyp, nasal dermoid, capillary hemangioma (most common frontonasal mass), nasopharyngeal tumors (rhabdomyosarcoma [RMS], lymphoma, juvenile nasopharyngeal fibroma, teratoma). DD for occipital cephalocele: cephalhematoma, caput succedaneum, cystic lymphangioma.

Dysraphism, Diastematomyelia, Tethered Cord

Spinal Dysraphism

General: spinal dysraphism = heterogeneous group of spinal anomalies characterized by incomplete closure of mesenchymal, osseous, and neural structures. Two main groups:

- **Open spinal dysraphism** (OSD) = incomplete neural tube closure. Ectoderm unfused over bony midline defect, allowing protrusion of structures from spinal canal
  - MMC—placode and meninges exposed at level of defect; placode extends past adjacent skin surface due to large anterior subarachnoid space
  - Myelocele as in MMC, but placode flush with adjacent skin—usually lumbosacral

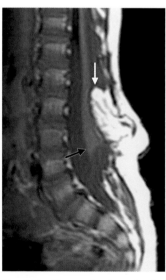

Fig. 4.13 Lipomyelocele and tethered cord in 14-month-old patient. T1-weighted sagittal MRI. Subcutaneous lipoma extends through posterior spina bifida into interior of spinal canal (white arrow). Club-shaped conus medullaris terminates at an abnormally low level (black arrow).

- **Closed dysraphism** = defect covered by skin
  - Lipomyelocele, lipomyelomeningocele, myelocystocele
  - Dorsal dermal sinus—epithelium-lined communication between skin and spinal canal without subcutaneous mass

Clinical features: MMC, myelocele = cord/meninges exposed, covered by rich vascular plexus. Closed dysraphism = subcutaneous mass, local nevi.

Imaging: MRI for MMC—**neurosurgical emergency** due to risk of infection/ulceration. Preoperative MRI: apply rigorous selection criteria and sterile technique! Prone position, sagittal and axial images/isotropic 3D sequence. Dehiscence of subcutaneous fat, muscles, bones. Low-sited cord herniates through defect, forms posterior wall of locally expanded CSF space. Dilated subarachnoid space. Nerve roots arise from anterior placode wall, run horizontal/ascending course. Lipomyelocele (**Fig. 4.13**).

> OSD is always associated with Chiari malformation type II. Hydrocephalus and hydromyelia are usually present after surgery.

Diastematomyelia

General: diastematomyelia = split cord malformation = longitudinal cleavage of spinal cord. Each hemicord has central canal and one ventral and one dorsal nerve root. Both parts may have separate dura or common dura; intact cord above and below that level. Septal partition may consist of connective tissue, cartilage, or bone. Location: 85% below level of T8 vertebral body.

Clinical features: pain, neurogenic bladder dysfunction, lower limb paralysis. Patients often have nevi, lipomas, and local increase in hair growth.

Imaging:

- **Radiographs:** bone spur, fusion/segmental anomalies, scoliosis
- **CT:** clearly defines bone spur and vertebral body anomalies
- **MRI:** T2-weighted axial and coronal—separate cord (**Fig. 4.14**). Isotropic 3D sequence may be helpful

> Neonatal hemicords clearly demonstrated by US (see also Sect. 4.2).

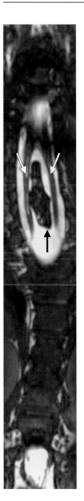

Fig. 4.14 Diastematomyelia in boy. T2-weighted coronal MRI demonstrates wide bony bridge (black arrow) and two separate spinal cords, each with its own central canal (white arrows).

DD: syringomyelia, vertebral body fracture with displaced intramedullary bone fragment.
Associated abnormalities: tethered cord, vertebral body malformations, scoliosis.

Tethered Cord

General: tethered cord = dorsal/caudal fixation of spinal cord/conus medullaris. Normal level of conus = T12–L2.
Clinical features: diverse; symptoms may appear at any age—pain, paresthesias, hyperactive reflexes, lower limb paralysis, neurogenic bladder dysfunction.
Imaging: MRI—abnormally low position of conus medullaris (below L3; **Fig. 4.13**). Conus thinned due to traction effect, indistinct junction of conus

and filum terminale. In severe cases, spinal nerves may run horizontally or even caudocranially.

> Cauda equina fibers normally sag with gravity in supine patient, which can mimic dorsal attachment in sagittal images. Resolve by also imaging in prone position.

Associated abnormalities: diastematomyelia, spinal lipomas, MMC, filum terminale syndrome.
Treatment: surgical (retethering is common after corrective surgery).

Metabolic Diseases

Leukodystrophies

General: dysmyelinating diseases primarily affecting white matter—intrinsically defective myelin broken down. Examples: adrenoleukodystrophy (ALD), metachromatic leukodystrophy (MLD), Pelizäeus–Merzbacher disease (PMD), Alexander disease, Canavan disease, Krabbe disease (globoid cell leukodystrophy [GLD]), Van der Knaap leukodystrophy.
Clinical features: vary with type of disease; often nonspecific, especially in early stage.

- ALD: progressive cognitive and neurologic impairment
- MLD: unsteady gait, behavioral abnormalities
- PMD: nystagmus, poor head control, spasticity, ataxia
- Alexander disease: megalencephaly, developmental delay
- Canavan disease: macrocephaly, epilepsy, developmental delay
- GLD: hyperirritability, diminished reflexes

Imaging:

- **CT:** hypodense white matter; megalencephaly in Canavan and Alexander diseases; early hyperdense basal ganglia in GLD (globoid cell accumulation and calcification); atrophy in later stages
- **MRI:** abnormal white matter signal intensity, usually diffuse and symmetrical (**Fig. 4.15**). Sites of occurrence: supratentorial white matter > cerebellar. Exceptions: GLD—early cerebellar involvement; Alexander disease—abnormal signal intensity and contrast enhancement of dentate nuclei. Characteristic distribution pattern seen in some leukodystrophies, such as Van der Knaap leukodystrophy = almost complete absence of subcortical white matter, swelling of gyri, subcortical cysts

4

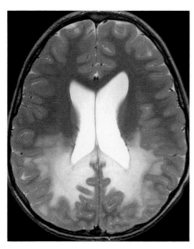

Fig. 4.15   Adenoleukodystrophy in 8-year-old boy. T2-weighted axial MRI shows patchy hyperintensity of parieto-occipital white matter in periventricular, central, and subcortical regions.

> FLAIR = best sequence for detecting demyelination in patients > 2 years of age. Difficult to evaluate white matter at < 2 years of age.

Metabolic Diseases of Gray Matter

Metabolic diseases primarily affecting gray matter are often difficult to differentiate—altered signal intensity and decreased volume also seen in white matter (Wallerian degeneration) but less pronounced than in leukodystrophy.

Examples: pantothenate kinase-associated neurodegeneration (PKAN), Nieman–Pick disease, neuroaxonal dystrophy.

Metabolic Diseases Affecting Gray and White Matter

Heterogeneous group of syndromes. Diagnosis = clinical/laboratory/biopsy.

Examples: Zellweger syndrome, Wilson syndrome, MELAS (mitochondrial encephalomyopathy, lactic acidosis, strokelike episodes), Leigh syndrome, and glutaric aciduria type 1.

Craniofacial Anomalies, Craniosynostosis, and Congenital Diseases of the Ear

Facial Clefts

General: classification based on interorbital distance.

- Simple cleft (normal interocular distance) > 99%. Affects upper lip and palate. Usually an isolated anomaly. Clinical diagnosis; imaging not indicated
- Complete cleft lip and palate (unilateral/bilateral)—impaired chewing, drinking, hearing, speech, respiration, facial growth
- Facial cleft with hypertelorism < 1%
- Facial cleft with hypotelorism—in some patients with HPE (very rare)

Imaging: 3D CT for evaluation of complex clefts (following adequate ossification), particularly for surgery planning.

Craniosynostosis

General: cranial/craniofacial dysmorphia caused by premature closure of one or more sutures (calvarium/skull base) (**Table 4.1**).

Imaging:

- **Radiographs:** skull film—controversial; some authors require it as initial study (slightly oblique projection); often unsatisfactory. Today, CT initial study of choice in cases of high clinical suspicion

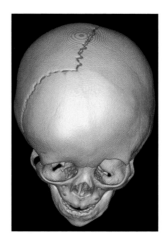

Fig. 4.16   Unilateral synostosis of left coronal suture (plagiocephaly) in 9-month-old boy. Anterior oblique surface display (3D spiral CT) documents premature closure of coronal suture on left side.

Table 4.1 Overview of primary craniosynostoses with affected suture, description of head shape, and usual designations for typical cranial configurations

Suture	Head shape	Designation
Sagittal	Long, narrow	Scapho- or dolicocephaly
Bilateral coronal	Short, broad, hypertelorism, small anterior cranial fossa	Brachy- or bradycephaly
Metopic	Pointed forehead	Trigonocephaly
Bilateral lambdoid	Shallow posterior cranial fossa, shortening of longitudinal diameter, prominent forehead	Turricephaly
Unilateral coronal	Unilateral frontal flattening, obliquity of orbit and nasal septum	Plagiocephaly
Unilateral lambdoid	Unilateral flattening of occiput	Plagiocephaly
All sutures	Small, round	Microcephaly

4

- **CT:** 3D CT; reduce dose but apply at least 100 kV. 3D surface display and reconstructions (**Fig. 4.16**)

Syndromes with craniofacial anomalies: Goldenhar, Apert, Crouzon.

Treatment: surgical (calvarial/suture osteotomy).

Congenital Diseases of the Ear

General: Diseases include congenital aural atresia (auricular deformities, absence of external auditory canal), congenital ossicular deformities (conductive hearing loss), inner ear malformations (sensorineural hearing loss), congenital cholesteatoma (develops from aberrant embryonic epithelial rests, similar to intracranial epidermoid). May be located in middle ear, mastoid, geniculate ganglion, petrous apex, external auditory canal, cerebellopontine angle cistern).

Imaging: CT—imaging modality of choice.

Syndromes with congenital abnormalities of the ear: Treacher–Collins syndrome (mandibulofacial dysostosis), Crouzon syndrome (craniofacial dysostosis), Apert syndrome (acrocephalosyndactyly), Goldenhar syndrome, Klippel–Feil syndrome.

Cerebral Diseases in Immature and Mature Newborns

Hypoxic-Ischemic Encephalopathy, Bleeding, and its Complications

General: brain responds in different ways, depending on maturity at time of hypoxic-ischemic insult (**Table 4.2**).

Periventricular leukomalacia: PVL = hypoxic-ischemic injury to periventricular white matter in premature infants. Reperfusion after ischemia in preterms often leads to periventricular or even intraventricular hemorrhage (IVH), which is particularly common in germinal matrix zone = germinal matrix hemorrhage (GMH = subependymal bleeding [SEB]). Germinal matrix zone (= site where "new" neurons are formed) = region between ventricle wall and brain parenchyma, very active between gestational weeks 8 and 28—highly susceptible to hypoxia and mechanical trauma/microvessel disruption. Longest-active portion near head of caudate nucleus.

Peri-/intraventricular hemorrhage: four grades of severity (see also Sect. 4.2): grade I = GMH/SEB; grade II = IVH; grade III = IVH and enlarged LV; grade IV (old term)—today, replaced by IVH III + "PVH" (periventricular hemorrhagic infarction =

Table 4.2 Typical findings and sites of involvement in diffuse hypoxic-ischemic encephalopathy as function of child age and grade of severity

Age	Mild to moderate hypoxia	Severe hypoxia
Premature infants (< 34 weeks)	Damage to periventricular white matter (PVL)	Thalamus, basal ganglia, brainstem
Term infants (> 36 weeks)	Watershed infarcts between MCA, ACA and PCA (parasagittal)	Brainstem, anterior cerebellar vermis, thalamus, basal ganglia, perirolandic cortex
> 4–6 postnatal months	Watershed infarcts between MCA, ACA and PCA (parasagittal)	Basal ganglia, diffuse cortical damage

Abbreviations: PVL, periventricular leukomalacia; MCA, middle cerebral artery; ACA, anterior cerebral artery; PCA, posterior cerebral artery.

venous infarction—caused by stasis in compressed draining veins running along dilated ventricle).

IVH, uncommon in term infants, usually has different cause/source: choroid plexus, vascular malformation, tumor, rupture of hemorrhagic infarction (usually thalamic) into ventricular system, coagulopathy, residual germinal matrix. Posthemorrhagic dilatation of fourth ventricle is poor prognostic sign.

HIE in term infants predominantly affects areas with high energy demand (lateral thalami, posterior portions of lentiform nucleus, hippocampus, perirolandic cortex).

Clinical features: hypotonia, epilepsy, irritability, falling hematocrit. Later results in variable motor development problems (spasticity) or mental retardation.

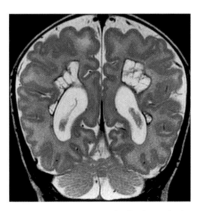

Fig. 4.17   Periventricular leukomalacia in 7-week-old former preterm infant. T2-weighted coronal MRI shows periventricular cystic lesions and mural hypointensities (blood residues).

Imaging:

- **Ultrasound:** see Sect. 4.2.
- **CT:** clearly displays hemorrhage. US/MRI preferred to avoid radiation exposure.
- **MRI:** germinal matrix—normally has high T1 and low T2 signal intensity
  - Acute GMH: T1- and T2-hypointense
  - IVH: often associated with secondary CSF flow obstruction and hydrocephalus
  - PVL: periventricular T1-hyperintense lesions, often linear; possible (later) "classic" cystic lesions (T1-hypointense, T2-hyperintense; **Fig. 4.17**). End stage: ventriculomegaly with irregular borders (mainly affecting posterior horns), periventricular hyperintensity in FLAIR and T2-weighted sequences (gliosis). Decrease in white matter volume, thinning of corpus callosum (**Fig. 4.18**)
  - Fresh watershed infarctions: hyperintense in diffusion-weighted sequences. Lactate peak on spectroscopy very sensitive indicator. Later gliosis, atrophy, ex-vacuo enlargement of LVs, Wallerian degeneration.
  - Acute stage of HIE in term infants: thalami and lentiform nuclei T1-hypointense/isointense, T2-hyperintense; increasing T1 signal intensity in 3 to 7 days (**Fig. 4.19**)

DD: choroid plexus cyst, ventriculitis, periventricular calcifications in TORCH infections.

> IVH, PVH, and PVL usually diagnosed with US in acute stage at bedside.

Complications: posthemorrhagic hydrocephalus, often requires shunting.

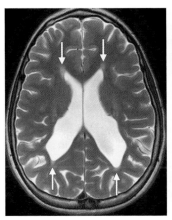

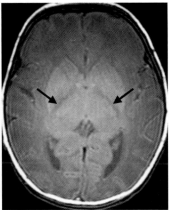

Fig. 4.18   Fig. 4.19

Fig. 4.18 MRI in 14-year-old former preterm infant with tetra-spastic cerebral palsy. T2-weighted axial MRI shows periventricular leukomalacia, thinning of supratentorial white matter, and hyperintensity of deep white matter (gliosis, arrows). Lateral ventices show ex vacuo dilatation with squared corners, extending partly to subcortical U-fibers.

Fig. 4.19 Hypoxic-ischemic encephalopathy in 6-day-old term infant. Axial T1-weighted MRI without contrast administration shows masking (hypointensity) of internal capsule (arrows) and hyperintensity of basal ganglia and thalamus.

4

Hydrocephalus

General: increased CSF with pressure effects on brain parenchyma due to imbalance between CSF production, circulation, and reabsorption.

- **Hypersecretory hydrocephalus:** choroid plexus papilloma
- **Obstructive hydrocephalus**
  - Noncommunicating hydrocephalus: aqueductal stenosis, Chiari malformation types I and II, DWM
  - Communicating or malabsorptive hydrocephalus: extraventricular obstruction of subarachnoid space, may occur after intracranial bleeding, meningitis, venous hypertension
- **Malformation-associated and normal-pressure hydrocephalus**

> Ventriculomegaly not synonymous with elevated-pressure hydrocephalus.

Clinical features: macrocephaly (with open cranial sutures), signs of increased intracranial pressure (with closed sutures).

Imaging:
- **Radiographs:** wide sutures, large tense/bulging fontanelle, thinning of dorsum sellae, increased craniofacial ratio
- **US:** modality of choice in newborns for initial diagnosis and follow-up—see Sect. 4.2
- **CT:** in noncommunicating hydrocephalus—large rounded ventricles, periventricular halo of de-creased density (impaired transependymal CSF flow), narrow basal cisterns, compressed sulci. In communicating hydrocephalus—enlarged basal cisterns and sulci.
- **MRI:** enlarged third ventricle, rostral bulge of lamina terminalis, dilated LVs including temporal horns, possible compressed sulci. FLAIR = most sensitive sequence for detecting impaired transependymal CSF drainage (accentuated around anterior and posterior horns, less along lateral wall)—may be absent in chronic/compensated obstruction

DD: benign widening of subarachnoid space in small children with/without macrocephaly, common between 6 and 24 months of age (no neurologic abnormalities), familial macrocephaly, ex vacuo ventriculomegaly (atrophy), hemimegalencephaly.

> Not always easy to distinguish ventricular enlargement in (elevated-pressure) hydrocephalus from atrophy. Data on head circumference and its growth essential for diagnosing hydrocephalus—excessive or too-rapid increase in head circumference favors hydrocephalus; small or diminishing head circumference suggests atrophy.

Treatment: shunt implantation, elimination of cause (whenever possible).

Infections of the Central Nervous System, Orbit, Sinuses, and Ear

Congenital and Neonatal Infections

General: if brain still developing at time of insult, pattern of injury varies from that in mature brain! **TORCH infections (transplacental):** toxoplasmosis, rubella, cytomegalovirus (CMV), herpes simplex virus (HSV-2 usually acquired during passage through birth canal), HIV, syphilis.

Clinical features: epilepsy, developmental delay, microcephaly.

Imaging:

- **US:** see Sect. 4.2
- **CT/MRI:** fairly specific patterns, mainly with calcifications and secondary changes
  - Toxoplasmosis: Ca^{2+} in basal ganglia, periventricular white matter, cortex
  - CMV: Ca^{2+} mainly periventricular; initial findings are polymicrogyria/LIS, white matter glial scars, myelination delay, frequent cerebellar hypoplasia (**Fig. 4.20**)
  - Rubella: Ca^{2+} periventricular, cortical, basal ganglia; microcephaly, dilated inner CSF spaces; myelination delay, patchy T2 hyperintensities (white matter)
  - Syphilis: leptomeningeal contrast enhancement extending into Virchow–Robin spaces
  - HIV: Ca^{2+} in white matter and basal ganglia; atrophy
  - Neonatal HSV: initially, areas of impaired diffusion (hyperintense); then T1-hypointense and T2-hyperintense; meningeal enhancement; multicystic encephalomalacia, atrophy

DD: TS (subependymal Ca^{2+}), chronic venous ischemia (AVF, venous malformation—subcortical Ca^{2+}, atrophy), congenital lymphocytic choriomeningitis, neurocysticercosis.

Acquired Infections

Bacterial Cerebritis, Brain Abscess

General: cerebritis = first stage of bacterial brain infection, may regress or form abscess. Main causative organisms in neonatal period: citrobacter, proteus. Routes of infection: contiguous spread (sinusitis, mastoiditis), hematogenous, postoperative (iatrogenic), cardiopulmonary anomaly.

Brain abscess = advanced stage of cerebritis. Usually large and periventricular in newborns/infants, may rupture into CSF spaces. Subcortical and basal ganglia sites common in older children.

Clinical features: headache, fever (in 50%), seizures, focal neurologic deficits, irritability, poor feeding.

Imaging:

- **CT:** cerebritis = hypodense area with indistinct margins (increased H_2O content); abscess = hypodense (more hypodense at center, less peripherally), rim enhancement, perifocal edema (**Fig. 4.21**)
- **MRI:** cerebritis = T1-hypointense and T2-hyperintense with slight mass effect. Patchy contrast enhancement. Thin enhancing abscess wall in "mature" abscess, T2-hypointense and T1-isointense. Center T2-hyperintense and T1-hypointense. Perifocal edema. Diffusion-weighted sequence with ADC map: diffusion restriction at

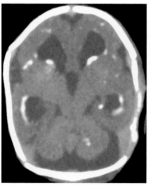

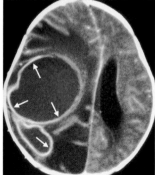

Fig. 4.20 **Intrauterine cytomegalovirus infection in newborn girl.** Unenhanced CT shows multiple, predominantly periventricular calcifications, and cerebellar hypoplasia.

Fig. 4.21 **Large hematogenous brain abscess in 3-month-old boy.** Axial CT after contrast administration shows intensely enhancing abscess wall with smooth inner borders (arrows), marked perifocal edema, contralateral midline shift, and dilatation of left lateral ventricle secondary to foramen of Monro obstruction.

Fig. 4.20   **Fig. 4.21**

center and hypointensity in ADC (DD: brain tumor).

DD: brain tumors, demyelinating diseases such as MS and ADEM, hematoma undergoing reabsorption.

Treatment: cerebritis usually responds well to antibiotics—close-interval follow-ups.

! Caution: development of brain abscess.

Brain abscess may be difficult to distinguish from tumor (clinical information, diffusion) → diagnostic–therapeutic aspiration/biopsy.

Encephalitis

General: herpes simplex encephalitis—almost always due to HSV-1 infection (affinity for limbic system).

Clinical features: fever, seizures, vomiting, altered level of consciousness, motor weakness.

Imaging:

- **CT:** unrewarding during initial days.
- **MRI:** shows early T1-hypointensity, increased signal intensity on T2-weighted and FLAIR sequences. Typically located in medial temporal lobe, insular cortex, cingulum (may occur anywhere in small children). Delay in treatment → later defects, so prompt diagnosis critical (CSF aspiration = lumbar puncture (LP)/laboratory; do not wait for imaging!).

Varicella zoster encephalitis, measles encephalitis, Rasmussen encephalitis, progressive multifocal leukoencephalitis (PML): relatively rare, imaging findings nonspecific.

Meningitis

General: bacterial or viral inflammation of meninges—diagnosed from clinical and laboratory (LP) findings, not by imaging. CT and MRI used to detect complications, or may precede LP in patients with signs of increased intracranial pressure.

Clinical features: headache, stiff neck.

Imaging: CT and MRI initially negative in most cases; occasionally show thickening and increased enhancement of meninges. Complications: hydrocephalus, venous sinus thrombosis, venous and arterial infarctions (vasculitis), ventriculitis, cerebri-

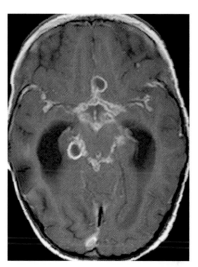

Fig. 4.22   Tuberculous meningitis in 4-year-old girl. T1-weighted axial MRI after contrast administration. Basal CSF spaces filled with markedly enhancing inflammatory material, and multiple inflammatory granulomas seen. Temporal horns dilated.

4

tis and abscess formation, septated cysts, localized defects, subdural hygroma.

Special form—tuberculous meningitis: insidious onset; predominantly affects basal cisterns that become filled with inflammatory–granulomatous material (**Fig. 4.22**). Cranial nerve deficits, hydrocephalus, tuberculomas in brain parenchyma have low T2 signal intensity, show inhomogeneous enhancement. Infarctions (vasculitis).

Treatment: specific antibiotic therapy, abscess drainage, shunting of hydrocephalus.

Sinusitis and its Complications

General: acute bacterial sinusitis complicates 5–10% of upper respiratory infections in children. Clinical diagnosis is difficult, imaging findings are not definitive.

Clinical features: acute sinusitis—headache, slight fever, cough, respiratory distress. **Complications**—frontal swelling, swollen eyelids, protrusio bulbi.

Imaging: evaluation by imaging is not routinely indicated for suspected acute bacterial sinusitis! Not even radiographs are taken, owing to low sensitivity and specificity (mucosal swelling, anatomic variants, sinuses not yet pneumatized).

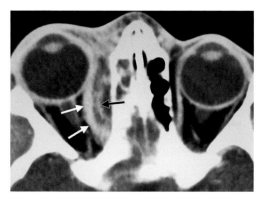

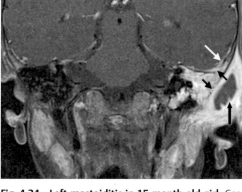

Fig. 4.23   Orbital complications of right ethmoid sinusitis in 8-year-old boy. Axial CT after contrast administration shows orbital invasion by postseptal extraconal abscess with enhancing membrane (black arrow). Note thickening and increased enhancement of displaced medial rectus muscle (white arrows). Protrusio bulbi also present.

Fig. 4.24   Left mastoiditis in 15-month-old girl. Coronal T1-weighted MRI after contrast administration demonstrates retroauricular subperiosteal abscess (thick black arrow), osteolysis (short black arrows), and dural enhancement (white arrow).

CT and MRI are used only to detect complications! Frontal osteomyelitis (Pott's puffy tumor), bone destruction, extracranial inflammatory mass, epidural/subdural empyema, meningitis, cerebritis, brain abscess, cavernous sinus thrombosis. Orbital complications: orbital cellulitis (inflammation/edema of orbital fat), subperiosteal and orbital abscess (also detectable by postcontrast axial and coronal CT or coronal reformatting; **Fig. 4.23**).

> MRI superior to CT for imaging orbital apex and detecting intracranial complications, poorer for bone destruction.

DD: polyps, juvenile nasoangiofibroma, Langerhans cell histiocytosis, RMS, lymphoma, juvenile nasopharyngeal fibroma.

> Sinusitis common in patients with cleft lip and palate, choanal atresia, Kartagener syndrome (hypo-/aplasia of paranasal sinuses, bronchiectasis, situs inversus).

Treatment: antibiotics; complications treated surgically.

Mastoiditis

General: mastoiditis = complication of otitis media.
Clinical features: ear pain, fever, retroauricular swelling, protruding ear, facial nerve palsy.
Imaging: CT/MRI—obliteration of middle and inner ear, mastoid cells, bone resorption. Complication: retroauricular subperiosteal abscess (**Fig. 4.24**). Abscess may break through at mastoid tip and track along sternocleidomastoid muscle ("Bezold abscess"). Intracranial rupture → meningitis, cerebritis, subdural/cerebral abscess, sigmoid sinus thrombosis.
DD: severe otitis externa with retroauricular spread.
Treatment: uncomplicated acute mastoiditis is treated with antibiotics. Surgery indicated for cases unresponsive to antibiotics and for complications.

Case Study 4.1

History: 7-week-old boy, former premature infant, with respiratory distress syndrome, epileptic seizures, irritability, and poor feeding.
Suitable modalities: US or MRI.

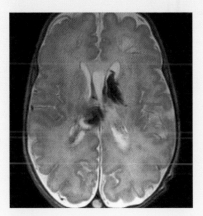

Fig. 4.25

Available images: T2-weighted axial MRI.
Findings: hypointense lesions—subependymal and in adjacent brain parenchyma on left side, also in thalamus on right side. Superior sagittal sinus filled with hyperintense material. Hyperintense (cystic) lesion in frontal white matter on left side.
Diagnosis: SEB and parenchymal hemorrhage on left side. Thalamic hemorrhage on right side, venous sinus thrombosis, PVL in left frontal region.

Case Study 4.2

History: abnormal fetal ultrasound (US); imaging ordered for postpartum confirmation and evaluation.
Suitable modalities: US or MRI.

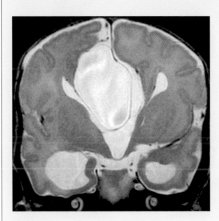

Fig. 4.26

Available images: T2-weighted coronal MRI in 3-day-old infant.
Findings: absence of corpus callosum, third ventricle communicates with interhemispheric fissure, steer-horn configuration of LVs, large interhemispheric lesion isointense to CSF.
Diagnosis: agenesis of corpus callosum with interhemispheric cyst.

4

▮ **Case Study 4.3** ▮

History: 18-month-old girl had been resuscitated after aspirating peanut.
Imaging: noncontrast CT.

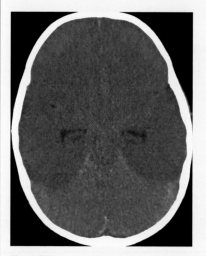

Findings: decreased gray–white matter differentiation, cerebellum hyperdense relative to diffusely hypodense cerebrum ("white cerebellum sign").
Diagnosis: diffuse hypoxic brain injury.

Fig. 4.27

▮ **Quiz Case 4.1** ▮

History: 13-year-old girl experienced an initial seizure.

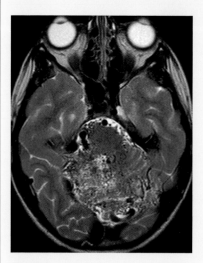

Fig. 4.28

Questions	Correct answers
What primary and subsequent studies are available?	MRI; if MRI contraindicated or unavailable, high-quality CT; DSA added if needed
What changes are present; what sequence was used?	Axial T2-weighted MRI showed multiple scalloped hypointensities in PCF and brainstem, sites of increased signal intensity in adjacent cerebellum
Interpretation and diagnosis?	Flow voids, sites of reactive gliosis/ischemia → AVM
Complications?	Brain hemorrhage, infarction
What modality should be added for planning and providing treatment?	Conventional catheter-based DSA with endovascular embolization

Quiz Case 4.2

History: 22-month-old boy with slight weakness on right side, predominantly affecting arm, and slight cranial bossing on left side.

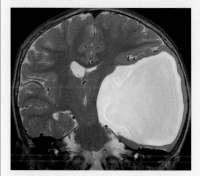

Fig. 4.29

Questions	Correct answers
What imaging modality should be used initially?	MRI; if MRI contraindicated or unavailable, high-quality CT
What changes are present, what sequence was used?	Coronal T2-weighted MRI. Large temporal intraventricular lesion isointense to CSF; compression and displacement of adjacent brain areas, midline shift; thinning and bulging of calvarium
How should radiologic signs be interpreted within the clinical context?	Cystic mass displaying no malignant features
Diagnosis?	Intraventricular neuroependymal cyst
Is further imaging necessary?	No
Treatment?	Size and clinical manifestations warrant shunt insertion

4

████ **Quiz Case 4.3** ████

History: 3½-year-old girl with growth retardation.

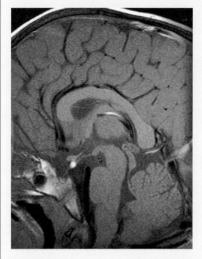

Questions	Correct answers
What imaging modality should be used initially?	MRI
What changes are present, what sequence was used?	T1-hyperintense structure in infundibulum, small anterior pituitary, small sella turcica; sagittal T1-weighted MRI without contrast
Diagnosis?	Ectopic posterior pituitary; hypoplasia of anterior pituitary
Is further imaging necessary?	No
Treatment?	Hormone replacement

Fig. 4.30

Bibliography

1 Barkovich AJ. Pediatric Neuroimaging. Philadelphia: Lippincott Williams & Wilkins; 2005: 659–703

2 Beitzke D, Simbrunner J, Riccabona M. MRI in paediatric hypoxic-ischemic disease, metabolic disorders and malformations—a review. Eur J Radiol 2008; 68(2): 199–213

3 Hetts SW, Sherr EH, Chao S, Gobuty S, Barkovich AJ. Anomalies of the corpus callosum: an MR analysis of the phenotypic spectrum of associated malformations. AJR Am J Roentgenol 2006; 187(5): 1343–1348

4 Janse van Rensburg P, Andronikou S, van Toorn R, Pienaar M. Magnetic resonance imaging of miliary tuberculosis of the central nervous system in children with tuberculous meningitis. Pediatr Radiol 2008; 38(12): 1306–1313

5 Lopes Ferraz Filho JR, Munis MP, Soares Souza A, Sanches RA, Goloni-Bertollo EM, Pavarino-Bertelli EC. Unidentified bright objects on brain MRI in children as a diagnostic criterion for neurofibromatosis type 1. Pediatr Radiol 2008; 38(3): 305–310

6 Phelan JA, Lowe LH, Glasier CM. Pediatric neurodegenerative white matter processes: leukodystrophies and beyond. Pediatr Radiol 2008; 38(7): 729–749

7 Simbrunner J, Riccabona M. Imaging of the neonatal CNS. Eur J Radiol 2006; 60(2): 133–151

8 Sorantin E, Robl T, Lindbichler F, Riccabona M. MRI of the neonatal and paediatric spine and spinal canal. Eur J Radiol 2008; 68(2): 227–234

9 Tortori-Donati P. Pediatric Neuroradiology Head, Neck and Spine. Berlin, Heidelberg, New York: Springer; 2005; 1551–1608

4.2   Neurosonography in Newborns and Children

Michael Riccabona

US = essential modality for imaging the pediatric (neonatal) neurocranium, eye, and spinal canal.
Advantages: no ionizing radiation, exquisite resolution, dynamic functional imaging with real-time or (color) Doppler sonography ([C]DS), bedside imaging capability; may be repeated as often as desired —ideal for follow-up.

3D US improves standardized documentation, conspicuous analysis of complex anatomy, and comparison to other sectional imaging or on follow-up.

Limitations: gray–white matter differentiation and evaluation of subcalvarial-peripheral areas, subarachnoid hemorrhage (SAH)/trauma are difficult particularly after initial months of life due to increasing ossification.

> Problem of dwindling knowledge and skills in (pediatric) neurosonography, rarely addressed in radiology as a whole. *But,* neurosonography is essential tool, especially in newborns and critical care settings → hence covered here in some detail, despite limited scope.

Technique of Pediatric Neurosonography

Approaches for Scanning

- **Newborns:** use physiologic, nonossified scanning "windows"; i.e., large/small/lateral fontanelles, open sutures, transoccipital, transtemporal, nonossified portions of spinal canal
- **Children:** transtemporal scanning through thin, minimally ossified portions of calvarium, similar to adults (TCI = transcranial imaging); transoccipital US

Transducer Requirements

- **Newborns:** high-frequency sector probes/microcurved (10-5 MHz), high-resolution linear probe (17-8 MHz) for near-field imaging and spinal US—with virtual convex mode also for deeper parts (up to 4 MHz)

- **Children** (TCI): low-frequency sector probes for transtemporal scans (5-1 MHz)

> ! Note vulnerability of brain, especially in premature infants → use low acoustic energy—always mechanical index (MI) 0.7; thermal index [TI] < 1 with Doppler sonography. May use higher MI/TI in children (TCI), as goodly portion of sound energy absorbed by calvarium.

Imaging Protocol

- **Transfontanellar** brain imaging: US probe angled in fan-shaped pattern in coronal, (para-) sagittal and coronal planes (**Fig. 4.31**). Axial scans from lateral side—important for evaluating peripheral CSF regions and occipital brain areas.

> ! Avoid transducer pressure on fontanelle → may compress superior sagittal sinus or underlying brain tissue (especially with microcurved probes). Copious US gel = good acoustic coupling without pressure.

- **TCI** = axial scans with probe rotated/angled over fixed application site (i.e., site of best sound penetration)—define central and skull-base structures (cerebral crura, circle of Willis), supratentorial ventricles and aqueduct, check for midline shift. Subcalvarial peripheral regions should be scanned whenever possible.

After essential structures have been surveyed in gray scale, and standard planes have been documented:

- Activate **CDS** (vascular anatomy, flow direction) and duplex Doppler sonography (DDS) for spectral analysis (arterial and venous flow patterns; **Fig. 4.32**). Typical DDS sampling sites:
    a) arterial limb: internal carotid arteries (ICAs) and middle cerebral arteries (MCAs) as well as posterior cerebral arteries (PCAs) on both sides (sides are compared), anterior cerebral artery (ACA)/pericallosal artery, basilar artery

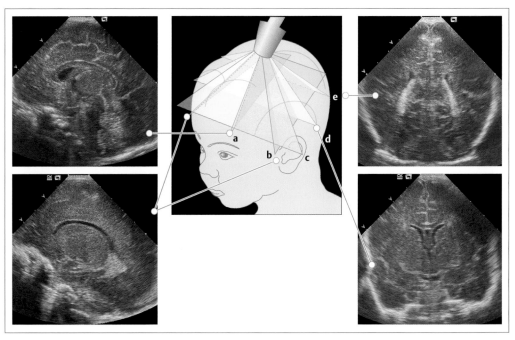

Fig. 4.31a–d Diagrammatic representation of transfontanellar neurosonography, with normal findings. Diagram shows classic scan planes for transfontanellar neurosonography. Images illustrate normal findings in sagittal (**a**), parasagittal (**b**), coronal (**c**, frontal; **d**, mid), and posterior occipital coronal (**e**) scan planes.

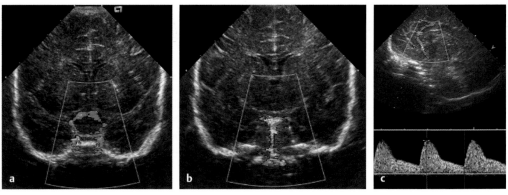

Fig. 4.32a–c Transfontanellar cerebral DS, normal findings. Normal findings in coronal (**a**, **b**) and sagittal (**c**) scans. CDS views of circle of Willis (**a**) (internal carotid artery and anterior cerebral artery [ACA]), basilar artery, and inflow from both vertebral arteries (**b**) and ACA (**c**). Doppler spectrum (**c**) is from ACA/pericalosal artery.

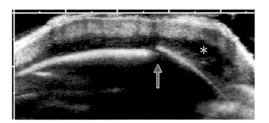

Fig. 4.33 Small-part US/calvarial sonography with high-resolution linear probe. The bone entry echo (→) is interrupted and displaced by skull fracture with associated hypoechoic hematoma (*).

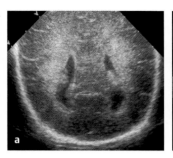
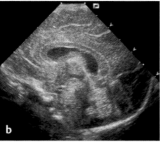

Fig. 4.34a, b Cranial US in premature infant, normal findings.
a Hyperechoic periventricular parenchyma (= immature white matter), broad posterior horns, and decreased convolutions (coronal image).
b Large cavum septi pellucidi and vergae and large extracerebral CSF space in posterior cranial fossa (sagittal scan).

b) venous limb: superior sagittal sinus, great cerebral vein, posterior fossa sinuses

- **Brain surface evaluation:** transfontanellar with linear probe (extracerebral CSF space, cerebral gyri, gray-white matter differentiation, etc.)—also useful for calvarial US (galeal hematoma, skull fracture, etc.; **Fig. 4.33**)
- **Cranio-cervical junction:** axial scans through lateral fontanelle, nuchal/occipital
- **Spinal US:** longitudinal and transverse scans, (para)median through nonossified posterior arch elements/spinous processes. Evaluate spinal canal contents/spinal cord, conus medullaris (level), bony boundaries (vertebral body margins)

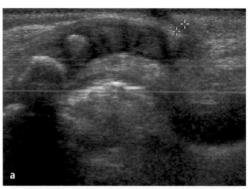

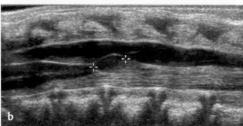

Normal Findings

Vary with age.
Premature infants: slightly wider LVs, decreased gyral pattern, less gray-white matter differentiation, physiologic periventricular echoes (= PVEs, signs of "immaturity"). Cavum septi pellucidi and vergae (may be large), slightly larger extracerebral CSF spaces (**Fig. 4.34**).
Term infants: LVs are narrower, considerable gray-white matter differentiation, distinct gyral pattern with deeper sulci (**Fig. 4.31**).
Spinal US: level of conus medullaris at L2 or higher. Physiologic lumbar/cervical cord thickening, visible central canal echo. Filum terminale < 2 mm in diameter. Mobile cauda equina. Hypoechoic CSF space with supporting ligaments and anterior/posterior nerve routes. Spinal cord and its coverings. Coccyx cartilaginous; last coccygeal vertebra may be angled backward (e.g., associated with sacral dimple, **Fig. 4.35a**).

Fig. 4.35a, b Normal spinal US findings, midsagittal scan from posterior side with child lying prone over pad.
a "Sacral pore." Lowest, cartilaginous coccygeal vertebra (hypoechoic) splayed slightly outward and connected to dimple by fine oblique channel (++).
b Conus medullaris at level of L2 vertebral body, with physiologic terminal ventricle (++), cauda equine/filum terminale.

Sacrum contains variable amount of moderately echogenic fat. Physiologic variant/embryological remnant: small cystic structure located at origin of or in filum terminale (= filar cyst) or in/on lowest part of conus medullaris (= terminal ventricle; **Fig. 4.35b**).

Common Neonatal Disorders

Hypoxia

General: see Sect. 4.1. US features depend on brain maturity. (C)DS should always supplement gray-scale imaging. Always schedule follow-ups (see below).

Term Infants

Initial US findings may be nonspecific. Otherwise **diffuse hypoxia** (e.g., peripartal asphyxia) may present with narrow/obliterated ventricles and diffusely echogenic parenchyma (= diffuse edema = "bright brain") or focal patchy parenchymal areas of increased echogenicity (= focal edema, e.g., in basal ganglia). Loss of gray–white matter differentiation, reversal of echo pattern (**Fig. 4.36a**). Focal hypoxia = infarction: regional edematous zone, hyperechoic area, often wedge-shaped with relatively sharp margins (not detectable initially!).

Course: increasing structural irregularities, necrosis/cyst formation, progressive enlargement of inner/outer CSF spaces (ex vacuo = atrophy due to diffuse global hypoxia; see **Fig. 4.58**). Focal hypoxia: necrotic area/cyst—especially with secondary hemorrhage or large defect (**Fig. 4.36b**).

(C)DS: initially normal spectral waveform (up to 24 hours after event). Then diastolic hyperemia and global rise in flow velocities (resistive index [RI] ↓; **Fig. 4.36c**) → increasing brain swelling and rising resistance = initial decline in diastolic perfusion (RI ↑) and potentially tent-shaped diastole, then diastolic flow reversal (RI > 1) → decrease in systolic flow velocity, culminates in undulating flow = reflects deficient antegrade perfusion (→ brain death; **Fig. 4.37**).

Improvement/normalization may occur at any stage from 3 to 5 days after the event. Similar DS waveforms/flow patterns also seen in older children (TCI) following hypoxic brain injury (e.g., near-drowning).

Premature Infants

Periventricular white matter vulnerable zone in immature brain. Initial appearance of edematous zones = echogenic, inhomogeneous structural irregularities, initially difficult to distinguish from physiologic zones of immaturity (PVEs). Follow-up will show whether irregularities mature to normal pattern or progress to periventricular zones of cystic necrosis (PVL; **Fig. 4.38** and **Fig. 4.60**). Also watch for zones of cerebellar hypoxia!

> Fine or subtle changes are difficult to detect sonographically—often only follow-ups diagnostic. Subtle structural transformation, white matter thinning, and gliosis are difficult or impossible to detect with US. If within diagnostic window (days 2–10 after event) and findings equivocal but might have therapeutic implications → diffusion-weighted MRI and MR spectroscopy (lactate peak detection, see Sect. 4.1).

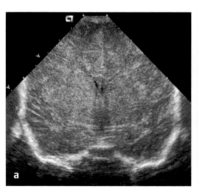 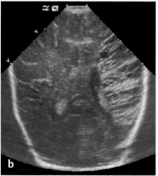 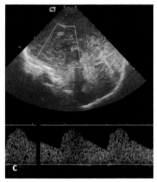

Fig. 4.36a–c B-mode and Doppler US findings in asphyxia/hypoxia/infarction.

a Coronal scan in severe asphyxia. Hyperechoic inhomogeneous brain parenchyma, accentuated basal ganglia, partially reversed echogenicity of cortex and white matter; ventricles almost obliterated.

b Older infarcted area in left middle cerebral artery territory. Lytic–cystic transformation, still some diffuse parenchymal echogenicity and ex vacuo dilation of left lateral ventricle (coronal scan).

c Sagittal scan, CDS, and spectral sampling of anterior cerebral artery: slightly increased diastolic flow velocity, slightly decreased resistance index—early "hyperemic" phase after asphyxia.

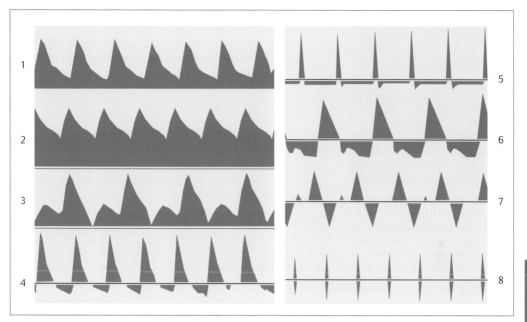

Fig. 4.37 Progression of Doppler waveforms in asphyxia. Typical evolution of Doppler flow spectrum after asphyxia. Initial normal flow (1), then (diastolic) hyperemia and tachycardia (resistive index [RI] ↓, 2), decreased early diastolic flow (tent-shaped diastole, 3), increasing diastolic flow reversal (RI ↑, 4), bradycardia and decreased flow velocities (5), diastolic reflux of all forward systolic flow (6), and finally undulating flow (7) or deficient pulsation of static blood column (= brain death, 8).

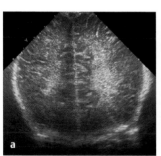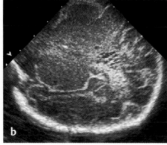

Fig. 4.38a, b   US findings in periventricular leukomalacia.
a Coronal scan in premature infant shows patchy, asymmetrical, inhomogeneously increased periventricular echogenicity.
b Parasagittal scan with probe angled toward periventricular region shows increasing cyst formation over time (= PVL).

Hemorrhage

Intracranial Hemorrhage in Premature Infants

Due to vascular immaturity in subependymal germinal matrix, minimal trauma, blood pressure variations, hypocapnia, etc. → vascular tearing and (intraventricular) hemorrhage (IVH). Simplest form = pure subependidymal bleed (SEB) = intraventricular hemorrhage grade I (IVH I) (**Fig. 4.39**).

Other stages: **IVH II** (slight bleeding into LV), **IVH III** (increasing LV dilatation, blood > 50% of LV), **IVH III and PVH** (periventricular hemorrhage, formerly called "IVH IV")—not caused by IVH burrowing into parenchyma but by secondary hemorrhagic infarction of periventricular tissue due to stasis of veins running along LVs (= venous infarction; **Fig. 4.40**).

Other hemorrhagic entities accessible to US imaging: **choroid plexus hemorrhage** (confined to plexus), intracerebral hemorrhage (**ICH**) = (traumatic) parenchymal bleeding, secondary hemorrhagic infarction, epidural hematoma (**EDH**) (axial

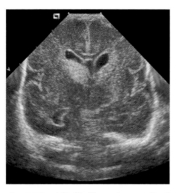

Fig. 4.39 US findings in cerebral hemorrhage. Coronal scan in premature infant shows large choroid plexus hemorrhage on the right side with associated obstruction of foramen of Monro.

scan = TCI), subdural hematoma (**SDH**) (plus linear transducer)—special form: **tentorial hemorrhage** (requires additional scan from lateral posterior fontanelle).

Subarachnoid hemorrhage (SAH) and contusional/shear hemorrhage difficult or impossible to detect and diagnose, and particularly to exclude, with US.

Term Infants

Intracranial hemorrhages less common than in premature infants; occur predominantly in basal ganglia/cerebral parenchyma and often take form of hemorrhagic infarction (**Figs. 4.41a** and **4.52**).

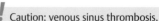

! Caution: venous sinus thrombosis.

Obstetric trauma—hemorrhage from tentorial tear, possible SAH/EDH (e.g., after forceps delivery, **Fig. 4.41b**).

EDH/SDH = targeted search (use linear US probe and TCI), detectable in first months of life (fall/child abuse). SAH difficult to detect with US.

Evolution of Hemorrhage

Clots become encysted, and are increasingly broken down (see **Fig. 4.59**). Cysts of variable size (cyst conglomerate) may form in choroid plexus, ventricle, or parenchyma (= porencephalic cyst), may coalesce with ventricular lumen (**Fig. 4.42**).

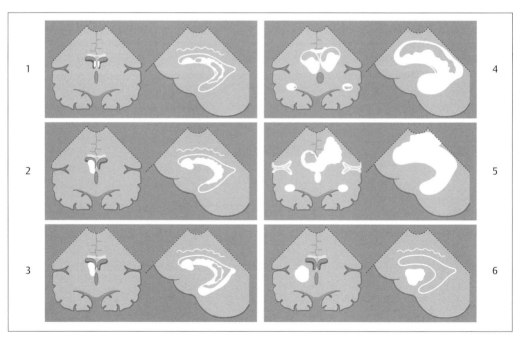

Fig. 4.40 Diagrammatic representation of US classification of typical intracranial hemorrhages. Choroid plexus hemorrhage (1), subependymal bleeding = intraventricular hemorrhage [IVH] I (2), IVH II (3), IVH III (4), IVH III and periventricular hemorrhage—formerly classified as IVH IV (5), intracerebral hemorrhage (illustrated for basal ganglia hemorrhage) (6).

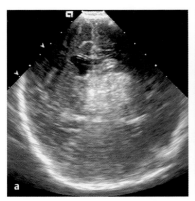

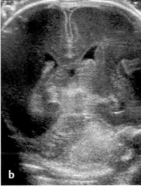

Fig. 4.41a, b   Other intracranial hemorrhages.
a Coronal scan of echogenic left basal ganglia mass (= hemorrhage) in mature newborn.
b Coronal scan with linear probe. Inhomogeneously hyperechoic left cerebellar region and tentorium after obstetric trauma in premature infant = tentorial and cerebellar hemorrhage.

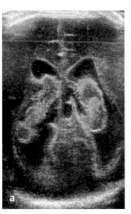

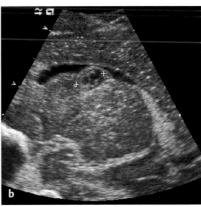

Fig. 4.42a, b   Older intraventricular hemorrhage with lytic and cystic changes.
a Coronal scan with linear probe in premature infant with bilateral IVH III shows marked cystic transformation of clotted blood plus double outlines of broadened, echogenic ventricular borders (= sign of posthemorrhagic ventriculitis).
b Magnified view of parasagittal scan with sector probe documents cystic transformation in IVH I (++).

4

After IVH—abacterial arachnoiditis/ventriculitis (= increased echogenicity of thickened ventricular wall) → impaired CSF circulation, production, absorption, and secondary hydrocephalus: US follow-up with standardized measurements (see section below and Sect. 4.1).

Hydrocephalus

General: see also Sect. 4.1. Enlargement of inner/outer CSF spaces. Causes: imbalance between CSF production/absorption or obstructed CSF drainage. Classification:

- Phenomenologic = internal/external/communicating;
- Functional = hypersecretory, obstructive, malresorptive, ex vacuo;
- Etiologic = posthemorrhagic, inflammatory, aqueductal stenosis, caused by mass/tumor, posttraumatic, caused by malformation), shunt failure.

Imaging:

- Role/indication: investigate clinical status, confirm clinical suspicion, antenatal findings; follow-up of ventriculomegaly/hydrocephalus after diagnosis and during treatment
- Imaging goals: classification, anatomic visualization (preoperative), differentiation of etiology and type, assessment of intracranial pressure (indirectly based on ventricular configuration and perfusion patterns)
- Capabilities of CT/MRI, see Sect. 4.1

Ultrasound in Hydrocephalus

General principles: CSF space enlarged (supra-/infratentorial, extracerebral, standardized ventricular measurements); diameter less accurate than cross-sectional area or ventricular volume. Ratio of LV diameter to parenchymal width often helpful (growth-concordant size increase without parenchymal damage?), measurement of occipital, tem-

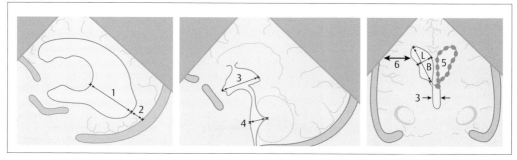

Fig. 4.43 Diagrammatic representation of standard US measurements in hydrocephalus in parasagittal, midsagittal, and coronal scans (coronal scan at level of foramen of Monro). Occipital ventricular width (1), occipital parenchymal width (2), third ventricle (3), fourth ventricle (4), lateral ventricle (LV) circumference/area (5), length of LV (L), depth of LV (B), coronal width of cerebral parenchyma (6).

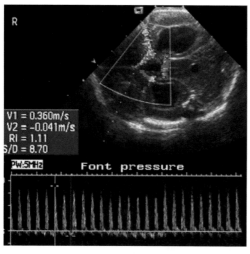

Fig. 4.44 DS in hydrocephalus, fontanelle compression test. Transtemporal DS in hydrocephalus during fontanelle compression test (same patient as in **Fig. 4.61**). Reversal of diastolic blood flow during test = intracranial pressure significantly increased. Maximum systolic flow velocity (still) normal but falls during compression test. Note: transtemporal scan displays only small section of lateral ventricle.

poropolar, and frontal parenchymal width particularly helpful (see **Fig. 4.61a, b**).

Ventricular width or dilatation does not equal elevated brain pressure; brain parenchyma width, sulzi shape, as well as cerebral perfusion assessment are clues for diagnosis.

Important aspects:

- Width assessment—requires standardized, reproducible scan planes (coronal scan at level of foramen of Monro, parasagittal scan through frontal, posterior, and temporal horn on both sides; **Fig. 4.43**).

Precise midsagittal scan used to define aqueduct and fourth ventricle (or TCI).

- Extracerebral CSF space evaluated with linear probe through fontanelle or by TCI (evaluate opposite side, also used for aqueduct visualization)
- Evaluate ventricular lumen (plexus? signs of posthemorrhagic changes? internal echoes as with hemorrhage or inflammation, etc.), ventricular lining (e.g., thick, echogenic ventricle wall in posthemorrhagic ventriculitis)
- Visualization of aqueduct (if necessary by TCI; see **Figs. 4.45** and **4.61c**)

Special form—isolated ventricle (isolated dilatation of one ventricle): for example, foramen of Monro obstruction = one dilated lateral ventricle; isolated fourth ventricle—obstruction of aqueduct and foramina of Luschka and Magendie (e.g., postinflammatory, posttraumatic); diagnosis: supratentorial hydrocephalus—aqueductal stenosis, but foramen of Monro patent.

DS: Locate essential vessels with CDS, targeted DDS = spectral analysis of flow pattern.

- **Increased intracranial pressure** → diastolic flow velocity initially decreased, then systolic velocity → diastolic flow reversal and increased RI values; also helpful:

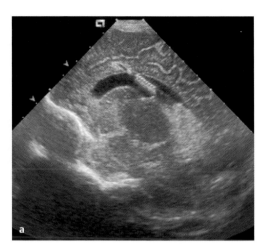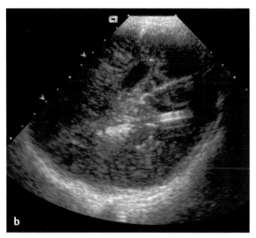

Fig. 4.45a, b   US imaging of the drain tip in shunted hydrocephalus. Transfontanelle (**a**) and transtemporal (**b**) US scans in shunted hydrocephalus. Transfontanellar scan clearly defines anterior portion and tip of drain (periventricular malposition). Transtemporal scan displays posterior portion of drain and its continuity.

– **DS of extra- and intracranial portion of ICA** at junction of extra-/intracranial artery segments—marked difference in extra-/intracranial waveforms without angle correction (normal intracranial ICA flow velocity ≤ extracranial velocity). With slightly elevated pressure = intracranial flow velocity ↑. With greatly elevated pressure (> 20 cm H_2O) = intracranial flow velocity ↓. Useful parameter = ratio of intra- to extracranial flow velocity (normal = 0.8–0.9, slight pressure increase > 1, marked pressure increase < 0.8)

– **Fontanelle compression test:** fontanelle gently compressed during DS imaging. With normally compliant brain → no significant change in Doppler spectrum. With slight pressure increase → deterioration of diastolic flow velocity (with increase in RI), when pressure gets more elevated decrease of systolic flow velocity with increase in RI (**Fig. 4.44**).

Transtemporal scanning (MCA) also used for fontanelle compression test → ensures constant position of sample volume, which is more difficult and challenging with transfontanellar scans.
Note: typical flow changes with result from (sub)-acute increased brain pressure. However, despite elevated intracranial pressure, practically normal flow pattern may be restored in chronically increased pressure.

- **CSF flow imaging/measurement:** possible only if particles present within CSF. Normal = bidirectional flow modulated by and synchronous with respiration, flow velocity = 1 to 10 cm/s

Findings in shunted hydrocephalus—follow-up: Evaluation of ventricular width, perfusion, shunt position/tip/course, valve (**Fig. 4.45**). Detection of possible CSF fistula, CSF leakage along drain, CSF pooling around exit site/valve.

Shunt failure = ventricular width ↑, parenchymal width ↓, decreased perfusion (see above).

Overshunting = ventricular collapse, torn bridging veins → SDH, slitlike ventricle.

! Caution: pressure may be increased or decreased.

With **ventriculoperitoneal shunt**—supplement imaging with abdominal US (CSF cysts at end of shunt, ascites = indirect evidence of patent shunt, provided lack of other abdominal condition). US can assess subcutaneous shunt continuity.

With stiff ventricles—significant pressure differences may exist with little or no dilation/volume changes.

Limitations of US: Scans are sometimes difficult to interpret with regard to:
- Assessing intracranial shunt continuity (especially with advanced ossification);

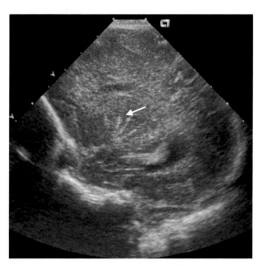

Fig. 4.46 Noncalcifying vasculopathy. Parasagittal scan reveals echogenic streaks (→) along basal ganglia vessels.

- Locating drain tip (especially with shunts in extracerebral CSF space);
- Evaluating extracerebral CSF space (e.g., temporopolar arachnoid cyst).

If findings equivocal → MRI (see continuous visualization of shunt) or CT (MRI not available, emergencies) and radiography (to trace shunt and check for disconnection or malposition).

Inflammation and Calcifications

Inflammation

General: see also Sect. 4.1.6. No typical sonomorphologic correlate for inflammatory conditions.
Congenital encephalitis: intrauterine, usually viral. Detectable postnatally by residua (noncalcifying

vasculopathy, parenchymal calcifications, cerebellar hypoplasia, etc.; **Fig. 4.46**).
Encephalitis: US can detect only secondary phenomena—regional edema zone/infarction with secondary hemorrhage (e.g., in herpes encephalitis), abscesses (bacterial meningoencephalitis, fungal), general diffuse hyperemia = indirect, nonspecific sign on DS (RI ↓, flow ↑).
Meningitis: widening of extracerebral CSF space with internal echoes (in **purulent meningitis**), on (C)DS meningeal hyperemia and hypervascularity —morphologic features indistinguishable from (sub)acute bleeding. Differentiate widened subdural space from subarachnoid space by CDS: numerous vessels in subarachnoid space, only few crossing bridging veins in subdural space.
Ventriculitis: broad, hyperechoic ventricle wall, internal echoes in ventricle—abacterial after hemorrhage (irritation by blood breakdown products).

> ❗ Caution: development of hydrocephalus—temporary external drainage? Serial lumbar puncture?

Brain abscess: a "complicated cyst" may be characterized by echogenic sediment, membranelike rim of perifocal change (= abscess membrane and perifocal edema); may be small or large, isolated or multiple (**Fig. 4.47**).

Other US criteria: posterior acoustic enhancement confirms liquid nature, CDS establishes vascular or avascular nature, and demonstrates hypervascular membrane.

Intracranial Calcifications

General: rare; may form after congenital infections (often perivascular = "noncalcifying vasculopathy," especially in basal ganglia, nonspecific). Sometimes

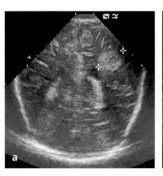
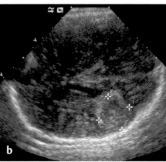

Fig. 4.47a, b Brain abscess. Note variable US morphology of rounded brain abscess (++), depending on extent of necrosis in transfontanellar (**a**) and transtemporal (**b**) scans.

found also after hemorrhage or trauma and in necrotic zones.

> Typical hyperechoic foci of calcification usually do not cast typical acoustic shadows (due to numerous reflective surfaces in neurocranium). Slightly calcified structures may escape detection on survey radiographs but often detectable with US. If findings uncertain and have therapeutic relevance → CT/MRI.

Cysts, Masses, Tumors

Cysts

See Sect. 4.1 and below.

General: dysontogenetic neuroepithelial (normal variant, periventricular/in choroid plexus), posthemorrhagic, posthypoxic, cystic malformations.

Cystic tumor components and liquefaction ("complicated cysts") are rare.

US appearance: round to oval, echo-free area with sharp margins and echogenic rim. Distal acoustic enhancement (**Fig. 4.48**). If mass liquid but does not meet all essential criteria = "complicated" cyst (e.g., internal echoes, ill-defined, thick, irregular borders, etc.)—consider DD: abscess, hematoma undergoing absorption, intralesional hemorrhage, etc.

> Use CDS to differentiate cyst from ectatic vascular malformation or aneurysm. Do not mistake physiologic cavities for cysts (e.g., cavum veli interpositi).

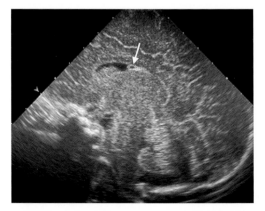

Fig. 4.48 Choroid plexus cyst. Transfontanellar parasagittal scan shows small cyst (++, →) in choroid plexus with relatively echogenic wall and no other plexus abnormalities—most likely dysontogenetic choroid plexus cyst (DD: prior choroid plexus hemorrhage).

Tumors

See also Sect. 4.1, 8.2.

General: rare in newborns, may be hamartomatous, syndromic (TS, NF). Very rare entities in first months of life (= accessible to US): medulloblastoma, primitive neuroectodermal tumor, teratoma, choroid plexus papilloma, choroid plexus carcinoma, ependymoma.

- **US appearance:** nonspecific—requires further investigation by MRI (CT)
- **Role of US:** detection (not exclusion!), secondary hydrocephalus? Cerebral hemorrhage? (Increased intracranial pressure? Urgent need for external drainage? etc.)

Malformations of the Brain

Classification and details, see Sect. 4.1.

General: Today, most brain malformations are detected and diagnosed prenatally with US and diagnosed/classified by fetal MRI.

Postpartum: US = first confirmatory modality. Use MRI for detailed evaluation (give therapeutic–prognostic rationale).

Typical US-accessible changes (useful for classification/identification):

- Enlargement of inner/outer CSF spaces, atypical ventricular anatomy (e.g., monoventricle)
- Disproportionate expansion of ventricular system (e.g., aqueduct stenosis, isolated fourth ventricle)
- Regional expansion, especially of extracerebral CSF spaces (arachnoid cysts—temporopolar affinity, midline cysts)
- Changes in midline structures (e.g., absent corpus callosum = agenesis of corpus callosum with associated syndromes, partial agenesis of corpus callosum, septum pellucidum agenesis = septo-optic dysplasia/DeMosier syndrome, MMC-associated Arnold–Chiari malformation, **Fig. 4.49**)
- Decreased/increased gyral pattern, decreased/flattened/increased sulci
- Changes in PCF (Dandy-Walker malformation, rhombencephalosynapsis, etc.)

4

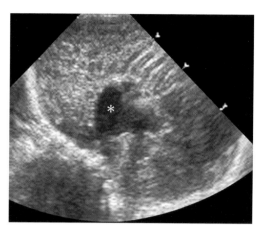

Fig. 4.49   US appearance of corpus callosum agenesis (Arnold–Chiari malformation). Midsagittal scan in newborn with myelomeningocele. Corpus callosum absent (= agenesis of corpus callosum), third ventricle dilated (*), radial gyri extend to ventricular roof.

US of limited value for imaging of:

- Atypical parenchymal structure (myelination-, migration-, maturation disorder)
- Cleft anomalies (schizencephaly)—open-lip schizencephaly better detectable, closed-lip schizencephaly difficult to depict
- Posterior fossa pathology, metabolic disorders, leukodystrophy, and so on

For malformations and syndromes → US imaging of neurocranium and spinal canal plus search for other manifestations (kidney, heart, eye, GI tract, etc.).

Vascular Malformations and Diseases

General: aneurysm and stenosis of cerebral arteries rare, as large AVMs. Further details in Sect. 4.1.

Vein of Galen Malformation

Significant in newborns = conglomerate of different vascular malformations with shunting of blood causing vein of Galen to enlarge (see Sect. 4.1).
US: gray-scale shows cystic midline structure at roof of tentorium; large, hypoechoic tubular structures may arise from it (afferent/efferent vessels; **Fig. 4.50**).

- **CDS** essential—demonstrates often turbulent and accelerated blood flow; targeted DDS can define arterial feeders and draining veins (**Fig. 4.51**)

Strategy: small vein of Galen aneurysms (VGAs) without cardiac decompensation (usually only one or few feeders, little shunt flow, relatively low flow velocity of draining vein with little arterialisation) = US follow-up, followed later by MRA/CTA.

Large VGA and/or cardiac decompensation = early additional dedicated sectional imaging (CTA/ MRA) for detailed vascular anatomy (interventional

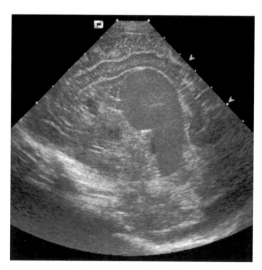

Fig. 4.50   Arteriovenous malformation with vein of Galen aneurysm. Precise midsagittal scan displays inhomogeneous hypoechoic, supratentorial cystlike mass.

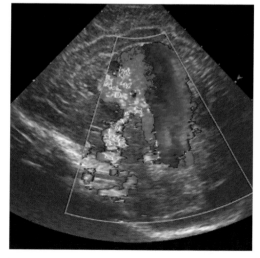

Fig. 4.51   CDS appearance of a vein of Galen aneurysm. Scan shows turbulent blood flow in aneurysm and hyperemic afferent artery.

planning). MRI indicated for parenchymal assessment, i.e., secondary hypoxic-hemorrhagic brain damage (by steal phenomenon).

Other Vascular Malformations/Pathology

General: can sometimes be detected by CDS. Contrast-enhanced TCI-CDS may be used in older children. Always use CTA/MRA for definitive diagnosis or exclusion, and preinterventional conventional catheter angiography.

Some rare changes in extracerebral arteries and veins important in children. Etiology: primary congenital (or with fibromuscular dysplasia/associated with syndromal conditions) or secondary (postinterventional/posttraumatic/postoperative/vasculitis):

- **Hypo-/Aplasia of one vertebral artery**: important in newborns; turning head to side may compromise dominant large-caliber vertebral artery supplying basilar artery → decreased blood flow to brainstem–possible link to sudden infant death; usually resolves after 1 year of age.
  US diagnosis in first months of life = targeted functional DS of basilar artery/proximal vertebral arteries (transfontanellar) → head turned 90° to right and left from neutral position while evaluating flow in both vertebral arteries and basilar artery.
- **Subclavian steal syndrome:** may be postoperative, may occur in aortic coarctation/interrupted aortic arch and heart disease; collateralization of extracranial vascular occlusion or decreased blood flow.
  CDS: reverse flow in affected collateralized vertebral artery, also possible decreased or reversed flow in the basilar artery (additional collateralization via anterior circulation)
- **ICA occlusion:** collateralization, mainly via anterior circulation → define intact circle of Willis (transfontanellar and transtemporal amplitude-encoded CDS scans) = prerequisite for arteriovenous ECMO (ICA cannulation/ligation). May also occur posttraumatic (dissection is most common in children).
- **Venous occlusion/congestion in neck veins**: postoperative, after central venous catheter placement; with heart defect–pathologic venous drainage = congestion of cerebral veins → dilatation of (extracerebral) CSF spaces.

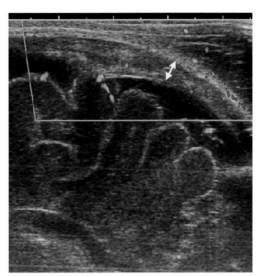

Fig. 4.52 Venous sinus thrombosis. Midsagittal US image acquired with linear probe scanning along open suture: echogenic thickening of superior sagittal sinus (++) with no color flow signals in venous sinus thrombosis.

(C)DS: intracranial venous flow slowed, does not show typical modulation.

- **Venous sinus thrombosis:** only superior sagittal sinus thrombosis reliably diagnosed with US (through fontanelle and open suture, during first months of life).
  US appearance = inhomogeneous echogenic masses in incompressible enlarged sinus, no detectable flow (CDS and DDS; **Fig. 4.52**). If prompt definitive diagnosis required and (C)DS equivocal → venous CTA; otherwise MRI and MRV (contrast-enhanced if needed; high-resolution fat-saturated isotropic T1-weighted 3D volume sequence helpful)
- **Sickle cell vasculopathy:** DS/TCI used to screen for overt/silent cerebral infarction or follow-up of at-risk sickle cell patients. Time averaged mean maximum velocity (TAMX) used to classify risk: normal < 170 cm/s, conditional/intermediate 170 to 200 cm/s, abnormal < 200 cm/s
- **Rare others:** Moya-Moya disease, other vasculitis, etc.–TCI may depict associated perfusion alterations in affected main arteries if severe; otherwise small vessel disease difficult to assess

4

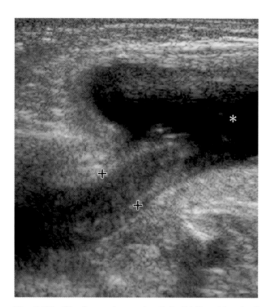

Fig. 4.53 Myelomeningocele. Spinal US, midsagittal scan from posterior side with child lying prone over pad. Image shows cystlike subcutaneous mass (*) and atypical cord termination extending into mass (++).

Spinal Ultrasound: Spinal Cord Pathology Accessible to Ultrasound

Spinal Dysraphism

See also Sect. 4.1.

General: closed/open, overt/occult. Terminology based on contents, anatomy and composition (meningocele, myelocele, myelomenigocele = MMC, myelocystocele = cystic opening of central canal, lipomeningomyelocele) or location (posterior, anterior, sacral, lateral).

Other entities: diastematomyelia, dorsal dermal sinus, spinal lipoma, tight or thickened/fatty filum terminale, hydromyelia, tethered cord, caudal regression syndrome.

Overt Spinal Dysraphism

Usually detected in utero.

Primary form with open defect, not an indication for local US (risk of infection!). May scan neurocranium and proximal spinal cord for additional findings (Chiari type II malformation, hydrocephalus, agenesis of corpus callosum, diastematomyelia, hydro-/syringomyelia).

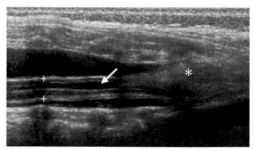

Fig. 4.54 Tethered cord. Spinal US, midsagittal scan from posterior side with child lying prone over pad. Spinal cord (++) extends to sacral level and is adherent to inhomogeneous echogenic intraspinal mass (= lipoma, *) with widening of central canal (= hydromyelia, →).

If closed or "covered"—typical "cyst" appearance with variable contents, depending on type (**Fig. 4.53**).

Postoperative US follow-ups, especially of neurocranium (development of hydrocephalus) and in cases with neurologic deterioration (retethering/tethered cord, epidermoid cyst, hydro-/syringomyelia).

Occult Spinal Dysraphism

US = primary neonatal imaging modality when external signs noted (**atypical** sacral dimple, cutaneous stigmata such as hairy nevus, hemangioma in midline, bulge suspicious for lipoma, etc.).

> Small sacral pore at normal location not associated with higher incidence of spinal malformations = no indication for US.

US findings:

- **Tethered cord:** low position of conus medullaris, straight and attached filum that may be thickened (tight filum terminale); limited mobility of nerve roots (**Fig. 4.54**)
- **Intraspinal lipoma:** echogenic structure, often associated with low position of conus medullaris and tethered cord (fixation of filum terminale/conus), possible dermoid cyst

> Do not confuse these cysts and hydromyelia with physiologic terminal ventricle!

- **Diastematomyelia:** double spinal cord, often separated at midline by cartilaginous/bony spur = two parallel cords → detected/excluded only by axial US scans; often associated with hydromyelia, intradural/filum terminale lipoma, MMC. Spinal radiographs to evaluate for bony changes

> Carefully assess location, length, and union to common cord. Also check for common or separate dural/arachnoid sheath.

- **Dorsal dermal sinus:** persistent epidermal communication between skin and spinal canal/spinal cord; runs obliquely upward from skin (usually with posterior stigmata) above S2, may be traceable to/into spinal cord/canal depending on size and fluid content. Axial and sagittal scans recommended

> Distinguish from physiologic sacral pore—sinus pilonoidalis may have hyperechoic bandlike connection (even with small unechoic tubular lumen) to end of coccyx, so it runs caudad—hence not dermal sinus. May become infected, but does not cause meningitis.

- **Caudal regression syndrome:** variable agenesis of coccyx/sacrum/lumbar spine leading to anomalies of caudal spinal cord—conus medullaris rounded, truncated, sometimes fixed, and often terminates at wrong level. Association with anterior meningocele (Currarino triad) → screen for anterior cystlike expansions with posterior, abdominal, and perineal scans

Spinal Tumors Accessible to Ultrasound

General: extremely rare. Primary imaging modality MRI (see Sect. 8.2).

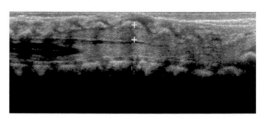

Fig. 4.55 Spinal US imaging of intraspinal epidural hematoma. Two composited posterior midsagittal scans with child lying prone over pad. Echogenic feature (++) after lumbar puncture = intraspinal EDH external to cord, indistinguishable from other masses (tumor) by its US appearance.

US = some applications: postoperative follow-up (access to spinal canal persists), tumor invasion of spinal canal (e.g., neuroblastoma—hourglass tumor, etc.), significant interspinal tumor components/deposits/metastases—before ossification of the bony walls.

Other Applications of Spinal Ultrasound

Vertebral body change: manifested indirectly by interruption of bone entry echo—accurately evaluate bone anatomy with radiographs/other sectional imaging modalities.

(Obstetric) trauma: US = useful for bedside evaluation of cord injury (cord avulsion, cord hematoma, EDH)—US also helpful after LP and failed (re-) puncture attempts → LP can be successfully accomplished with US guidance (slightly upright position to allow CSF to descent to puncture level) avoiding hematoma (**Fig. 4.55**).

- **Spinal EDH:** moderately echogenic mass occupying spinal canal and compressing subarachnoid space, potentially displacing cord. Possible compression/displacement of spinal cord. Older hematomas become increasingly hypoechoic.
- **Spinal cord injuries:** change in typical hypoechoic appearance of cord. Edema and hemorrhage = increased echogenicity of cord → cannot be differentiated with US, although cord continuity can be assessed—for early bedside imaging and initial evaluation after severe obstetric trauma with injury to cervical cord. Detailed evaluation = MRI.

Ultrasound of the Orbit and Eye

Method: high-resolution high-frequency (10–17 MHz) linear/sector US probe, scan through closed upper eyelid. Use low sound output energy, plenty warm US gel, avoid transducer pressure!

Normal findings: eyelid, cornea, anterior chamber, iris, ciliary body, lens, vitreous, papilla, optic nerve exit point. Behind globe—eye muscles (hypoechoic bandlike structures) = muscle cone, optic nerve, and nerve sheath, accompanying vessels.

Ocular pathology:

- **Microphthalmia/anophthalmia:** with empty eye socket or occluded lid—good opportunity to evaluate for size/presence of eyeball

4

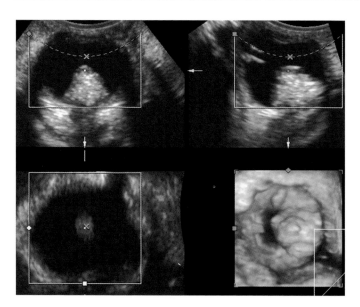

Fig. 4.56   Retinoblastoma. 3D US study of eye. Three orthogonal scans and rendered image demonstrate hyperechoic intraocular mass (= retinoblastoma).

- **Coloboma:** findings range from slight ectatic bulge to large cystlike deformity, caused by defective closure of optic vesicle; easily detected and demonstrated
- **Persistent hyperplastic primary vitreous:** persistence of primary vitreous and hyaloid vasculature (Cloquet canal)—may be difficult to evaluate clinically and ophthalmologically due to leukocoria and cataract. US = cone-shaped sonodense masses on posterior surface of lens, echogenic cord leading to optic nerve papilla with persistent hyaloid artery (on CDS)
- **Retinal detachment:** curved double lines in vitreous body, sometimes folded; moderately echogenic inhomogeneous texture. Pediatric cases usually occur in retinopathy of prematurity
- **Optic disk drusen:** echogenic deposits in optic nerve papilla, calcifications—may cast acoustic shadows
- **Papilledema:** occurs in setting of increased intracranial pressure; bulging of the papilla, swelling of optic nerve sheath

Eye tumors: see Sect. 8.2 for more details.

- **Retinoblastoma:** most common malignant eye tumor in children. US shows variable-sized intraocular globular or oval echogenic masses, sometimes multicentric, some showing marked hypervascularity, may be associated with small calcifications (**Fig. 4.56**). Use MRI to detect spread behind eye and to optic nerve

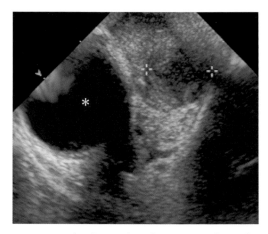

Fig. 4.57   Orbital cystic lymphangioma with intralesional hemorrhage. US shows slight indentation of globe (*) by septated, confluent, inhomogeneous mass of variable echogenicity. Mass includes cystlike area (++) of variable size (= orbital cystic lymphangioma with intralesional hemorrhage).

- **Other rare tumors:** astrocytoma, metastasis (e.g., leukemia, neuroblastoma)

Orbital pathology:

- **Retrobulbar abscess:** arises from sphenoid cells/orbital septum. Easily scanned with US through eye. US findings: typical abscess formation with inhomogeneous hypoechoic swelling of adjacent (rectus) muscle, echogenic double lines

Quiz Case 4.4

History: microcephalic infant after complicated perinatal course. Prematurity, protracted difficult neonatal period (IRDS and long-term ventilation, short bowel syndrome after severe NEC and long-segment bowel resection), feeding problems, nutritional osteopenia.
Clinical findings: neurologic abnormalities, lack of head growth, open fontanelle.

Fig. 4.58a–d

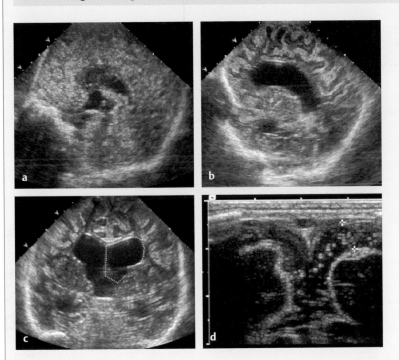

4

Question: Neurologic abnormalities and developmental delay referable to organic brain damage?

Questions	Correct answers
What are the imaging options?	US, MRI
What images are available?	US scans of neurocranium through large open fontanelle
Findings?	Sagittal, parasagittal, and coronal scans: dilated ventricular system; broad, flat gyri with wide subarachnoid space. US of brain surface with linear probe = broad extracerebral CSF space
Diagnosis?	Cerebral atrophy with internal and external hydrocephalus ex vacuo

History: intubated, ventilated premature infant (delivered in week 28), 2 weeks old. Complicated pregnancy and delivery. Referred for investigation of peri- and postnatal problems.
Laboratory findings: (hemorrhagic?) anemia, hyperbilirubinemia.
Clinical findings: neurologic abnormalities.

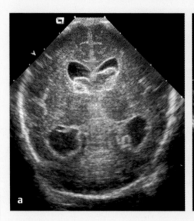 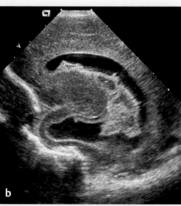

Fig. 4.59a, b

Question: Neurologic abnormalities referable to organic brain disease?

Questions	Correct answers
What are the imaging options?	US (MRI)
What images are available?	Transfontanellar US
Findings?	Coronal and parasagittal scans: bilateral dilatation of LVs with inhomogeneous echogenic masses in/around choroid plexus consistent with early lytic clots, sediment in posterior horn (blood), echogenic ventricle walls, signs of immaturity (poor gyral development)
Diagnosis?	Bilateral IVH III, not fresh, with encysted clots, signs of posthemorrhagic ventriculitis

along ethmoid cell boundary. US also useful for follow-up during antibiotic therapy

- **Tumors of the orbit:** see also Sect. 8.2. Hemangioma, lymphangioma, RMS, teratoma, neuroblastoma, metastases. US findings nonspecific, aside from potentially marked hypervascularity with hemangioma (DD: RMS) and septated multicystic lymphangioma (possible echogenic sediment and fluid–fluid levels due to intralesional hemorrhage) = US-guided puncture and instillation of sclerosing agents feasible (**Fig. 4.57**)
- **FB localization:** US not established for this indication, though it can clearly detect many FBs

- **Dacrocystocele:** congenital mucocele = circumscribed cystlike expansion of lacrimal saccule and duct, collection of mucoid and cellular debris; result of distal mechanical occlusion of nasolacrimal duct → bulge/swelling atcanthus. US = complex cystic mass with tubular structure continuing toward nasolacrimal duct. Gentle pressure evokes floating internal echoes = proof of complex liquid nature. Findings diagnostic— no need to add MRI or other imaging studies.

Quiz Case 4.6

History: newborn girl, 3 weeks old. Complicated perinatal course after premature twin birth.
Clinical findings: subtle neurologic abnormalities.

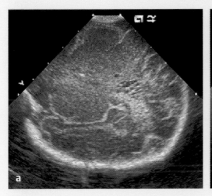 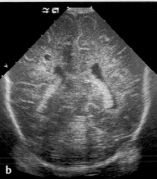

Fig. 4.60a, b

Question: morphologic cause for abnormal findings?

Questions	Correct answers
What are the imaging options?	US, (MRI)
What images are available?	Transfontanellar US scans
Findings?	Coronal and parasagittal scans: bilateral periventricular cysts in inhomogeneous echogenic periventricular parenchyma
Diagnosis?	Periventricular leukoencephalomalacia (PVL)

Bibiliography

1 Bulas D. Screening children for sickle cell vasculopathy: guidelines for transcranial Doppler evaluation. Pediatr Radiol 2005; 35(3): 235–241

2 Coley BD, Siegel MJ. Spinal Sonography. In: Siegel MJ, ed. Pediatric Sonography, 4th ed. Philadelphia: Lippincott Williams & Wilkins; 2011: 647–674

3 Coley BD, Murakami JW, Koch BL, Shiels WE II, Bates G, Hogan M. Diagnostic and interventional ultrasound of the pediatric spine. Pediatr Radiol 2001; 31(11): 775–785

4 Deeg KH. Zerebrale Dopplersonografie im Kindesalter. Berlin, Heidelberg: Springer; 1989

5 Deeg KH, Lode HM, Gassner I. Spinal sonography in newborns and infants—Part I: method, normal anatomy and indications. Ultraschall Med 2007; 28(5): 507–517

6 Deeg KH, Lode HM, Gassner I. Spinal sonography in newborns and infants—part II: spinal dysraphism and tethered cord. Ultraschall Med 2008; 29(1): 77–88

7 Deeg KH. Gehirn. In: Hofmann V, Deeg KH, Hoyer PF, eds. Ultraschalldiagnostik in Pädiatrie und Kinderchirurgie. 3rd ed. Stuttgart: Thieme; 2005: 1–180

8 Gassner I, Mair M. Bulbus oculi und Orbita. In: Hofmann V, Deeg KH, Hoyer PF, eds. Ultraschalldiagnostik in Pädiatrie und Kinderchirurgie. 3rd ed. Stuttgart: Thieme; 2005: 191–202

9 Mair MH, Geley T, Judmaier W, Gassner I. Using orbital sonography to diagnose and monitor treatment of acute swelling of the eyelids in pediatric patients. AJR Am J Roentgenol 2002; 179(6): 1529–1534

10 Riccabona M. Pediatric neurosonography. In: Riccabona M, ed. Pediatric Ultrasound, Requisites and Applications. Heidelberg: Springer; 2014

▬ **Quiz Case 4.7** ▬

History: newborn girl, 3 weeks old. Prenatal suspicion of hydrocephalus.
Clinical findings: large head, slightly tense fontanelle; no other abnormalities.

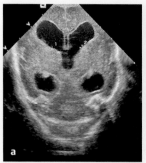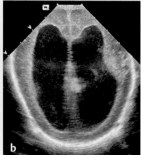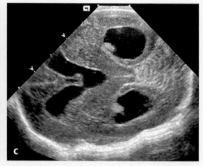

Fig. 4.61a–c

Question: hydrocephalus?

Questions	Correct answers
What are the imaging options?	US, MRI (CT)
What images are available?	Transfontanellar and transtemporal US scans of neurocranium
Findings?	Coronal scans (**a, b**): dilatation of supratentorial ventricular system. Transtemporal scan (**c**): nonvisualization of aqueduct
Diagnosis?	Supratentorial hydrocephalus secondary to aqueduct stenosis

11 Riccabona M, Resch B, Eder HG, Ebner F. Clinical value of amplitude-coded colour Doppler sonography in paediatric neurosonography. Childs Nerv Syst 2002; 18(12): 663–669

12 Riccabona M, Nelson TR, Weitzer C, Resch B, Pretorius DP. Potential of three-dimensional ultrasound in neonatal and paediatric neurosonography. Eur Radiol 2003; 13(9): 2082–2093

13 Simbrunner J, Riccabona M. Imaging of the neonatal CNS. Eur J Radiol 2006; 60(2): 133–151

14 Siegel MJ. Brain. In: Siegle MJ, ed. Pediatric Sonography, 4th ed. Philadelphia: Lippincott Williams & Wilkins; 2011: 43–117

15 Unsinn KM, Geley T, Freund MC, Gassner I. US of the spinal cord in newborns: spectrum of normal findings, variants, congenital anomalies, and acquired diseases. Radiographics 2000; 20(4): 923–938

16 Veyrac C, Couture A, Saguintaah M, Baud C. Brain ultrasonography in the premature infant. Pediatr Radiol 2006; 36(7): 626–635

5 Pediatric Uroradiology

Michael Riccabona

5.1 Development and Embryology

Pronephros regresses → metanephros (becomes Gartner duct in females, seminal vesicles, etc. in males) → metanephros: metanephric blastema becomes glomeruli and tubules. Ureteric buds (mesonephric duct) sprout from endodermal cloaca (**Fig. 5.1**).

Buds grow upward and meet with metanephros, inducing normal renal parenchyma formation → parenchyma derived from blastema, pelvicalyceal system (PCS) and ureter from ureteric bud. Next comes longitudinal growth and ascent/rotation of kidney with "rope ladder" arrangement of renal arterial supply.

- Normally, vessels regress spontaneously, eventually forming single renal artery

Urinary bladder splits off from cloaca by urorectal septum, also forming urethra.

- Development of male urethra is complex. Allantois normally regresses to form urachus by 15th week of gestation; may persist longer
- Obliterated urachal duct remnants may be detectable postnatally

The three fetal duct systems (Müllerian, Gartner, Wolffian) are precursors of genital organs.

- Uterus, ovary, adnexa, vagina/testis, seminal vesicle, and vas deferens

Primary or secondary (e.g., vascular) disturbances in these developmental processes → urogenital malformations, cyst formation, dysplasia, ectopia, etc.

5

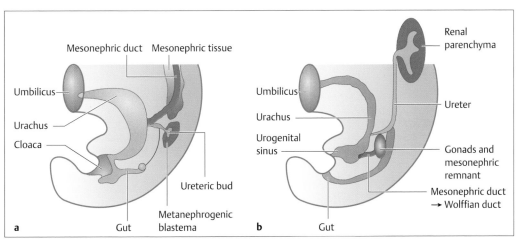

Fig. 5.1a, b Simplified diagrams showing embryonic development of urogenital tract. Early phase (**a**) and late phase (**b**). The mesonephric duct develops into genital structures while sprouting ureteric bud (blue) meets with blastema and induces renogenesis → differentiation into ureter and pelvicalyceal system.

Ultrasound and Basic Aspects of Doppler Ultrasound

See also Sect. 1.4.

Prerequisites: good hydration, full bladder, transducer (probe) appropriate for patient age and targeted area/access.

Procedure:

- Apply warmed US gel. Start with bladder, survey completely in longitudinal and transverse scans.
- Optimize image: set focus, gain, output/input, adjust TGC curve (especially when imaging lower abdomen/bladder), etc.
- Locate ostia and distal ureters, evaluate floor and neck of bladder:
  - Evaluate internal genitalia with adequately distended bladder (mandatory in females)
  - Possibly add perineal scans (for assessing urethra, vagina, cloacal malformation, anal atresia)
- Take standard measurements of bladder, bladder wall and ureter, with volumetry:
  - S^{Bl} (correction factor, varies for different bladder shapes); e.g., use $S^{Bl} = 0.7$–1.1 for square shaped bladder, $S^{Bl} = 0.5$ for spherical or elliptical bladder.
- Survey both kidneys completely in longitudinal and transverse scans (anterior/lateral/posterior approach), take standard measurements of PCS (if dilated) and kidney (**Fig. 5.2**). Record any other abnormalities (see Extended US Criteria, **Table 5.1**). Always include evaluation of perirenal

(adrenal, etc.) and perivesical space (internal genitalia, etc.).

- Kidney volumetry essential: Vol = L × W × H × 0.52
- Compare measured volumes with tables of normal values for age/weight
- Renal symmetry (relative renal volume in %, left + right vol = 100%)
- Always image entire urinary tract before and after voiding.

Table 5.1   Extended ultrasound criteria

Essential US criteria helpful in assessing likelihood of pathology
▪ Dilatation of pelvicalyceal system and ureters
▪ Bladder and renal volume (symmetrical? tables of normal values for age/weight, etc.)
▪ Bladder wall thickness and configuration
▪ Urachus? Diverticulum?
▪ Bladder neck and proximal urethra?
▪ Appearance of renal parenchyma (differentiation, thickness, echogenicity, focal abnormalities, cysts, etc.)
▪ Residual urine, post-voiding dilatation
▪ Urothelial width
▪ Renal vascular anatomy: perfusion abnormalities? asymmetric ureteral jet?
Pathology by these criteria → further investigation or at least follow-up

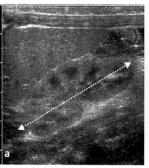 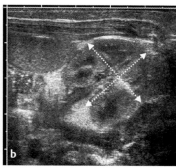

Fig. 5.2a, b   Normal neonatal kidneys: US appearance and volumetry. Longitudinal scan of right kidney (**a**), transverse scan of left kidney (**b**). Note typical sonographic features of neonatal kidney, including echogenic cortex, accentuated corticomedullary differentiation, and echogenic (pre)papillary distal medullary pyramid. Arrows = standard axes for renal measurements.

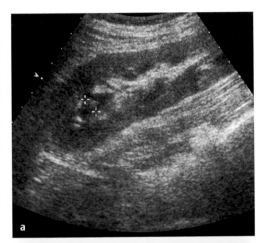

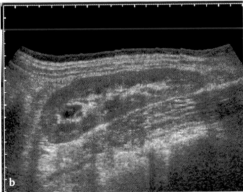

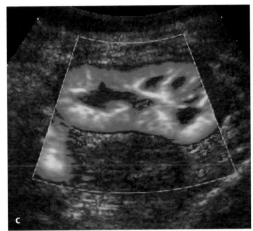

Fig. 5.3a–c Panoramic US evaluation of renal transplant (RTx).
a Renal allograft imaged with standard transducer—RTx too large for full-length measurement with standard probe. Altered upper calyx (++) documented along with organ dimensions.
b Panoramic image depicts true length of RTx, allowing for accurate measurement.
c Power Doppler scan in same patient shows homogeneous peripheral vascularity and physiologic areas of decreased color in medulla, which normally has less blood flow.

5

- "US genitography" may add information = instill NaCl into bladder and vagina (and rectum) via catheter before/during scan
- Testes: always use high-resolution linear probe; always compare both sides and evaluate inguinal canal

> All parts of examination (all scanned organs) should be adequately documented.

Modern Methods in Urosonography

- **HI, compounding:** especially useful for evaluating urine-filled structures
- **Extended FOV/panoramic US:** for measuring enlarged structures (bladder, larger tumor, renal allograft; **Fig. 5.3a, b**)
- **CDS:** for defining vascular anatomy and ureteral jet, urolithiasis (twinkling artifact)

- **Power Doppler:** peripheral renal parenchymal vascularity/perfusion, acute segmental pyelonephritis (APN), infarction, contusion, laceration, scar, diffuse decrease in blood flow (renal failure, renal vein thrombosis, etc.; **Fig. 5.3c**)
- **PW-DDS** (pulsed-wave duplex Doppler scanning): spectral analysis for flow velocity, flow spectrum, resistive index (RI) and acceleration index (renal artery stenosis [RAS], increased resistance, acute renal failure [ARF], etc.)

Conventional Radiography and Fluoroscopy

Additional studies: voiding cystourethrography, contrast-enhanced voiding urosonography (ce-VUS). Other studies (intravenous pyelography/urography [IVP/IVU], plain radiographs) rarely or less often used today.

Voiding Cystourethrography

Evaluation of bladder and urethra, vesicouretal reflux (VUR). See also Sect. 1.2 and 1.3.

Technique: pulsed digital FL with last-image-hold documentation (radiation hygiene!).

Procedure: suprapubic/transurethral catheterization (normal urinalysis!), latex-free, etc.

- Instill radiographic contrast medium into empty bladder, fill with physiologic pressure
- Image bladder during contrast instillation (bladder neck, early low pressure VUR? diverticulum?)
  - Observe contrast drip infusion → additional functional information (infusion halted by raised intravesical pressure? VUR episode? unstable bladder? etc.). Aids in detecting VUR and bladder dysfunction
- When contrast medium instilled: take oblique projection to show both distal ureters (VUR, diverticula, etc.)
- Evaluate urethra during voiding (AP for females, lateral for males), include both kidneys
- Document and grade any VUR that is found (**Fig. 5.4a, b**)
  - with VUR into PCS—image kidney (intrarenal reflux?)
- Obtain final postvoid image (residual urine? contrast outflow dynamics in VUR, etc.; **Fig. 5.4c**)

> Cyclic (2–3) contrast instillations recommended in first year(s) of life to increase detection rate of VUR.

Standard evaluation, see Sect. 5.5; see also European society (ESPR and ESUR) recommendations.

Ultrasound Voiding Cystoureterography

Also called contrast-enhanced voiding urosonography (ce-VUS). Offers same or better VUR detection rates than voiding cystourethography (VCUG) without radiation exposure; *however,* yields less anatomic information on urethra and ureters, may miss diverticula, gives poorer survey view than VCUG.

Technique, procedure: Bladder catheterization followed by instillation of NaCl and US contrast medium. Methodology same as VCUG but without radiation exposure. Continuous US visualization of bladder, retrovesical space, and PCS of both kidneys before, during, and after contrast instillation and voiding. VUR = any contrast medium visible in ureter/PCS (**Fig. 5.4 d, e**).

> Presently, no US contrast medium available that is approved for pediatric imaging; current use is off-label. If necessary, urethra can be imaged on perineal scans and observed during voiding (potentially needs repeated instillation and some patience).

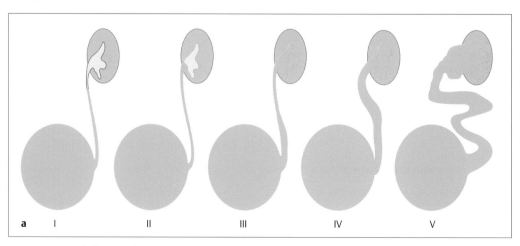

a   I   II   III   IV   V

Fig. 5.4a–e   Radiologic evaluation of vesicouretal reflux (VUR).

a Grades I–V of VUR based on international radiologic classification of reflux.

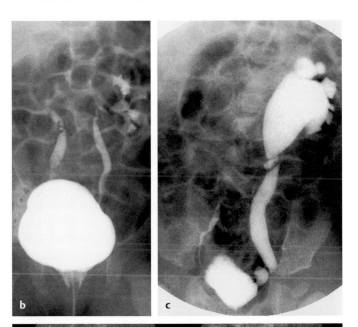

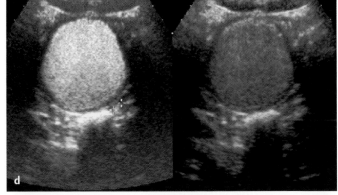

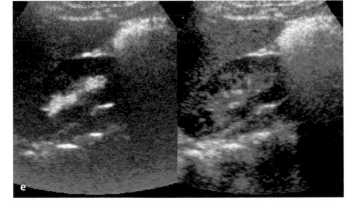

Fig. 5.4a–e   *continued*

b, c   VCUG. Typical findings in low-grade bilateral VUR (**b**). Left side shows high-grade VUR with proximal diverticulum and secondary ureteropelvic junction stenosis that restricts contrast drainage. Post-void image shows low-grade VUR on right side (**c**).

d, e   Side-by-side image display, ce-VUS. Scan shows bladder (bright) filled with contrast medium (Levovist) and, behind bladder, contrast-filled refluxing ureter (++), definable only with special contrast visualization technique (**d**). Later image shows contrast medium in nondilated pelvicalyceal system (PCS) (**e**). The classification of VUR by ce-VUS is like conventional VCUG but adds width of ureter/PCS before contrast instillation into bladder (grading: a = narrow, b = dilated).

5

Plain Abdominal Radiographs

May be used to check for urolithiasis (adjunct to US). Same applies to IVP. Used very rarely after contrast-enhanced CT.

- Collimate image to targeted region (kidney-ureter-bladder radiograph [KUB]); include pelvic floor!
- Use age-appropriate dose parameters and film–screen systems; follow **ALARA** principle (see Sect. 1.2, 1.3)
  - Image plates/digital systems with adequate resolution and pediatric (electronic) filtering/postprocessing, adjusted for age/weight

Intravenous Pyelography

IVP rarely used in modern pediatric imaging, has been mostly replaced by US and MRI.
Technique, procedure: same technical factors as KUB; possible to use lower X-ray dose.

- Only few (2 or 3) images taken at specified predefined intervals after IV contrast administration
- Protocol adapted to clinical question, e.g., pre-/postoperative, after trauma, urolithiasis
  - Potentially an additional film may be taken after administration of a diuretic drug, after voiding, after position change (postoperative), etc.
  - Adjust contrast dose for age! Note hydration, creatinine. Infusion-IVP contraindicated/outdated
  - Tomograms never obtained in children

Nuclear Medicine Imaging (Urinary Tract Scintigraphy)

Principle: (serial) images of target organ activity acquired with gamma camera following intravenous/intravesical administration of tracer labeled with radioactive technetium (mostly ^{99m}Tc).

- **Direct radionuclide cystography (DRNC)** = radiotracer administered through bladder catheter (for VUR detection)
- **Static renal scintigraphy** = images tracer excretion (^{99m}Tc-DMSA [dimercaptosuccinic acid]) and accumulation in renal parenchyma. Used to evaluate renal parenchyma, (relative) size, and

scarring. Rewarding in patients with adequate renal function and no significant obstruction
  - SPECT (single-photon-emission computed tomography) can improve anatomic resolution

> ! Caution: dose, motion artifacts.

- **Dynamic/diuretic renography (renal scintigraphy)** = ^{99m}Tc-MAG3 (mercaptoacetyltriglycine) administered intravenously. Tracer dynamics observed over time and plotted as time–activity curves
  - Elimination and excretory dynamics, differential kidney function
  - Indications: obstructive uropathy, renal function tests
  - Indirect VUR evaluation: delayed imaging in cooperative children with mature bladder function = **indirect RNC** → allows VUR detection without catheterization (VUR = reappearance of activity in PCS/ureter after outflow of activity from those sites, e.g., after voiding)

Magnetic Resonance Imaging

See also Sect. 1.6.

Plain Magnetic Resonance Urography (MR Urogram)

The excretory portion of urinary tract is imaged completely with heavily T2-weighted sequences (RARE [rapid acquisition with relaxation enhancement], HASTE, PACE [prospective acquisition correction], with diaphragm/respiratory gating, etc.).

- Good diuresis essential, so diuretic should be given (furosemide 1 mg/kg, to maximum of 20 mg) with adequate hydration at beginning of examination to distend PCS. Small children need sedation.
- MR urogram gives detailed anatomic information without radiation exposure or contrast administration. Even newborns and children in renal failure (relative contraindication to contrast use owing to risk of nephrogenic systemic fibro-

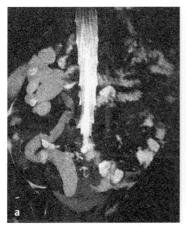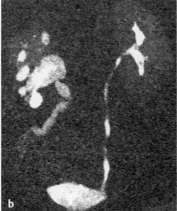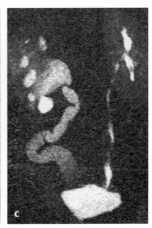

Fig. 5.5a–c   Magnetic resonance urography.

a 3D reconstruction of T2-weighted MRU (e.g., HASTE, RARE, PACE, etc.) for noncontrast imaging of (dilated and urine-filled) pelvicalyceal system (PCS) and right ureter. Of course, other fluid-filled structures (bowel, spinal canal, gallbladder, etc.) are also visualized.

b 3D reconstruction of later phase after Gd administration (T1-weighted GRE, VIBE, etc.) shows variable contrast filling of PCS and ureters.

c 3D GRE after furosemide (same patient as in **b**) now shows fully opacified megaureter with massive hydronephrosis on right side. Left kidney and ureter appear normal.

5

sis [NSF]) can be imaged without contrast medium (**Fig. 5.5a**).

- Limited ability to evaluate renal function and renal parenchyma.
- Inversion recovery (IR) sequences improve detection of scars.
- DWI and BOLD (blood oxygenation level dependent on contrast) as well as MR-spectroscopy widen MR potential.

Dynamic Diuretic Magnetic Resonance Urography (MRU)—Dynamic Functional Magnetic Resonance Renography

Rapid T1-weighted (3D) GRE sequences acquired before, during (serial scans), and after Gd administration to visualize and quantify parenchymal enhancement and dynamics of contrast excretion and drainage (**Fig. 5.5b, c**).

- Arterial and cortical enhancement; may include visualization of renal vessels (MRA)
- Parenchymal phase, excretion (transit time) and accumulation in PCS, drainage into ureter and bladder

- Modern MR technology and software allow quantification of renal function and urinary outflow similar to scintigraphy

Advantages: avoids radiation exposure, yields exquisite information on vessels, parenchyma, PCS, ureters, bladder, excretory dynamics, and surrounding structures ("one-stop shop" imaging).

Disadvantages: somewhat tedious, requires sedation in small children, limited in patients with urolithiasis. Quantification software not commercially available, validation yet restricted.

Computed Tomography of the Child's Urinary Tract

See also Sect. 1.5.

High radiation exposure limits indications for urogenital CT in children.

> CT should not be used for routine stone detection in children!

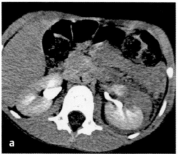

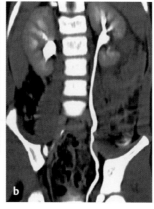

Fig. 5.6a, b Urinary tract CT in (multiply) injured child.
a Axial scan.
b Coronal reformatted image along left ureter, reconstructed late-phase CT with suspected ureteral injury (not confirmed—anterolateral segmental laceration of lower left ureter).

Technique: if indicated (see **"Justification"** in Sect. 1.1); protocol should be adjusted for age/weight.

- Hydration, prevention of contrast-induced nephropathy (creatinine, etc.)

> Normal creatinine values vary with age. Example: normal creatinine for newborns ca. 0.2 mg%. Normal GFR values also adjusted for age.

- X-ray dose: e.g., mAs = (b.w. +5) × 3; kV = 80–120, slice thickness, increment, pitch, kernel, etc. (see also Sect. 1.5)
- Contrast dose (2.5–1 mL/kg; flow rate = 1–2 mL/s) and scan delay (= Vol^{CM}: flow rate × F; $F^{art} = 0.6$; $F^{Pa} = 1.8$; $F^{Py} = 2.5$)—vary with acquisition time and type of equipment (see also Sect. 1.5)

> Avoid multiphase acquisitions.

Indications:
- Severe or multiple injuries (**Fig. 5.6**)
- Complications of various nephro-urologic diseases that cannot be evaluated by other methods
  - e.g., abscess, stone-related pyonephrosis (MRI not available, US inconclusive, etc.)
- Complicated urolithiasis that cannot be adequately assessed by other means
- Tumor diagnosis and staging (if MRI unavailable or inadequate for clinical question)
- CTA for evaluation of vascular pathology (individual timing important)
- Pre-/postoperative imaging in selected cases (if US/VCUG/MRI/scintigraphy not adequate)

> Always precede with detailed US examination. Order CT only if it will have therapeutic implications!

See recommendations of European societies (ESUR and ESPR).

Basic Aspects of Angiography and Interventional Uroradiology

Diagnostic Angiography

Procedure basically the same as in adults.
- Rarely necessary in pediatric age group (AVM, RAS, AVF—with facilities ready for an interventional procedure)

> ! Higher complication risk—small vessels (risk of dissection), ↑ risk of vasospasm, kidney more mobile and elastic parenchymal, higher risk of AVF when large core-biopsy needles used (**Fig. 5.7b**).

Interventions

Interventional procedures such as renal biopsy (**Fig. 5.7a**) guided with US whenever possible (see European recommendations). CT-guided biopsies rare and basically/nearly obsolete (few exceptions exist).
- Percutaneous nephrostomy (PCN): US-guided, supplemented by FL, depending on need/clinical question, e.g., FL for defining ureteral anatomy, fistula, perforation—extravasation
- Use of child-appropriate pulsed FL systems, dose adjusted for body weight
- Mandatory postinterventional follow-up (US including CDS) and monitoring! Liberal use of peri-/postinterventional analgesia/sedation

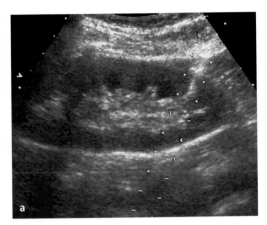

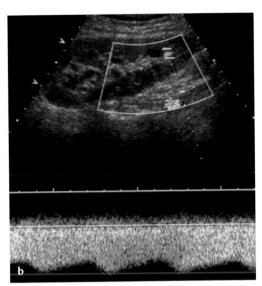

Fig. 5.7a, b US-guided renal biopsy.
a US image during renal biopsy displays proposed biopsy tract (:::::) and needle, which appears as bright
linear echo.
b CDS after procedure reveals postbiopsy arteriovenous
fistula with associated spectral waveforms indicating
arteriovenous shunting.

5.3 Age-Dependent Normal Findings in the Pediatric Urogenital Tract

5

General: the older the child, the more closely normal findings will resemble those in adults. Here
we will consider only relevant differences rarely
touched upon in adults.

Urethra: typical anatomy (VCUG)—do not confuse
physiologic constrictions with valves (**Fig. 5.8**)!
Tightening of pelvic floor during micturition can
mimic anatomical obstruction—essential to have
good image quality and detailed knowledge of
anatomy.

Bladder: capacity varies with age. Rule of thumb:
bladder volume = (age in years) +2 × 30 mL. Normal
bladder wall thickness varies little with age but
does vary with bladder distention—approximate
upper limits are > 2 mm with full bladder, > 4 mm
with empty bladder. Initially increased frequency
and physiologic immaturity—residual urine can be
meaningfully determined and bladder function assessed only after child has learned bladder control;
before that, micturition observed and bladder re-
cord/image kept.

Urachus: may normally be demonstrable during
first weeks of life (**Fig. 5.9**). If it persists → cord, urachal cyst (forms in cord, may become inflamed),
patent duct (weeping umbilicus)—may be diagnos-

able only with full bladder or during micturition
(**VCUG**, ce-VUS).

> ! Caution: (non)neurogenic bladder dysfunction/in-
> fravesical obstruction with increased intravesical pres-
> sure (impairs closure of urachus).

> ! Nodular expansion of bladder roof: normal finding
> at base of urachus. (Do not mistake for bladder wall
> tumor!)

Kidney: normal neonatal parenchymal pattern different from adults. Cortex hyperechoic to liver parenchyma. Other differences: accentuated corticomedullary differentiation, fetal lobulation,
rounded hyperechoic papillae and distal medulla
(= physiologic deposits, formerly called "Tamm–
Horsefall syndrome") (**Fig. 5.2**).

> Persistent/progressive in children with significant co-
> existing problems (dehydration, medication, etc.) →
> papillary calcinosis, nephrolithiasis.

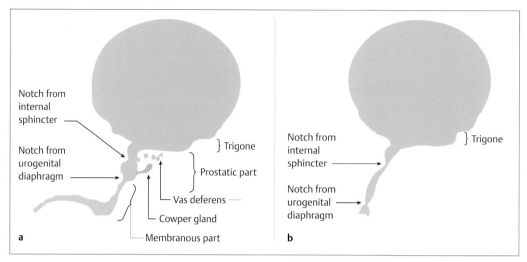

Notch from internal sphincter

Notch from urogenital diaphragm

} Trigone

Prostatic part

Vas deferens

Cowper gland

Membranous part

a

Notch from internal sphincter

Notch from urogenital diaphragm

} Trigone

b

Fig. 5.8a, b Urethral anatomy distinguished from abnormal urethral findings. Typical normal anatomy of male (**a**) and female (**b**) urethra by VCUG, lateral projection → do not mistake physiologic constrictions ("notches") for stenosis, stricture, or valve (e.g., trigone, internal sphincter, pelvic floor, suspensory ligament, etc.).

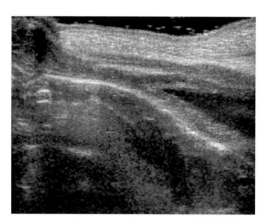

Fig. 5.9 Urachus. Sagittal midline US scan through lower abdomen. Urachal remnant in newborn appears as cordlike structure passing from bladder to umbilicus —may still be normal in newborns.

- PCS: mild distention detectable today by improved imaging capabilities may not have definite pathologic significance (for DD: other US abnormalities such as thickening of renal pelvic wall—extended criteria, see **Table 5.1**)
- Renal size: volumetry—table of normal values for age/weight (see Sect. 5.2)
- Doppler scan: RI values and $V^{systmax}$ vary with age. Initially, RI ↑ (70–80%) and $V^{systmax}$ ↓ (40 cm/s). Both gradually approach adult values (RI earlier than $V^{systmax}$)

Physiologic immaturity during first months of life = decreased contrast excretion and concentration → DMSA, MAG3, IVP, MRU problematic and potentially unrewarding. Use different normal values for creatinine (different muscle mass, etc.—for example, upper normal limit in newborns about 0.4 mg/dL) and for GFR (0.33–0.5 mL/min/1.73 m^2 during first 2 years, about 0.55 mL/min/1.73 m^2 by 3 years of age).

5.4   Inflammatory Urinary Tract Diseases

General: urinary tract infections (UTIs) are subdivided into upper and lower tract. Renal damage and associated long-term effects occur only in upper UTIs (= renal involvement) → imaging focuses increasingly on detection of renal involvement (long-term effects) and risk factors—new imaging algorithm for pediatric UTI (see recommendations of ACR, ESUR, ESPR, etc.).

Be alert in newborns—for equivocal clinical findings, nonspecific symptoms. UTIs may reflect occult urinary tract anomaly → imaging studies ordered more freely (including VCUG in boys) during first year of life.

Risk factors for renal involvement: type of causative organism, treatment (start, duration, and nature); genetic, immunologic, socioeconomic, and habitual factors, bladder dysfunction, urinary tract malformation or dysfunction (including VUR).

UTI diagnosed from laboratory tests (urinalysis, blood count, CRP level)—reliable clinical diagnosis essential = entry criterion for imaging.

Imaging:

- **US:** used to evaluate renal involvement, detect any malformations or signs of complications. Recommended in 24 to 48 hours during first 2 years (full bladder, good hydration)

  US findings: bladder changes = thickened bladder wall, atypical bladder tone, particles floating in the bladder (usually do not settle out), bladder wall hypervascular by (a)CDS or power Doppler. Lax ureter with thickened wall, possible slight dilatation, internal echoes, may show sluggish peristalsis (**Fig. 5.10a**). Kidney: enlarged, altered echo texture (diffusely increased echogenicity, regional or diffuse loss of corticomedullary differentiation, patchy inhomogeneous echo pattern, decreased echogenicity due to incipient necrotizing component), thickened renal peripelvic echo band, echogenic renal pelvis with thickened wall ("urothelial sign"), internal echoes in PCS (**Figs. 5.10b** and **5.11a**). Vascularity may show regional/segmental decrease (power Doppler) or diffuse asymmetrical inhomogeneity (diffuse involvement) (**Fig. 5.10c**; see Case Study 5.1, **Fig. 5.42**)
- **Radiographs, IVP:** not indicated

5

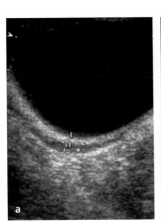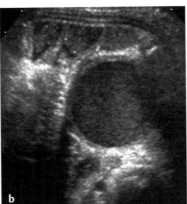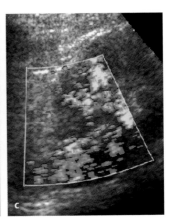

Fig. 5.10a–c   US findings in urinary tract infection (UTI).

a Nondilated, lax distal ureter (++^{1}) with thickened wall (++^{2}) in acute UTI.
b Axial scan shows ballooning of renal pelvis with thickened pelvic wall (urothelial sign) and internal echoes (pyuria due to ureteropelvic junction stenosis).

c Power Doppler shows segmental hypoperfusion in region with increased echogenicity and loss of corticomedullary differentiation due to acute segmental pyelonephritis.

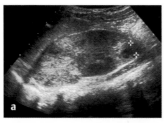
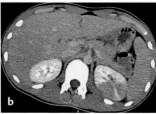
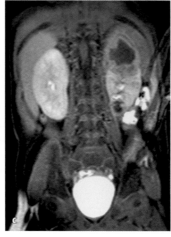

Fig. 5.11a–c Complications of urinary tract infection.
a Multiple hypoechoic zones of liquefaction (one marked ++) in suppurative pyelonephritis.
b Contrast-enhanced CT in suppurative pyelonephritis of left kidney.
c Contrast-enhanced coronal T1-weighted MRI. Fat-saturated sequence shows multiple renal abscesses of left kindney in pyelonephritis.

- **DMSA scintigraphy:** evaluates renal involvement in patients with equivocal US and clinical findings. Renal involvement = (focal) area of decreased tracer uptake. Standard test for evaluating differential kidney function and scarring after UTI (the latter at earliest 3–4 months after UTI)
- **VCUG:** after UTI—indicated in small children with documented renal involvement or US-signs indicating pathology; may be used in every (male) infant with UTI (to assess urethra). Urine should be sterile; optimum timing = 4 to 6 weeks after UTI
- **MRI:** to detect complications (if US equivocal) and complex malformations (**Fig. 5.11c**)
- **CT:** for severe complications and for DD if MRI unavailable (e.g., suspected xanthogranulomatous pyelonephritis [XPN]; **Fig. 5.11b**)

Follow-up after UTI: initial imaging study = US. Use DMSA to detect renal scarring (or MRI). VCUG as defined above.
Complications: pyonephrosis, necrosis, abscess formation, UTI-related lithiasis. Can usually be adequately evaluated with US—MRI another option (**Fig. 5.11a, c**). Pyonephrosis—PCN may be performed under US guidance.
Special forms: XPN, tuberculous pyelonephritis, hemorrhagic cystitis, schistosomiasis (= typical bladder changes), collecting system infection due to obstructive uropathy, candidiasis (most common in immunocompromised patients, preterm infants, antibiotic therapy, megaureter). CT or MRI may be used for DD and confirmation (**Fig. 5.11b, c**).

5.5   Vesicoureteral Reflux

General: retrograde flow of urine from bladder into ureter toward kidney, usually result of congenital ostium immaturity or malformation (= primary congenital VUR). Postnatally not damaging to kidney per se—potential aggravating factor in UTI whereby bacteria ascend from bladder.

Secondary VUR results from bladder dysfunction due to raised intravesicular pressure (decompensation of ostium) or ectopic ureteral insertion (e.g., into diverticula, common with duplex kidney)—anatomic component also present.

Only VUR with recurrent UTIs requires treatment; up to 90% resolve spontaneously. Traditional long-term antibiotic prophylaxis increasingly questioned. Indications for surgical treatment more restrictive—some children with VUR and recurrent UTIs are treated with subureteral injections ("kidney protection," "antibiotic sparing").

Bladder dysfunction—should be specifically looked for, diagnosed, and treated. Essential for healing VUR and preventing postoperative recurrence.

Imaging:

- **VCUG** and **ce-VUS:** see Sect. 5.2 (**Fig. 5.4**)
- **RNC** (direct, indirect): see Sect. 5.2
- **Typical findings:** reflux of contrast medium/radiotracer into ureter and kidney. Standard grading (I–V) and classification systems (high-/low-pressure, uni-/bilateral, primary/secondary, etc.) (**Fig. 5.4**). Conventional VCUG most widely used, recommended in infants and for urethral evaluation (in males). RNC and ce-VUS for follow-up

VCUG should always precede surgery; can define entire ureter (anatomy) and detect any intermittent bladder diverticula (paraostial diverticulum, ostial diverticulum, Hudge diverticulum; Case Study 5.2, **Fig. 5.43f**). US without contrast medium can detect only indirect VUR signs (lateralized/gaping ostium, atypical course of distal ureter, bladder trabeculation, urotehlila sign, changing PCS distention, etc.). Direct detection by CDS is rare.

- **DMSA scintigraphy:** used after VUR diagnosis to evaluate renal function, detect scarring, or dysplasia.

5.6 Congenital Hydronephrosis

General: routine prenatal US screening often detects dilatation of PCS. The term "hydronephrosis" (HN) dates from time when any detectable fetal PCS was considered evidence of urinary tract obstruction. Modern high-resolution US may show physiologic cavities, so low-grade HN is no longer considered pathologic in all cases.

Fetal HN is usually associated with obstructive uropathy (megaureter [MU], ureterovesical junction stenosis [UPJS]) or VUR (especially high-grade), alternatives are megacalycosis, ampullary renal pelvis (RP). DD = mainly includes renal cysts, multicystic dysplasia (MCD), hypoechoic medullary pyramids.

Imaging:

- **US:** initial imaging study. Timing depends on fetal grade of severity—high-grade bilateral HN in males should be investigated on first day of life. Moderate to low-grade unilateral HN should be investigated no earlier than 1 week. Scans obtained before and after voiding should cover whole urinary tract.

  US findings: variable dilatation of PCS (±ureters). Standard grading system takes into account shape of calyces and parenchymal thickness (HN grades I–IV, **Table 5.2**). Adequate renal function and hydration essential (see recommendations of ESUR and ESPR—Grading of Hydronephrosis)

Table 5.2 Ultrasound grading of hydronephrosis. (Adapted from fetal grading HN I–IV [V] according to Riccabona et al. 2008)

HN 0	No pelvicalyceal system visible
HN I	Renal pelvis visible, but with small axial diameter
HN II	Renal pelvis and calyces visible, normal shape of fornix and papillae
HN III	Calyces dilated, fornices rounded, papillae flattened, no parenchymal thinning
HN IV	Gross dilatation of calyces, fornices rounded, papillae flattened, with parenchymal thinning
HN V	Used in some places to denote massive dilatation of pelvicalyceal system with only thin residual rim of renal parenchyma (extreme HN IV)

Dilatation depends on hydration, bladder distention, and position (supine/prone imaging yield different values!). Kidneys evaluated not only for axial PCS width in millimeters but other criteria as well (see extended US criteria, **Table 5.1**). Standardized measurements are essential (see **Figs. 5.2** and **5.12**).

5

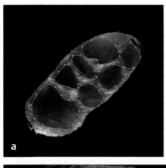

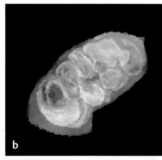

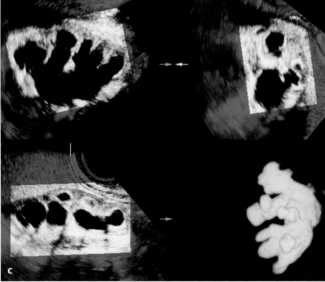

Fig. 5.12a–c   3D US of hydronephrosis and ureteropelvic junction stenosis. 3D US options for determining renal parenchymal volume and surveying dilated pelvicalyceal system (PCS).
a Semiautomated calyceal segmentation. Rendered image.
b Parenchyma (reduction) minus calyces (whitish).
c Multiaxial and rendered views of dilated PCS (different patient).

- **Other imaging studies:** VCUG, scintigraphy, MRU, depending on presumptive diagnosis and grade of PCS dilatation

> IVP no longer used in investigating HN. Every detectable mild "collecting system dilatation" does not justify trouble and expense of further imaging studies.

Follow-ups—primarily US with good hydration (see ESUR and ESPR recommendations—Postnatal Imaging in Fetal Hydronephrosis). Findings dictate need for further tests.

Obstructive Uropathy

Definition: urinary outflow obstruction by some sort of stenosis. Anatomic sites of predilection = ureteropelvic junction, ureterovesical junction, urethra.

Clinical definition: any type of outflow obstruction that jeopardizes renal function and renal growth potential. Dilatation alone, with normal function, is not an indication for treatment ("urinary tract cosmetics"). Currently, however, there is no imaging study that can provide definitive assessment and prognosis—we cannot predict which children will need surgery → underscores importance of follow-up under standardized and comparable conditions.

Ureteropelvic Junction Stenosis

Definition: stenosis at junction of upper ureter and renal pelvis. Causes urine retention in kidney with PCS dilation—unlike acute obstruction, often causes greater expansion of extrarenal RP (very compliant in neonates = *windkessel* effect), so degree of dilatation does not necessarily correlate with degree of obstruction.

> In some cases, decreasing dilation over time does not signal improvement but deterioration with decline in urine volume due to impaired renal function. Conversely, persistent dilatation may signify well-functioning kidney with good urine production. Dilatation does not equal obstruction!

Imaging: goal = prompt identification of patients who will benefit from surgery helps to assess infection and monitor for possible decompensation of obstruction.

- **US:** standard measurements (parenchyma and PCS) and regular follow-ups with good hydration—comparable body position and scan planes essential. Difficult to measure and compare relative renal parenchymal volumes between sides with 2D US. Volumetry based on 3D US yields

values comparable to scintigraphy (**Fig. 5.12**). CDS essential (atypical vascular anatomy, e.g., accessory renal artery or lower pole artery crossing ureteropelvic junction). Possible association with UPJS = important preoperative information (**Fig. 5.13a**).

> Evaluate renal parenchyma (thinning? intact corticomedullary differentiation? increasing parenchymal echogenicity?), PCS (ureteropelvic junction, shape of calyces, etc.), and perfusion (asymmetric RI in acute decompensation; progressive, diffuse decrease in vascularity by power Doppler due to chronic parenchymal damage; **Fig. 5.13b, c**).

- **IVP:** original gold-standard, no longer used today, to investigate UPJS; superseded by scintigraphy and MRU. Lasix diuretic IVP may be done in selected cases for preoperative anatomic visualization (e.g., if no MRI available, one or two

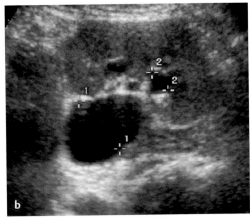

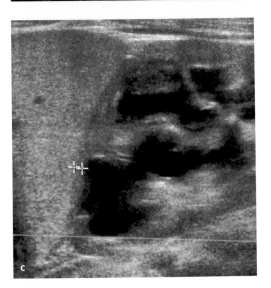

Fig. 5.13a–c   US findings in hydronephrosis and ureteropelvic junction stenosis (UPJS).
a CDS in UPJS—accessory renal artery crossing UPJ.
b Standardized axial measurements (++) in 2D US—dilated pelvis, only mildly dilated calices.
c Narrowest site in thinned renal parenchyma (++) in grade IV hydronephrosis.

5

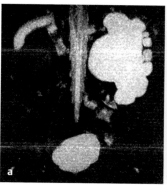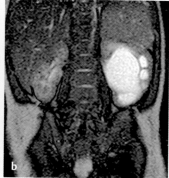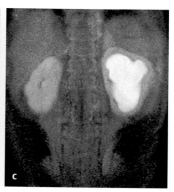

Fig. 5.14a–c   Standard MRU capabilities in ureteropelvic junction stenosis.

a, b Gross hydronephrosis of left kidney due to UPJS in 4-month-old infant. T2-weighted MRU (HASTE) as 3D reconstruction (**a**) and single coronal image (SSFP) (**b**).

c Late T1-weighted image after Gd and furosemide administration (single coronal slab) shows dilated left pelvicalyceal system with opacified urine. Parenchyma shows symmetrical enhancement but definite thinning.

well-timed images sufficient) or postoperative investigation of suspected recurrent or residual stenosis (done in some places as functional pyelography with decompression catheter)

- **Scintigraphy:** dynamic MAG3 scintigraphy with furosemide-induced diuresis. Various protocols in use. Scintigraphy can evaluate relative renal perfusion and function (including excretion) and outflow dynamics (normal, dilated and nonobstructive, partially obstructive, complete/decompensate obstruction = O'Reilly grades I–IV)
  Decompensated obstruction and partial obstruction with asymmetric or deteriorating partial renal function = indication for surgery
- **MRU:** static MR-urogram for anatomic evaluation (complex malformation, preoperative, DD: see Sect. 1.6 and Sect. 5.2). Dynamic functional MRU currently practiced at just few centers—will become standard method for evaluating anatomy and function ("one-stop shop imaging," will probably replace MAG3—see Sections 1.6 and 5.2; **Figs. 5.5** and **5.14**)
- **PCN:** today used only occasionally for pyonephrosis unresponsive to conservative treatment or high-grade bilateral UPJS and elevated renal markers/global renal function impairment (bridging measure till surgery)
- **Follow-ups:** primary study = US. PCS width measurements of limited value! With equivocal

findings/deterioration → dynamic scintigraphy. "Short IVP"/MRU may be used postoperatively (see recommendations of ESUR, ESPR, Working Group for Pediatric Nephrology, etc.).

Ureterovesical Junction Stenosis—Primary Obstructive Megaureter

General: ureterovesical junction obstruction (causing megaureter [MU]) is common in patients with thickened bladder wall (e.g., posterior urethral valve [PUV]) or duplex kidney (ureteral orifice too low = MU opens close to bladder neck). Or, primary dysplasia and dysperistalsis of a ureteral segment → dilation and obstruction (= primary obstructive megaureter). MU may occur in severe VUR or as mixed obstructive and reflexive form. Degree of intrarenal dilatation highly variable—from minimal to massive. Latter occurs with high-grade or secondary upper obstruction at ureteropelvic junction (kinking) with secondary UPJS or in upper moiety of duplex kidney (usually with dysplastic tissue, volume overload due to polyuria from dysplastic upper system).

Imaging:
- **US:** defines lower part of MU and any associated ureterocele (orthotopic/ectopic, single/duplex system), permits evaluation of peristalsis (can be documented by B-mode US; **Fig. 5.15**)

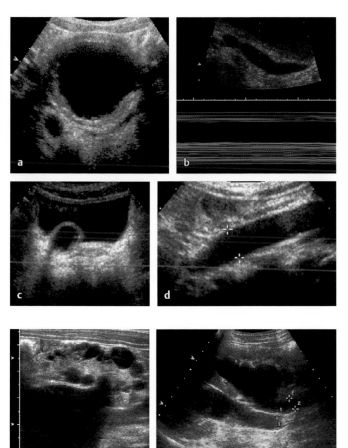

Fig. 5.15a–d US findings in megaureter (MU): evaluation by US of all relevant aspects.
a Bladder and thickened bladder wall, with MU imaged in cross-section.
b Longitudinal scan through distal atonic MU with M-mode assessment and documentation of peristalsis.
c Ureterovesical junction region with apparent uterocele.
d Midportion of MU (++).

Fig. 5.16a, b Possible US renal findings associated with megaureter.
a Pronounced MU with cystic dysplasia of renal parenchyma.
b Duplex kidney with two MU, one arising from upper system (++^{1}) and the other from dilated lower pelvicalyceal system (++^{2}) with apparent loop (kinking? secondary proximal stenosis?).

5

Specifically evaluate ureteropelvic junction, degree of intrarenal dilatation, and renal parenchyma (signs of dysplasia?) (**Fig. 5.16**).

- **IVP:** preoperative imaging option in highly selected cases (a well-timed delayed image with stimulated diuresis, usually sufficient) if no MR available
- **MRI(U):** both techniques are used and may suffice for anatomic preoperative imaging
- **MRU:** has replaced IVP and complicated anatomy indicates additional sectional imaging (complex relationships, atypical ureteral orifice, etc.) (**Fig. 5.5**; see Case Study 5.2, **Fig. 5.43**).
- **Scintigraphy:** DMSA—for renal function assessment, especially in duplex systems. Another option is MRU. Dynamic scintigraphy can quantify outflow dynamics and ureteral peristalsis

Helpful for evaluating patency of bladder catheter (not balloon-type!).

- **VCUG:** differentiate refluxive from obstructive forms
- **PCN:** for pyoureter/pyonephrosis that cannot be treated conservatively

Treatment and course: most cases managed conservatively with regular US follow-ups and intermittent MRU/scintigraphic follow-up. Prerequisite for primary reimplantation = good ureteral peristalsis, adequate (partial) renal function (> 10%). Otherwise ureterocutaneostomy—give ureter time to recover, acquire better tone. Ureter reimplanted after prolonged closure of stoma. May precede surgery with stoma catheterization and antegrade ureterography (FL).

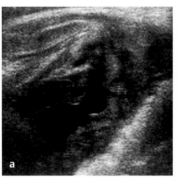
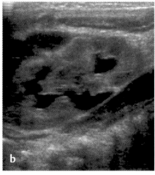

Fig. 5.17a, b   US in posterior urethral valve.
a Perineal US shows typical valvular configuration of posterior urethra with thickened, trabeculated bladder wall.
b Longitudinal scan of right kidney shows hydronephrosis and perirenal fluid collection (urinoma after forniceal rupture). Renal parenchyma slightly hyperechoic and dysplastic, lacks typical differentiation.

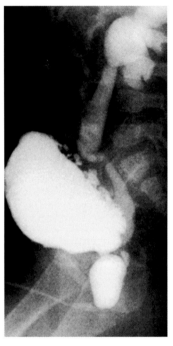

Fig. 5.18   VCUG in posterior urethral valve.
Lateral projection during attempted voiding shows valve-like configuration of posterior urethra, trabeculation with pseudodiverticulum, and high-grade vesicoureteral reflux.

Infravesical Obstruction

General: posterior urethral valve (PUV) most frequent cause of obstruction. Other causes: urethral hypoplasia (prune belly syndrome), partial/other valvular anomalies, double urethra, functional (e.g., MMC with neurogenic bladder dysfunction). Early treatment necessary to prevent potentially disastrous UTI/bladder decompensation. Usually, prenatal abnormalities found. Common findings: primary renal parenchymal dysplasia (intrauterine high-pressure VUR and renal maldevelopment—essential for further prognosis) and congenital reflux nephropathy (cRNP).

Imaging:

- **US:** prenatal scans may show megacystis, wall thickening, open bladder neck, urine ascites, oligohydramnios. Early postnatal US, including transperineal scans, should be done in first 24 hours. Typical US findings = widely open bladder neck, trabeculated bladder, wall thickening, and residual urine; also possible: dilatation of PCS and ureter (uni-/bilateral), renal dysplasia, urinoma, persistent urachus (**Fig. 5.17**). Perineal US (during voiding) will directly demonstrate valve, penile scanning may show other urethral anatomic changes.

> Infravesical obstruction not always associated with VUR or MU/HN/upper tract dilatation. With bladder wall thickening, dilatation of upper system may be obstructive (ureterovesical stenosis).

- **VCUG:** mandatory study using transurethral or suprapubic approach to confirm diagnosis (**Fig. 5.18**). Obtain lateral image during attempted voiding. Leave catheter in place to establish drainage!
- **Scintigraphy:** DMSA to evaluate (residual) renal function—delay after 4 to 6 weeks
- **MRU:** only in highly selected cases with complex changes or coexisting malformations of upper urinary tract
- **PCN:** only temporary measure in patients with high-grade bilateral upper obstruction not relieved by catheterization/vesicostomy

Duplex Kidney

General and etiology: see Embryology. Duplication may be unilateral or bilateral.

Definition: one kidney having two separate, fully formed pelvicalyceal systems. Different degrees recognized with double ureters (complete duplication) or bifid ureters, or bifid intrarenal system with septated renal pelvis and one ureter (partial duplication). Complete duplication associated with upper system obstruction (distal stenosis, ureterocele, MU); may be accompanied by dysplasia of upper parenchyma, and VUR into lower system (dysfunctional ostium in high lateralized position, possible cRNP/dysplasia).

> Duplex kidneys do not always have pathological significance. Forms not associated with urinary obstruction or parenchymal dysplasia considered a variant.

Imaging:
- **US:** central parenchymal band, interruption of central echo complex (**Fig. 5.19**). Kidney enlarged, may have notched outline at junction of upper and lower systems. Dysplasia = parenchymal structural abnormalities, potentially also associated with UTI disproportionate dilation of upper versus lower PCS. Two renal pelves, ureters, ostia (two ureteral jets at different sites). Possible accessory renal vascular pedicle.
  Meyer–Weigert rule: upper system is obstructive and drains distally, lower system is refluxive and drains into upper and lateralized ostium.

> Accessory renal vessels are not necessarily associated with duplication, and not every duplication has an accessory vascular pedicle.

- **VCUG:** with VUR in lower moiety—VCUG indicated only in patients with clinical symptoms or complex urinary tract anomaly. Possible bifid ureter with reflux into both moieties (**Fig. 5.20**)

> Not every (asymptomatic) duplex kidney does require investigation by VCUG.

- **IVP:** former gold standard for documenting duplex system and both ureters with mandatory postvoid images. No longer practiced today (availability of MRU, no treatment implications, hypofunction of one moiety due to reflux nephropathy [RNP]/dysplasia/high-grade obstruction with poor depictability, etc.)

5

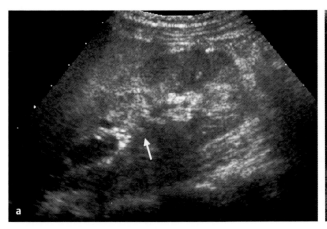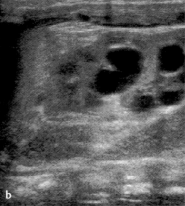

Fig. 5.19a, b   US appearance of duplex kidney.

a Central parenchymal band (↑) of duplex kidney with disproportionately large upper pelvicalyceal system. Parenchyma of upper moiety slightly thinner and less distinct due to obstructive dysplasia (Meyer–Weigert rule).

b Disproportionate dilatation of lower pelvicalyceal system in duplex kidney due to high-grade vesicoureteral reflux.

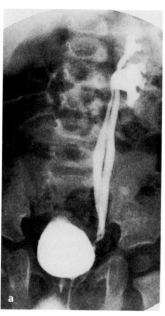
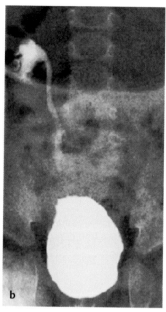

Fig. 5.20a, b   VCUG of duplex kidney. Patient had duplex kidney (detected by US) and recurrent febrile urinary tract infections. VCUG shows refluxing bifid ureter on left side, whose segments join at low level (**a**), and grade III vesicoureteral reflux into lower system of right duplex kidney (Meyer–Weigert rule) (**b**). In panel **b**, note absence of opacification of upper calyceal group and lily-like sag of pelvicalyceal system as indirect evidence of duplex kidney on VCUG.

- **Scintigraphy:** tracer uptake in parenchyma and tracer excretion depend on degree of dysplasia and associated urinary obstruction, with corresponding discrepancy between upper and lower systems. Scintigraphy allows discriminatory evaluation of outflow dynamics in obstructive systems with determination of relative functional status of upper and lower systems. Anatomical correlation (e.g., with US) essential for interpretation
- **CT:** not used for this indication—obsolete
- **MRI:** modality of choice, permits anatomical and functional evaluation of complex double systems (e.g., suspected ectopic ureter insertion). Diuretic T2-weighted MRU allows detailed evaluation of outflow system and will detect any (cystic) parenchymal dysplasia. Contrast-enhanced dynamic sequence = evaluation of renal parenchyma, excretion, and outflow (**Fig. 5.21**). Allows for quantitative renal function assessment/determination of relative function of both moieties by modern methods

DD: prominent Bertin column, infundibular stenosis, regional megacalycosis/calyceal anomaly, blunted calyces, triple or quadruple kidney, (extrarenal) cysts (e.g., at upper pole = suprarenal cyst)

Ectopia

General: ectopic kidney, ectopic ureteral insertion, ectopic urethra. In broadest sense, ectopia includes forms of hypospadias. Higher grades of ureteral ectopia often associated with gross abnormalities of renal development.

Renal Ectopia

Ectopic kidney may be intra-abdominal or intrathoracic, always associated with atypical PCS (megacalycosis—dilatation ≠ obstruction). Malrotation is usually present.

Inability to find kidney in renal bed at US → detailed imaging search from retrovesical area to lower thorax (US; other options are MRI or DMSA scintigraphy—the latter in prone position with open bladder catheter). May be only cystic-dysplastic ectopic remnant with minimal residual function (= silent on scintigraphy) (**Fig. 5.22a**). Patient may still be symptomatic, however (e.g., dribbling due to ectopic ureteral insertion into vagina). Ectopic kidney often associated with hypodysplasia and atypical multivessel supply and dysplastic PCS. Horseshoe kidney = both kidneys fused together; one part may be ectopic or malrotated (= crossed ectopia).

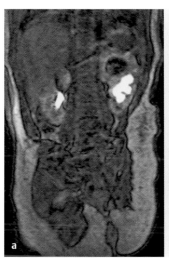
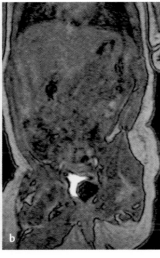

Fig. 5.21a, b Dynamic contrast-enhanced MRU of duplex kidney.
a Image shows enhancement of right and lower pelvicalyceal system of left duplex kidney. Upper left moiety shows faint, minimal enhancement.
b Bladder filled with opacified urine except for cystlike filling defect on left side = ureterocele draining left upper moiety via megaureter, still without contrast due to delayed excretion and slower urine flow.

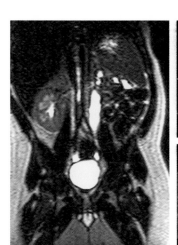
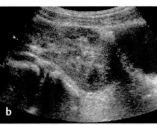
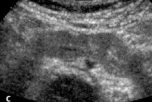

Fig. 5.22a–c US and MRI of renal variants (single kidney, ectopia, horseshoe kidney, etc.).
a MR investigation of single kidney suggested by US. Coronal T2-weighted MRU (SSFP) shows large, functioning single right kidney and flaccid, unusually large proximal left megaureter. Left kidney appears as small remnant with cystic dysplasia.
b Longitudinal midabdominal scan in midline shows malrotated ectopic kidney with atypical configuration occupying prevertebral location in pelvis. Kidney extends to roof of distended bladder.
c Axial midabdominal US scan shows horseshoe kidney with prevertebral parenchymal isthmus between medially displaced lower poles.

5

Horseshoe kidneys are at risk for injury to prevertebral isthmus (**Fig. 5.22c**). Possible ureteral obstruction at level of isthmus—always make detailed search for isthmus or document normal position and contours of lower renal pole in all planes.

tures (seminal vesicle, vagina, etc.). Associated renal segment is usually dysplastic. Detailed search for ureteral insertion is often time-consuming → high-resolution US with full bladder including transperineal scans, VCUG, (US) genitography, high-resolution MRI, endoscopy.

Ureteral Ectopia

Atypical course/insertion of ectopic ureter, e.g., retrocaval (leading to obstruction). Intravesical ectopia = ureter inserts too low (at bladder neck); or may open into posterior urethra or genital struc-

Hypospadias

Even in severe forms, hypospadias are not usually an indication for urethral imaging. Imaging may be done for postoperative complications (stenosis, fistula, etc.). Severe forms of hypospadias or ectopic urethra → high-resolution detailed US of upper urinary tract (associated or secondary changes). US findings may warrant further imaging studies.

Single Kidney

Failure of one kidney to form. In some cases, kidney may shrink in utero, becomes nonfunctional and not detectable postnatally, owing to underlying malformation (e.g., ureteral atresia, vascular event, high-grade obstruction, shrunken multicystic dysplastic kidney, etc.). Possible associated VUR into ureteral stump. Higher incidence of VUR into contralateral single kidney that has undergone compensatory hypertrophy. Ipsilateral genital malformations (Wunderlich syndrome).

> Prenatal/neonatal diagnosis of single kidney warrants early, detailed evaluation of internal genitalia, especially in girls (double uterus, uterus didelphys with an atretic hemivagina, etc.) (see Case Study 5.3, **Fig. 5.44**).

Imaging:

- **US:** presence of solitary, enlarged kidney (accurate volumetry!) with absence of contralateral kidney. Associated genital anomalies?
- **VCUG:** may show VUR into ipsilateral/contralateral ureter. Indication for VCUG without therapeutic implications is questionable. Possible alternative: RNC or ce-VUS/US-genitography
- **IVP/CT:** obsolete
- **DMSA scintigraphy:** can detect possible ectopic renal remnants, confirm parenchymal function (evidence of dysplasia?). Procedure requires adequate level of residual function
- **MRU:** can evaluate internal genitalia, screen for ectopic renal remnant (**Fig. 5.22a**); use high resolution (isotropic 3D) sequences

Bladder Exstrophy

Most severe malformation, associated with changes in lesser pelvis and pelvic skeleton. Imaging indicated for upper urinary tract (associated dysplasia, other malformations) and pelvic skeleton (for planning reconstructive measures in selected cases); should be reserved for specialized centers.

5.8   Urolithiasis and Nephrocalcinosis _____

General:

- **Urolithiasis** = stone/conglomerate in kidney or ureter with/without obstruction. Relatively rare in children, especially in Western countries. Association with predisposing factors such as hypercalciuria, oxaluria, cystinuria, diet. May be secondary to UTI and inflammation, drug therapy, or systemic diseases (CF, long-term intensive care, especially in newborns)
- **Nephrocalcinosis** (NC) = calcium deposition in renal parenchyma. May occur in renal parenchymal diseases (e.g., distal renal tubular acidosis [dRTA]), may be secondary to overdosage, abnormal parathormone levels, etc.
  - **Types of NC:** medullary, cortical, global. Three medullary stages distinguished by US

DD: urolithiasis (secondary?), regional papillary medullary calcification (e.g., after papillary necrosis, segmental medullary sponge kidney, hyperuricemia, prepapillary tubular deposits during/after furosemide therapy and intensive care), physiologic hyperechoic medullary pyramids in newborns.

Clinical features: urolithiasis—typical = colic and hematuria. Atypical symptoms may occur in small children, e.g., during gradual formation of large bladder stones (then think of metabolic disorders such as cystinosis).

NC—often asymptomatic initially, depending on underlying disease/complications.

Imaging—urolithiasis:

- **US:** initial study, usually diagnostic. Requires full bladder → scan distal ureter, make detailed search for (more or less) echogenic structure in urinary tract including papillae and medullae. Definite calcification = acoustic shadow. CDS = twinkling artifact (between closely spaced, highly reflective interfaces; **Fig. 5.23**)

> Not every stone casts acoustic shadow! Every stone does not twinkle, and not everything that twinkles is a stone (DD: air bubble, uncalcified papillary-medullary deposit, renal or pelvic wall calcification).

Acute obstruction = swollen kidney, hyperechoic parenchyma, remarkably little dilatation of intrarenal collecting system (including renal pelvis; if dilated = chronic/recurring, may be related to infection or malformation). (Mild) ureteral dilatation, possible internal echoes. CDS (ureteral jet) = asymmetric ureteral inflow into bladder. DDS: RI ↑ in affected kidney, asymmetric. Stones (especially bladder stones) move with position changes (distinguishes them from [intra-]mural calcifications)

- **Plain radiography:** large opacities of variable density projected over urinary tract. Slight calcification difficult/impossible to detect. X-ray localization sometimes useful for planning lithotripsy and other treatments (**Fig. 5.24a**)
- **IVP:** rarely necessary today for routine testing. May be used in cases with high clinical suspicion not adequately evaluated by US, where therapeutic implications exist

> Good image timing = fewer images needed. Two to three IVP images are often sufficient.

- **CT:** used very rarely and reluctantly in children. May offer problem-solving method for selected complicated cases or preoperative planning (percutaneous litholapraxy, **Fig. 5.24b**)

> Always adjust CT protocols for children. If dose too low → small, poorly calcified stones may be missed.

- **MRI:** currently used only on limited basis

5

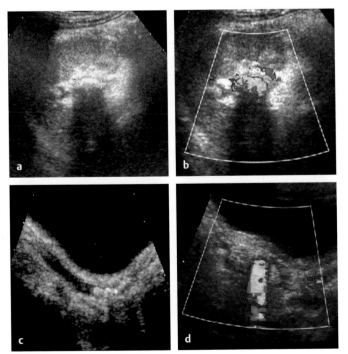

Fig. 5.23a–d US findings in urolithiasis.

a Staghorn calculus in renal pelvis with acoustic shadow (++). Kidney swollen and hyperechoic with hazy echo pattern.

b Prominent twinkling artifact on CDS.

c, d Distal ureteral stone with small acoustic shadow—can be imaged only through well-distended bladder. CDS again shows marked twinkling artifact.

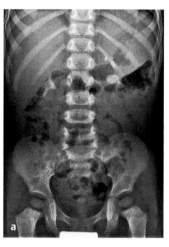

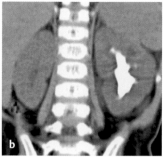

Fig. 5.24a, b   Radiographic and CT findings in urolithiasis.

a Plain abdominal radiograph shows bilateral renal pelvic stones (same patient as in **Fig. 5.23**), defines true extent better than US.

b Coronal image reformatted from unenhanced CT aids in planning lithotripsy for staghorn calculus in renal pelvis.

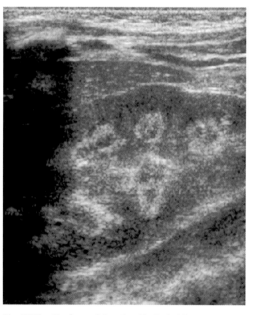

Fig. 5.25   Nephrocalcinosis. Typical US appearance with hyperechoic corticomedullary junction in infant with grade I–II medullary nephrocalcinosis.

Imaging—nephrocalcinosis:

- **US:** initial, adequate study. Shows echogenic corticomedullary junction in early phase (stage I), followed by increasing medullary echogenicity of medullary NC (stage II) (**Fig. 5.25**) and increasing calcification of renal cortex (stage III = global NC) → PCS cannot be evaluated at this stage. Deeper renal areas and possible stones at those sites difficult/impossible to detect with US. Staghorn calculus more difficult to distinguish (typical = normal-appearing papilla/medulla, sound stops at echogenic renal pelvic wall, does not penetrate into deeper renal areas due to acoustic shadowing)
- **Plain radiography/CT:** incidental finding. CT indicated in selected cases with pronounced calcification/equivocal obstructing stones, where therapeutic implications exist
- **MRU:** may find greater utilization in the future

5.9 (Poly)cystic Kidney Diseases and Nephropathies

Cystic Kidney Diseases

General: many cystic kidney diseases have genetic/familial/hereditary etiology. Renal cysts may also be acquired (postinflammatory, posttraumatic, dysfunctional, dysplasia-associated in obstructive uropathy/polyneuropathy [PNP], neoplastic). Necessary imaging depends on underlying cause and entity.

> Every renal cyst in children, including "simple" cysts, should at least be monitored. Enlargement or other changes warrant further investigation and detailed family history, as they often signify other (polycystic, renal, syndromic) disease.

Classification of cysts: simple/complicated, single/multiple, congenital/acquired, familiar and genetic/nonhereditary. Signs of complications: thick, irregular walls/outlines, size > 3 cm, internal septa, internal echoes/sedimentation, solid elements, aggregated cysts, mass effect, calcifications, hyperperfused areas in cyst walls. Family history compulsory for proper classification.

> The system for grading cysts basically follows adult model (Bosniak classification)—applicable to US (except for enhancement pattern), CT, and MRI.

Imaging:
- **US:** shows echo-free lesion with smooth margins (simple cyst), provides anatomical localization (medullary, cortical, parapelvic, exophytic, etc.)—helpful for classifying entities (**Fig. 5.26**). CDS can differentiate cysts from vascular ectasia (use adequate Doppler angle!) and from hypoechoic medullary pyramids or nodular masses based on posterior acoustic enhancement and bright peripheral echo. Further details depend on specific entity (see below)

5

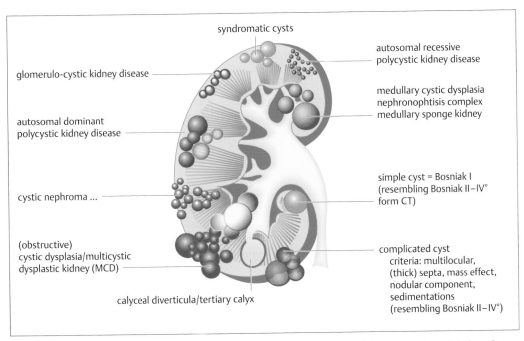

Fig. 5.26 Diagrammatic representation of renal cysts. Renal cysts can be differentiated by their typical arrangement, size, configuration, location, and appearance. Autosomal recessive polycystic kidney disease (ARPKD), autosomal dominant polycystic kidney disease (ADPKD). DD also includes aneurysms, lymphoceles, etc. (After Riccabona 2008 and Avni et al. 2012, adapted from Morcos SK.)

- **VCUG:** may be used to investigate renal cystic dysplasia, with corresponding therapeutic implications
- **IVP/CT:** obsolete. Exception: CT investigation of complicated cyst (suspected tumor, unexplained inflammatory process and MRI not available). Use child-appropriate protocols. Usually no need for multiphase CT (except to distinguish calyceal diverticulum from urinoma)
- **DMSA scintigraphy:** used to assess relative renal function in selected cases
- **MRI:** exquisite study, excellent for defining small cysts with heavy T2 contrast. DD of complicated cysts (fat-saturated sequence, dynamic, and contrast-enhanced). Delayed images acquired easily and without risk. MRI allows follow-up of multi-/polycystic kidney disease without radiation exposure—likely to assume greater role as treatment options for cysts (enzyme therapy, etc.) become available (detailed quantification, assessment of treatment response, etc.)

Important Entities

Simple Renal Cyst

US shows isolated, well-circumscribed, echo-free cyst with posterior acoustic enhancement and no wall or wall thickening—less common in children (**Fig. 5.27a**).

Dysplastic Cyst

Morphology = simple cyst of variable size, often associated with regional parenchymal dysplasia (atypical corticomedullary differentiation; **US** shows hazy parenchymal structure with increased echogenicity). Regional, segmental, diffuse—number and size of cysts do not always correlate with degree of dysplasia (**Fig. 5.27b**).

Associated with syndromes, familial/genetic/hereditary occurrence, obstructive uropathy.

Usually diagnosed by US. Scintigraphy/MRI may be used to evaluate (residual) renal function.

DD: other types of cyst. Exophytic mass of aggregated cysts = lymphangioma, (very rare). Hemorrhagic complicated cyst—think of cystic Wilms tumor.

Functional Cyst

(US) morphology = dysplastic/simple cyst. Often develops in chronic nephropathy/renal failure

(during dialysis, after transplantation, etc.). May grow in size, rarely undergoes malignant transformation → follow-up (US, possibly MRI).

Autosomal Dominant Polycystic Kidney Disease (ADPKD)

Hereditary renal disease usually characterized by multiple macrocysts. Rare in newborns, often manifested in children/young adults. Starts with appearance of individual regional cysts/dysplastic areas. Progression of disease → chronic renal failure. Associated with extrarenal cysts (liver, spleen, pancreas, etc.) and vascular changes (aneurysms, etc.).

Imaging: primary study = US. MRI used in selected cases (equivocal findings, DD: cystic mass).

> Check for extrarenal manifestations. Conduct regular follow-up. With asymmetric involvement, scintigraphy may be used to assess relative renal function.

Autosomal Recessive Polycystic Kidney Disease (ARPKD)

Often manifested in newborns; characterized by multiple microcysts and progressive renal insufficiency → early renal failure. Extrarenal manifestation = hepatic fibrosis of variable degree. (Hepatic fibrosis may be main presenting symptom in some cases).

Imaging: typical "salt-and-pepper" appearance of kidney at US—globular swelling with atypical, inhomogeneous parenchymal pattern (tiny microcysts, often too small to resolve, especially initially; **Fig. 5.27c**). Periportal fibrosis may be difficult to diagnose with US → MRI—used also for follow-up.

Medullary Sponge Kidney—Medullary Cystic Dysplasia

MSK = familial-hereditary cystic ectasia of renal tubules leading to urinary retention and stone formation/calcification. Unilateral, bilateral, diffuse, segmental. Usually diagnosed from secondary phenomena—urolithiasis, calcifications (in abdomen plain film), detected incidentally, familial examination for known risk.

Imaging:
- **US:** shows only advanced changes with significant irregular tubular ectasia and calcifications/deposits in medullary pyramids. Later stages may be indistinguishable from NC

- **CT:** not indicated despite typical findings of medullary precipitate
- **IVP:** can diagnose early stages based on stasis of contrast medium in ectatic tubules
- **MRU:** less sensitive to small calcifications, limited resolution—not used at present

Medullary Cystic Kidney Disease and Nephronophtisis Complex, Glomerulocystic Renal Dysplasia

Rare hereditary conditions, usually characterized by microcystic changes and progressive renal failure.

Multicystic Renal Dysplasia

End stage of severe renal dysplasia, usually associated with ureteral atresia—multiple cysts of variable size permeate parenchyma. Possible residual function (DMSA, MR, US, and CDS). Associated with ipsilateral genital anomalies. Cysts may regress spontaneously or may grow → mass effects.

Complications: inflammation, mass, rupture, hypertension, malignant transformation—latter controversial.

Imaging:

- **US:** many peripheral cysts of varying size. Scans may show small central area of residual parenchyma and residual signs of previous ballooning of obstructed PCS (**Fig. 5.28**)
- **Plain radiography:** sometimes detected incidentally on plain films (peripheral balloon-shaped calcifications projected over renal bed)
- **VCUG:** role increasingly questioned in diagnosis of MSK
- **CT:** not indicated
- **DMSA:** to evaluate possible residual function

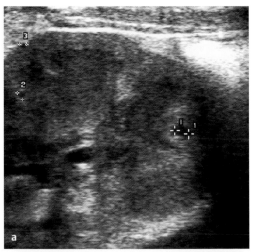

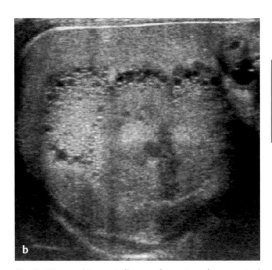

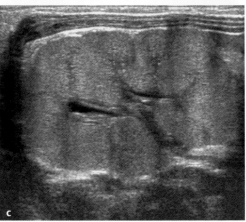

Fig. 5.27a–c (Neonatal) renal cysts, documented with high-resolution linear probe.
a, b Syndromic (**a**) and dysplastic (**b**) simple cysts (++).
c US in newborn with autosomal recessive polycystic kidney disease shows enlarged, hyperechoic kidney with loss of corticomedullary differentiation. Microcysts too small to be individually resolved ("salt-and-pepper kidney").

5

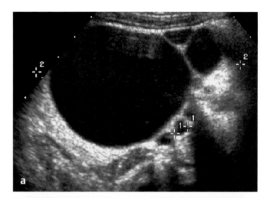

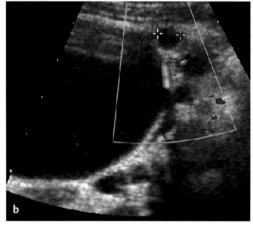

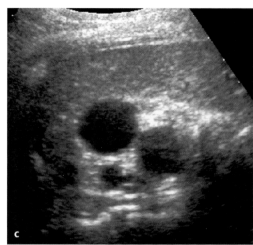

Fig. 5.28a–c Multicystic dysplasia (MCD).
a Typical US appearance. Longitudinal right flank scan shows large neonatal MCD with noncommunicating cysts of varying size and residual dysplastic renal parenchyma with predominantly central location.
b CDS shows residual septal vascularity.
c Spontaneous regression of MCD on follow-up (axial US). Cysts ↓, hyperechoic residual parenchyma still detected.

■ **MRU**: to evaluate associated genital tract anomalies, contralateral kidney, and residual parenchyma. Used also to investigate complications and for DD of equivocal findings

> Especially, residual function/perfusion in multicystic renal dysplasia requires US follow-up, owing to greater potential for complications. At some centers, persistent dysplasia that does not shrink over time is treated by early nephrectomy.

Syndromic Cysts

Many syndromic conditions include renal cysts/dysplasia → make targeted search for other syndromic changes (e.g., tuberous sclerosis [TS], von Hippel–Lindau disease, chromosome abnormality), especially in children with unexplained bilateral cysts or cysts in other organs.
Imaging: US morphology variable, ranging from simple cyst to gross polycystic–dysplastic changes or ARPKD-like features.

Other Cysts

Complicated (secondary) cysts after infection, surgery, trauma.
    Pararenal cysts (DD: duplex kidney, adrenal cyst, lymphangioma, teratoma, etc.).
Imaging: primary study = US. Shows highly variable morphology, often with irregular outlines, sedimentation, possible change in size.
DD: calyceal diverticulum, megacalycosis, calyceal ectasia, urinoma, duplex kidney, pararenal cysts. DD can be narrowed by dynamic contrast-enhanced MRU with delayed images.

Cystic Nephroma

Benign cystic renal tumor with progression to cystic nephroblastoma. Not always distinguishable from cystic Wilms tumor by imaging. May affect whole kidney or segments. Difference from multicystic renal dysplasia = small cysts with septa. Regional wall thickening, large atypical parenchymal areas, marked vascularity of septa, solid elements —increase likelihood of malignancy.

Imaging: variable findings. Usual initial study = US, sometimes VCUG (to differentiate from cystic dysplasia secondary to VUR; **Fig. 5.29**). Useful adjunct for DD = MRI. Follow-up = US and MRI (if latter not available and malignancy suspected = may consider CT) to avoid primary nephrectomy. For further DD and other malignant tumors, see Sect. 8.4.

Nephropathies

Hematuria

General: different implications in children than in adults—neoplasms less common as underlying disease (but possible). Hematuria usually has different cause (inflammatory, obstructive uropathy, VUR, familial, retroaortic renal vein, orthostatic proteinuria/hematuria, nephritis and nephropathies, renal vein thrombosis, hemolytic uremic syndrome, trauma, coagulopathies, urolithiasis, tumor, etc.) → always supplement clinical examination and urinalysis (erythrocyte morphology—renal?) by detailed US survey of entire urinary tract and abdomen.

Imaging: US shows more or less specific changes, may be diagnostic—e.g., renal/bladder tumor, renal injury, hemorrhagic cystitis and schistosomiatic bladder wall changes, urolithiasis/NC, renal vein thrombosis, PCS/ureteral dilatation, retroaortic left renal vein (= nutcracker/SMA syndrome, corresponding flow change in DDS = arterialized waveform with stenotic flow at site of renal vein compression). Reliable detection and evaluation of all changes requires targeted search utilizing all US capabilities. Further imaging/actions depend on ini-

5

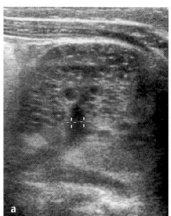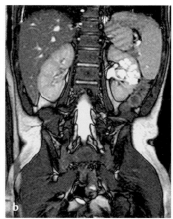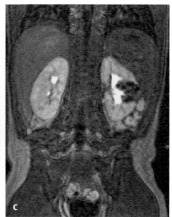

Fig. 5.29a–c   Cystic nephroma.

a   US scan of left kidney shows segmental, complex microcystic mass bordering on pelvicalyceal system (++).

b, c   Coronal MRU. T2-weighted TrueFISP (true fast imaging with steady-state precession) (**b**) and T1-weighted GRE after contrast administration (**c**)—multicystic mass in middle third, closely related to pelvicalyceal system, nonenhancing. Histology confirmed cystic nephroma.

tial findings (rarely IVP/VCUG, possible MRU/CT, renal biopsy, etc.).

> The many indications for primary CT urography in adults with hematuria are not applicable in children—only in exceptional cases.

Nephropathies, Nephrotic/Nephritic Syndrome

General: many congenital, hereditary/familial, acquired diseases. Detailed descriptions → specialized literature. Main imaging goal = (early) detection of signs of renal parenchymal disease (in screening examinations, US for nonspecific complaints, tests ordered for different reasons). Another goal = narrow DD in patients with clinical urologic–nephrologic symptoms, minimize risk of biopsy by pre-/peri-/postinterventional imaging support, detect secondary and accompanying changes.

Imaging:

- **US:** most widely used study. Key interpretive criteria = renal size, parenchymal structure (echogenicity, architecture, cystic dysplasia, segmental/diffuse, uni-/bilateral, etc.). (Power) Doppler = renal vascularity/perfusion (**Fig. 5.30**)

> DDS changes often correlate more with degree of renal failure and systemic components (medication, volume status) than with (severity of) underlying nephropathy/renal disease.

- **IVP/CT/VCUG:** not indicated
- **Scintigraphy, MRU:** used in selected cases to evaluate renal function, can narrow DD in complex situations

Benign Urinary Tract Tumors

See Sect. 8.4.

Most common benign forms: cyst, hamartoma, angiomyolipoma (AML). Less common: teratoma, lymphangioma, and many more (**Fig. 5.31**).

Imaging: findings typical in some cases (e.g., cyst, hyperechoic = AML), nonspecific in others. Primary US diagnosis and follow-up. MRI (CT) useful adjunct in equivocal cases.

> **!** Even benign tumors (especially AML) may hemorrhage and become acutely threatening when they reach certain size → follow-up, possible prophylactic embolization.

Note: renal tumors may be part of syndrome (TS, chromosome abnormality, etc.).

DD: other renal tumors/masses (see Sect. 8.4).

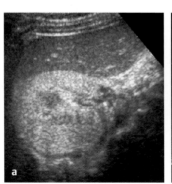 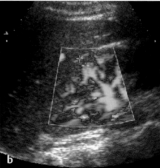

Fig. 5.30a, b   US appearance of various nephropathies and renal failure.

a Increased echogenicity of renal parenchyma in enlarged, swollen kidney. Nonspecific finding, may be seen in glomerulonephritis, acute nephropathies, or acute renal failure due to other causes (posthypoxic, toxic, etc.).

b Power Doppler shows hypovascular halo (++) plus a diffuse decrease in vascularity due to decreased perfusion/increased renal resistance.

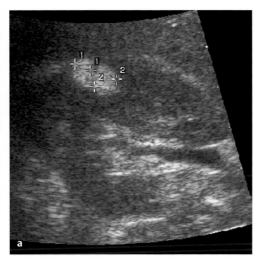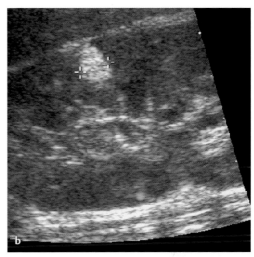

Fig. 5.31a, b Renal angiomyolipoma. Transverse (**a**) and longitudinal (**b**) US scans of right kidney. Hyperechoic neoplastic architectural distortion (++) typical of angiomyolipoma.

Renal Failure

General: acute/chronic, often with clinically presumed/known cause (chronic, postoperative, posttraumatic, postasphyxic, etc.).

Imaging goals:

1. Help to differentiate three main subgroups (pre-, intra-, postrenal renal failure):
   - **Prerenal renal failure:** systemic cause (e.g., hypoxia, decreased blood flow, congenital heart disease, vascular problem, hypovolemia, etc.)
   - **Intrinsic/intrarenal renal failure:** nephropathies due to various causes (e.g., toxic, drug-induced, other chronic renal disease, glomerulonephritis, glomerulo-/tubulopathy, metabolic disease, hemolytic uremic syndrome, renal vein thrombosis, etc.)
   - **Postrenal renal failure:** severe urinary tract obstruction (bilateral! single system!) = obstructive uropathy → oligo-/anuria, persistent renal damage
2. Monitoring and support treatment: image guidance for interventions (drainage, vascular access) investigation/management during renal failure (volume status, ascites, secondary changes in other organs). Subsequent monitoring also extrarenal (renal size/perfusion, treatment complications such as corticosteroid-induced aseptic necrosis, etc.)

Imaging:

- **US:** most widely used study, usually adequate, even at bedside (ICU, etc.). Can evaluate PCS and parenchymal morphology. (Power) Doppler and general status assessment (other organs, vessels, volume status, pleural effusion, ascites, etc.) essential. *Also*, placement of large CVCs, drainage of ascites/pleural effusion, biopsy investigation of underlying nephropathy, and follow-up.

> Doppler findings in particular are often nonspecific, not definitely related to entity or prognosis (numerous systemic factors are in play). May contribute to diagnosis/prognosis in selected cases (e.g., renal vein thrombosis—thrombus growth or resolution, follow-up of hemolytic uremic syndrome—return of normal Doppler waveform precedes clinical and laboratory improvement).

- **VCUG/IVP/CT:** not indicated or contraindicated (contrast administration! nephrotoxicity!)
- **Scintigraphy:** usually unrewarding—not used
- **MRI:** used in selected cases, especially to assess complex complications. Use with caution (risk of NSF—use only stable, macrocyclic Gd chelates!).

5

5.10   Urinary Tract Involvement by Systemic Disease, Bladder Dysfunction

Renal/Urinary Tract Involvement by Systemic Disease

Numerous systemic/extrarenal diseases may be manifested in the urogenital tract or lead secondarily to renal/urinary tract problems.

Examples:

- Glomerulonephritis with renal failure in lupus erythematosus
- Cysts and hypodysplasia in various syndromes
- Urinary tract anomalies in patients with congenital heart disease, syndromes, genetic diseases, nephropathies, parainfectious-paraneoplastic changes in other (systemic) diseases
- Nephropathy in metabolic diseases
- Increased risk of renal tumors in various syndromes (Denys–Drash syndrome, Beck–Wiedemann syndrome, von Hippel–Lindau disease, etc.)
- Renal failure due to hypoxia, severe hypotension and shock
- Renovascular hypertension in patients with systemic vascular disease
- Urinary obstruction by retroperitoneal mass, bladder dysfunction due to vertebral/spinal cord/CNS pathology

Symptomatology and imaging vary with manifestations (see specific subheads). Role of imaging = detection/"exclusion" of renal involvement, follow-up, DD.

> Urinary tract symptoms/findings may prompt further investigation and diagnosis (e.g., lupus erythematosus revealed by renal biopsy, spinal cord pathology by bladder problems, etc.).

Functional Bladder Disorders

General: importance increasingly recognized (cause of UTI, etc.). Decompensating bladder function = secondary problem (diverticulum, trabeculation, urinary reflux or obstruction). Early detection and prompt treatment = essential for good outcome. Causes and classification: neurogenic or habitual, disturbance of micturition and/or capacity/storage, neurogenic, or nonneurogenic bladder dysfunction.

Imaging:

- **US:** shows indirect signs (patent bladder neck, thickened bladder wall, bladder shape, residual urine)
- **VCUG:** modified technique (low contrast infusion pressure), observation of contrast drip infusion = semimanometric evaluation, allows for targeted FL imaging (bladder and bladder-neck configuration)
- **Video urodynamics:** special type of VCUG = combination of VCUG and urodynamics, with imaging focused on specific urodynamic change
- **Urodynamic tests:** pelvic floor EMG, Uroflow, simultaneous measurement of intra-abdominal and intravesical pressure and pelvic floor activity in relation to bladder-filling flow and pressure (see specialized literature)

> Initial US/VCUG examination may show indirect signs of dysfunction based on bladder shape (high tone, atypical outline and configuration), bladder wall thickening and trabeculation (possible pseudodiverticulum, definite diverticulum), residual urine (postvoiding), and bladder neck abnormalities → direct further exploration.

5.11   Imaging of the Pediatric Female Genital Tract _____

Postnatal Development

Uterus and ovaries initially large (maternal hormones) = prominent cervix, almost cystlike follicles, mobile ovaries (may be located far anterosuperiorly in abdomen)—followed by involution during subsequent weeks. Puberty characterized by size increase (mainly in the uterine corpus); ovaries also grow and follicles become more distinct.

> Optimum time for early detection of female genital anomalies = first month of life. Afterward, anomalies may be undetectable until (peri-/pre-) puberty.

Imaging:

- **US:** modality of choice. Transabdominal scans through full bladder can clearly define internal genitalia, may be supplemented by transperineal scans and (US) genitography (vagina, intersex, urogenital sinus, etc.). Neonatal linear probe is helpful (**Fig. 5.32a**). Typical uterine morphology varies with age (**Fig. 5.33**).
- **MRI:** limited indications; sometimes helpful for complex pathology, suspected tumor, or peripubertal imaging (US limited, no endovaginal scans). Use high-resolution sequences, possible isotropic 3D sequence. Angle images to conform to organ axes.

Ovarian Pathology

Ovarian Cysts

General: common, usually without pathologic significance. Large cysts—risk of torsion/hemorrhage.

   Imaging:
- **US:** typical cystic features = thin wall, echo-free lumen. With intracystic hemorrhage = internal echoes ("complicated cyst") (**Fig. 5.32a, b**)

> Normal follicles have same US appearance as small cysts (**Fig. 5.32c**).

- **MRI:** cystic cavities = T2 hyperintense, T1 hypointense, often detected incidentally. Intracystic hemorrhage → sedimentation with internal echoes. More common in newborns, especially common around puberty.

DD: prominent/dysfunctional follicle, cystic tumor, especially teratoma (solid elements? contains fat/calcium?).

Ovarian Torsion

Acute emergency that requires immediate surgery. Presents clinically with severe abdominal pain, nausea, abdominal rigidity (DD: appendicitis, urinary tract problem). Peak incidence in perinatal/neonatal and peripubertal periods.

5

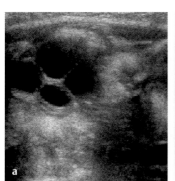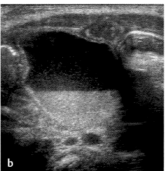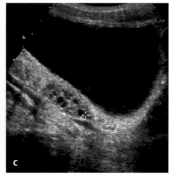

Fig. 5.32a–c   Neonatal and pediatric ovary.

a Normal neonatal ovary, located just beneath abdominal wall, has physiologically large follicles (high-resolution linear probe).

b Giant neonatal ovarian cyst with intracystic hemorrhage and sedimentation.
c Normal pediatric ovary (++) can be imaged behind full bladder, contains prominent follicles.

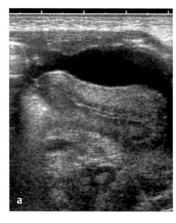

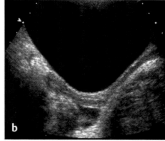

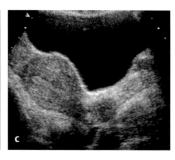

Fig. 5.33a–c   Examples of age-dependent uterine morphology. Newborn (large prominent cervix, **a**), infant (small, **b**), and pear-shaped organ in adult (also around puberty; large corpus, smaller cervix, **c**). Note: uterus can be clearly imaged with US only through a well-distended bladder!

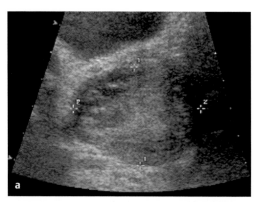

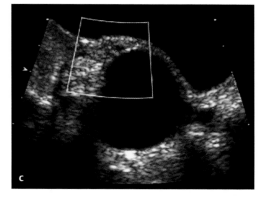

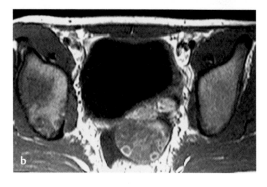

Fig. 5.34a–c   Ovarian torsion.
a Typical US appearance of ovarian torsion. Affected ovary large and hyperechoic with atypical structure (++, 5 × 4 cm!) and small, peripheral follicles largely obscured by internal echoes (= intraovarian hemorrhage and hemorrhagic infarction).
b Axial T1-weighted MRI shows swollen, edematous ovary with peripheral, partly hemorrhagic follicles.
c Pediatric ovarian torsion. A large cyst with slightly irregular margins capped by echogenic nodular structure (teratoma). CDS shows no detectable perfusion in hyperechoic, unstructured residual ovarian tissue.

Ovarian torsion in "latent" phase suspicious for underlying ovarian pathology (e.g., leukemic infiltration, teratoma, etc.).

Imaging:
- **US:** ovary rounded, enlarged, and hyperechoic, usually displaced medially. Ascites around ovary and in cul-de-sac. Multiple small follicles in peripheral radial pattern with internal echoes, may contain fluid levels (hemorrhagic infarction!)—may be masked by underlying ovarian disease (infiltration, cystic tumor, intracystic hemorrhage, etc.; **Fig. 5.34**)

CDS of is limited value, especially with partial torsion. Ovarian torsion may be slight, and ovary has a two-vessel blood supply = residual perfusion still present → suspicious/equivocal findings = immediate laparoscopic exploration! Exception: torsion in neonates probably occurred in utero or during birth = ovary cannot be salvaged.

Neonatal ovarian cysts may reach monstrous proportions and contain internal echoes (**Fig. 5.32b**). Wait-and-see approach usually justified; however, only large mass would warrant US-guided biopsy/surgery. May be difficult to distinguish from other cystic abdominal masses (enteric duplication, mesenteric cyst, etc.).

- **MRI/CT:** not indicated, unless available for **immediate** investigation of suspected tumor or DD of masses (**Fig. 5.34b**)

Pelvic Inflammatory Disease

Extremely rare in children. Inflammation may spread from perforated appendicitis or other nearby processes. Presentation after puberty same as in adults.

Pelvic inflammatory disease in children is always suspicious for a complex urogenital malformation with fistula formation or abuse—investigate accordingly!

Ovarian Malformations

Usually revealed by targeted search that was prompted by urinary tract anomaly or investigation of abnormal pubertal development and syndromic conditions.

Mayer–Rokitansky–Küster–Hauser syndrome: intact ovaries, failure of Müllerian duct development → absence of uterus and vagina. Bilateral enlarged ovaries with multiple cysts and pseudoprecocious puberty.

Absence of ovaries or hypoplastic/nonfunctioning rudimentary ovaries seen in various conditions such as Ulrich–Turner syndrome, testicular feminization, McCune–Albright syndrome, hypopigmentation, and fibrous ovarian dysplasia/streak gonads.

Diseases and Malformations of the Uterus and Vagina

Inflammations and tumors (see Sect. 8) are rare. Inflammatory conditions are most common in association with malformation/dysfunction/vaginal influx or abuse. Only other significant cause = intravaginal FB (e.g., inserted accidentally during play)—explore vagina (transabdominal and perineal US) for FB in small children with unexplained lower abdominal symptoms.

Malformations

Typical malformations: hymenal/vaginal atresia and double uterus/vagina (**Figs. 5.35** and **5.36**). Often undetected until puberty, require specific search (in children with risk factors). Classic manifestation = hydrocolpos/hydrometrocolpos (vagina ± uterus filled with complex fluid due to vaginal/hymenal atresia = retrovesical pseudocystic tubular structure). Vagina topped by uterus, which is usually fluid-filled but less dilated (see Case Study 5.4, **Fig. 5.45**).

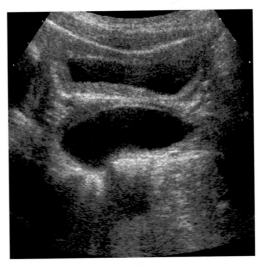

Fig. 5.35 Vaginal pathology in newborn. Longitudinal US scan of lower abdomen through full bladder shows fluid-filled retrovesical vagina. DD: fistula, urogenital sinus, vaginal influx during micturition (e.g., due to labial synechiae), artificial (during US genitography, etc.).

5

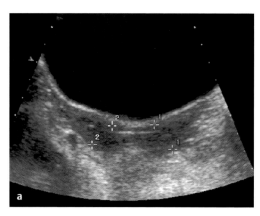
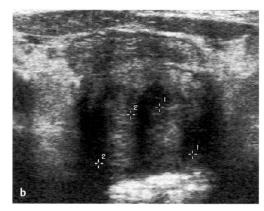

Fig. 5.36a, b   Double uterus in children. Lower abdominal transverse US scan through full bladder shows complete double uterus (uterus didelphis, ++) (**a**) and septate uterus with two cavities (++) (**b**).

Imaging:

- **US:** retrovesical fluid-filled structure = distended vagina filled with complex fluid. Obstruction visualized with transperineal scan. Lumen of uterus, containing variable amount of fluid, appears at upper end of tubular structure. Duplication anomaly—combination of vaginal atresia and double uterus (Wunderlich syndrome and renal agenesis). Try to define coronal and axial plane to evaluate uterine configuration (3D US with coronal reconstruction extremely helpful). Fluid instillation into vagina may occasionally improve anatomic orientation and DD (scan through NaCl-filled bladder = "US genitography")
- **FL:** conventional study for diagnosing genital anomalies—catheterization of bladder and vagina, contrast instillation into catheterized cavities → more or less typical impressions/outlines which allow indirect evaluation of structures not directly opacified (may be correlated with US findings). Often combined with US genitography —especially to aid visualization of small fistulae
- **CT:** not indicated
- **MRU:** anomalies detected incidentally during MRU (investigation of urinary tract malformation), otherwise/most for cases detected around puberty or later with restricted US access. Requires proper plane selection (axial and coronal in uterine/vaginal long axis, also sagittal images), possible isotropic 3D acquisition. NaCl instillation into vagina may be helpful. Usually, no need for contrast administration.
  Special indication: search for ectopic vaginal ureteral orifice = contrast drainage into vagina on delayed MRU, provided functionally competent residual renal tissue

5.12   Imaging of the Pediatric Male Genital Tract

General: diseases of prostate and seminal vesicle rarely of importance. Tumors discussed in Sect. 8.4. Problems relating to testis and its appendages of prime concern.

Imaging: US = adequate stand-alone study—except for tumors. Always use linear probe plus CDS, include evaluation of inguinal canal and spermatic cord (e.g., funiculocele, perfusion, inguinal hernia, retractile testis, etc.; **Fig. 5.37**), potentially also urinary tract.

Diseases and Malformations of the Testis

Anorchism, Polyorchidism

General: rare indication. Anorchism always requires differentiation from undescended testis or high-grade testicular hypoplasia. Polyorchidism can usually be diagnosed by palpation. Imaging (US) can confirm findings and differentiate from other masses.

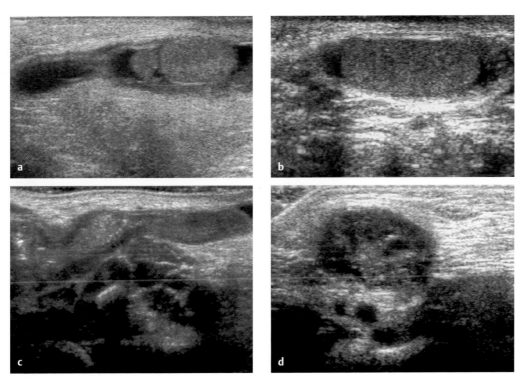

Fig. 5.37a–d   US appearance of inguinal canal in child with suspicious genital pathology.

a Testicular and funicular hydrocele. Scan shows peri-testicular fluid in scrotum, continuing into inguinal canal.
b Inguinal testis.

c Inguinal hernia. A bowel loop has herniated into patent inguinal canal. Slightly hypodysplastic retractile testis also visible, currently within inguinal canal.
d Female infant with painful groin swelling → US → ovary herniated into inguinal canal!

Undescended Testis, Retractile Testis, Inguinal Hernia

Typically, testes symmetrical and descended (= in scrotum). Physiologically still mobile during first months of life; may retract intermittently toward inguinal canal (especially with crying).

Abnormalities of testicular descent = testis retained in inguinal canal or abdominal cavity → impairs testicular maturation, increases risk of secondary tumors.

Palpable retractile testis, undescended testis—US (dynamic) can confirm hypodysplasia.

Imaging:

- **US:** targeted search with linear probe in scrotum, along inguinal canal, at entrance to inguinal canal, and within abdominal cavity. Intra-abdominal testis: usually hypodysplastic, some-times difficult to find (may be located anywhere along ureter, even at inferior border of liver/spleen, rarely fused). Dynamic sonopalpation can assess mobility/reducibility of testis in inguinal canal (size and vascularity/CDS and DDS). Undescended testis: often dysplastic (= small, hyperechoic, atypical-asymmetrical echo texture, decreased vascularity). Urinary tract exploration recommended in children with undescended testis (associated malformation?)

> Even after orchidopexy, testis often asymmetrically small/hypovascular, may show postoperative scar.

- **MRI:** cannot definitely exclude dysplastic-ectopic testis. Hypodysplastic undescended intra-abdominal testis may also elude MRI → therapeutic implications may warrant surgical/laparoscopic exploration

Testicular and Funicular Hydrocele

General: fluid collection between tunica vaginalis and tunica albuginea—thin fluid layer is physiologic in infants. Incomplete closure → larger fluid collection that communicates with inguinal canal/abdominal cavity. Concomitant reactive hydrocele due to inflammatory process, testicular tumor, ascites, ventriculoperitoneal shunt, trauma, varicocele, perfusion disorder, etc. = nonspecific.

Imaging: US—uncomplicated fluid, easily detected with linear probe. Scans will also detect any communication with abdominal cavity (**Fig. 5.38**).

> Focused search for cause and evaluation of testicular perfusion (e.g., large hydrocele with increased intrascrotal pressure) plus symmetry issues (always include evaluation of contralateral testis!).

Varicocele

General: dilatation/tortuosity of veins of pampiniform plexus. Rarer before than after puberty. Usually occurs on left side—associated with atypical termination of spermatic vein in left renal vein, incompetent venous valves, or retroaortic left renal vein. Right-sided hydrocele—suspicious for compression by tumor or other mass leading to venous stasis. All varicoceles in children should be investigated by abdominal US. Higher stages associated

Table 5.3 Clinical grading of varicocele

Grade I	Not visible to the eye. US shows slightly thickened spermatic cord, marked increase in vein lumen/venous markings during Valsalva maneuver
Grade II	Palpable dilatation of visibly large venous plexuses even without Valsalva maneuver; flow reversal on (C)DS during Valsalva maneuver
Grade III	Massive venous dilatation and tortuosity, visible to the eye ("bag of worms"); constant flow reversal on (C)DS even without Valsalva maneuver

with infertility → require treatment. Graded as shown in **Table 5.3**.

Imaging:

- **US:** shows mass of tangled, dilated veins with slow flow on CDS (DDS)

> Watch for flow reversal during Valsalva maneuver by CDS and DDS (grade II) or constant flow reversal (grade III). Flow reversal = absolute indication for treatment.

- **Venography:** in selected cases—aids in planning/conducting therapeutic embolization. Otherwise rarely used owing to radiation exposure risks.

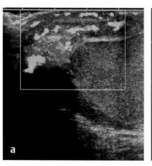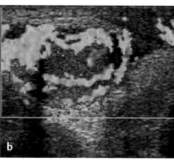

Fig. 5.38a, b Testicular inflammation.
a Epididymitis. CDS shows hyperperfusion of slightly prominent, hyperechoic epididymis.
b Posttraumatic orchitis. CDS shows hyperperfusion after minor trauma as evidence of postcontusional orchitis.

Acute Scrotum

! Urgent indication for imaging!

Causes: inflammation/torsion/incarcerated inguinal hernia.

 Imaging: US with high-resolution linear probe, CDS, and duplex scanning; always evaluate inguinal canal and both sides. Side-to-side Doppler waveform comparison is essential.

Typical findings:

- **Orchitis:** US = enlarged testis, markedly increased perfusion (CDS)—usually asymmetrical (**Fig. 5.38**). Focal forms inhomogeneous, often posttraumatic. Secondary abscess formation may occur. If recurrent, consider urogenital/urethral malformation (may add VCUG). MRI sometimes used for DD

 Rare DD: splenogonal fusion or intratesticular splenic and adrenal ectopia.

- **Epididymitis:** US = normal-appearing testis, often with associated hydrocele. Swollen epididymis with marked hypervascularity (CDS) (**Fig. 5.38**)
- **Testicular torsion:** US = swollen testis of variable echogenicity, depending on duration—initially echogenic, then increasingly hypoechoic and inhomogeneous. Concomitant hydrocele. Asymmetric decrease in vascularity/perfusion. Initial cessation of venous flow, then decreased arterial diastolic flow, culminating in absence of systolic arterial flow (compare sides! hemorrhagic infarction!)

! Caution: watch out for partial torsion with residual flow or spontaneous (partial) reduction as well as intermittent torsion (**Fig. 5.39**).

! Any indeterminate finding requires immediate surgical inspection. May attempt manual reduction of torsion under US guidance (improved perfusion?), but surgery always indicated.

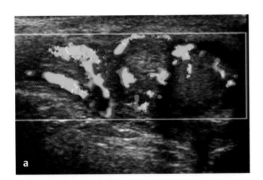

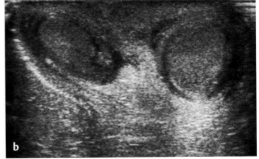

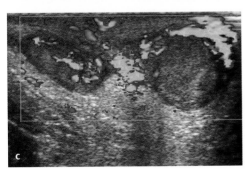

Fig. 5.39a–c DD of acute scrotum using US.
a Torsion of testicular appendages. Demarcation of swollen, hyperechoic paratesticular region without vascularity, reactive hyperperfusion of epididymis, increased perifocal perfusion. Testis itself appears normal.
b Testicular torsion. Right testis appears normal. Left testis enlarged and hyperechoic.
c CDS in testicular torsion. Unlike normal right testis with definable intratesticular vessels, left testicular parenchymal perfusion is not visualized (same patient as in panel **b**). Note: with definable intraparenchymal vessels on both sides, always add duplex US and waveform analysis—only symmetrical parenchymal waveform in normal and suspicious testes with equal arterial and venous spectra will definitely exclude (partial) torsion! Reactive hyperperfusion may develop after spontaneous reduction!

5

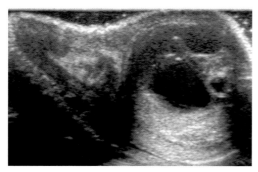

Fig. 5.40   Testicular tumors, role of (power) Doppler. Scan demonstrates complex cystic mass in testis with solid elements—testicular teratoma.

■ **Torsion of testicular appendages:** similar clinical presentation, but without perfusion changes in testis itself. US = enlarged, swollen, nonperfused testicular appendages that later calcify and shrink in size. Associated hydrocele, potentially reactive epedidymitis.

It is important to exclude other changes—as listed above.

■ **Incarcerated inguinal hernia:** intrascrotal structure, separate from testis, which can be traced through inguinal canal to abdomen. Perfusion may be intact, decreased, or absent depending on degree of incarceration. Accompanying ascites or hydrocele. Sometimes difficult to detect/identify due to collapsed bowel lumen and pain. Reduction may be attempted under US guidance

Other abdominal structures besides bowel may herniate through the inguinal canal (mesentery, bladder tissue, ovary, etc.; **Fig. 5.37**).

■ **Testicular trauma/tumor:** see Sect. 8.4 and **Fig. 5.40**.

5.13   Intersex, Urogenital Sinus, and Anogenital Malformations

Urogenital Sinus and Anogenital Malformations

Malformations show continuum of severity—from simple fistula and stenosis to complex urogenital sinus. May be associated with intersex, sacral agenesis, VACTERL syndrome, etc.
Imaging: (US) genitography and VCUG. Irrigoscopy possible option (search for fistula/sinus tracts)—should be reserved for specialized centers. Initial evaluation should include whole abdomen and spinal column (other changes, syndromic?—US, possible survey radiographs).

Intersex

Numerous causes—chromosomal, hormonal, dysgenetic, biochemical. Cases with equivocal clinical findings require chromosome analysis, hormone status, and US including US genitography—latter during first weeks of life (before involution of possible rudimentary female internal genitalia).
Imaging: goals of imaging (US with transperineal scans often adequate) = identification of uterus and ovaries/testes, urethral and vaginal assessment, and detection of rudimentary gonads (scrotum/labia/lower abdomen). Also evaluate any other changes (adrenal, etc.) that may cause (hormonal) disorders.
  ■ **US:** includes transperineal scans and US genitography (= document internal structures after catheterization/fluid instillation into urethra, vagina or vaginal rudiment, possibly rectum). Give special attention to visualization of (streak) gonads (= undifferentiated rudiment with fibrotic tissue and no typical differentiation along testicular or ovarian lines; US morphology usu-

ally resembles dysplastic testes more than typical ovaries; may be located at typical ovarian site or elsewhere in abdomen, groin, scrotum, labia)

> With equivocal soft-tissue structures in labialike skin folds, try to evaluate inguinal canal and look for possible rudimentary spermatic cord.

- Other possible imaging options: genitography, MRI

5.14   Other

- Adrenal diseases and tumors in children: see Sect. 8.3 and 9.2
- Urogenital tumors in children/tumors: see Sect. 8.4

- Imaging of urogenital trauma: see Chapter 6 (Trauma) and Sect. 1.6 (CT) (**Fig. 5.41a–c**)

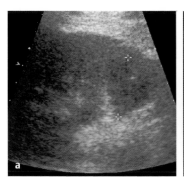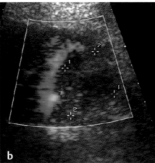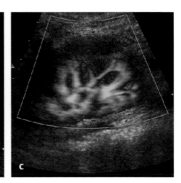

5

Fig. 5.41a–c   Renal trauma, role of (power) Doppler US.

a B-mode US shows slight, rudimentary regional change in renal parenchymal echo texture (sometimes absent, especially in early posttraumatic setting) as result of renal trauma.
b Same patient as in **a**. Power Doppler discloses renal injury (++).

c Demarcation of wedge-shaped traumatic parenchymal lesion with no definite change in parenchymal texture. A perirenal-subcapsular hematoma, almost isoechoic to renal parenchyma, more clearly delineated on near side of organ.

Case Study 5.1

Clinical findings: very sick infant with fever, abnormal urine, and leukocytosis.
Suitable modalities: US, possibly DMSA scintigraphy.

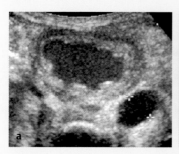 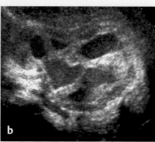

Fig. 5.42a, b

Findings: internal echoes in wall-thickened, trabeculated bladder, left MU (++). PCS of left kidney dilated, filled with internal echoes due to sedimentation. Renal parenchyma hazy and hyperechoic.
Diagnosis: UTI with HN and MU (refluxive? PUV?).
Additional tests: VCUG, possibly MRU or scintigraphy (after UTI subsides).

Case Study 5.2

Clinical findings: newborn with antenatal bilateral grade III HN.
Suitable modalities: US, VCUG, possibly MRU.

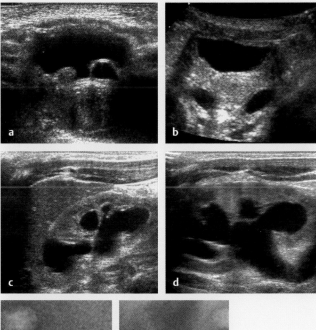

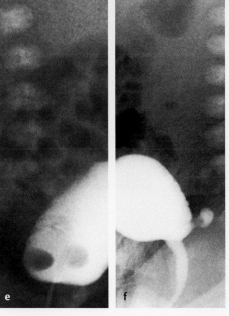

Fig. 5.43a–f

Available images: US (bladder, ureters, both kidneys), VCUG.
Findings: transverse bladder scan shows collapsed right ureterocele and distended left ureterocele (**a**), bilateral MU (**b**), grade III–IV HN of both kidneys (**c, d**). Unilateral VCUG during filling phase displays both ureteroceles (**e**) with diverticulumlike eversion of one ureterocele during micturition (**f**).
Diagnosis: MU with orthotopic ureterocele and HN on both sides.
Additional tests: further options are MRU, MAG3 scintigraphy.

5

Case Study 5.3

Clinical findings: girl with previous UTI.
Possible modalities: US, VCUG, DMSA.

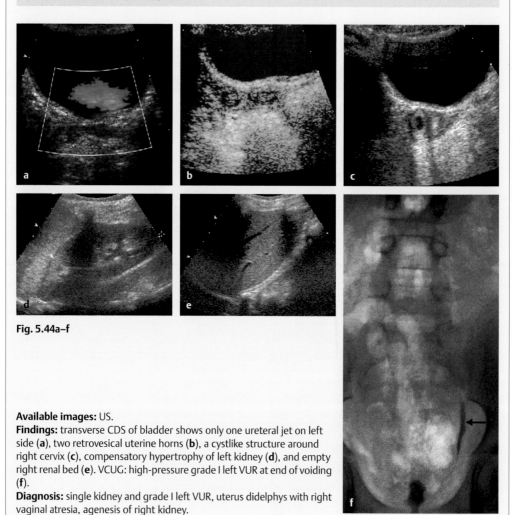

Fig. 5.44a–f

Available images: US.
Findings: transverse CDS of bladder shows only one ureteral jet on left side (**a**), two retrovesical uterine horns (**b**), a cystlike structure around right cervix (**c**), compensatory hypertrophy of left kidney (**d**), and empty right renal bed (**e**). VCUG: high-pressure grade I left VUR at end of voiding (**f**).
Diagnosis: single kidney and grade I left VUR, uterus didelphys with right vaginal atresia, agenesis of right kidney.

Case Study 5.4

Clinical findings: 13-year-old girl with abdominal pain and "suspected lower abdominal tumor."
Possible modalities: US, CT, MRI.

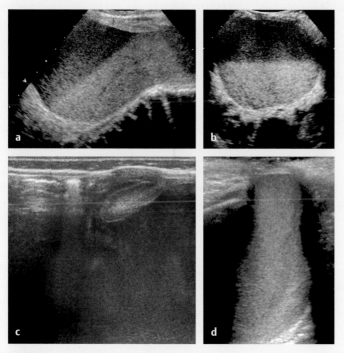

Fig. 5.45a–d

Available images: US.
Findings: midsagittal (**a**) and transverse (**b**) scans of lower abdomen show very large, distended, complex tubular structure with fluid level behind bladder. A uteruslike knob visible atop structure (**c**). Transperineal scan shows thick septum at vaginal outlet (**d**).
Diagnosis: hydrometrocolpos in vaginal atresia.

Bibliography

1 Avni FE, Garel C, Cassart M, D'Haene N, Hall M, Riccabona M. Imaging and classification of congenital cystic venal disease. AJR Am J Roentgenol 2012; 198(5): 1004–1013

2 Chapman SJ, Chantler G, Haycock GB, Maisey MN, Saxton HM. Radionuclide cystography in vesicoureteric reflux. Arch Dis Child 1988; 63(6): 650–651

3 Darge K, Troeger J, Duetting T, et al. Reflux in young patients: comparison of voiding US of the bladder and retrovesical space with echo enhancement versus voiding cystourethrography for diagnosis. Radiology 1999; 210(1): 201–207

4 Darge K, Troeger J. Vesicoureteral reflux grading in contrast-enhanced voiding urosonography. Eur J Radiol 2002; 43(2): 122–128

5 European Society of Paediatric Radiology (ESPR). http://www.espr.org

6 European Society of Urogenital Radiology (ESUR). http://www.esur.org

7 Fernbach SK, Maizels M, Conway JJ. Ultrasound grading of hydronephrosis: introduction to the system used by the Society for Fetal Urology. Pediatr Radiol 1993; 23(6): 478–480

8 Fernbach SK, Feinstein KA, Schmidt MB. Pediatric voiding cystourethrography: a pictorial guide. Radiographics 2000; 20(1): 155–168, discussion 168–171

9 Fotter R, Kopp W, Klein E, Höllwarth M, Uray E. Unstable bladder in children: functional evaluation by modified voiding cystourethrography. Radiology 1986; 161(3): 811–813

10 Fotter R, Riccabona M. Functional disorders of the lower urinary tract in children. [Article in German] Radiologe 2005; 45(12): 1085–1091

11 Fotter R, ed. Pediatric Uroradiology. 2nd ed. Berlin, Heidelberg, New York: Springer; 2008

12 Gassner I, Geley TE. Ultrasound of female genital anomalies. Eur Radiol 2004; 14(Suppl 4): L107–L122

13 Gordon I, Riccabona M. Investigating the newborn kidney: update on imaging techniques. Semin Neonatol 2003; 8(4): 269–278

14 Grattan-Smith JD, Jones RA. MR urography in children. Pediatr Radiol 2006; 36(11): 1119–1132, quiz 1228–1229

15 Grattan-Smith JD, Little SB, Jones RA. MR urography in children: how we do it. Pediatr Radiol 2008; 38(Suppl 1): S3–S17

16 Hofmann V, Deeg KH, Hoyer PF, eds. Ultraschalldiagnostik in Pädiatrie und Kinderchirurgie. Thieme, Stuttgart, 2nd ed. 1996; 382 p.

17 Lebowitz RL, Olbing H, Parkkulainen KV, Smellie JM, Tamminen-Möbius TE; International Reflux Study in Children. International system of radiographic grading of vesicoureteric reflux. Pediatr Radiol 1985; 15(2): 105–109

18 Maudgil DD, McHugh K. The role of computed tomography in modern paediatric uroradiology. Eur J Radiol 2002; 43(2): 129–138

19 Morcos SK. Non-neoplastic cystic renal lesions. In: Morcos SK, Thomsen H, eds. Urogenital Imaging: a Problem-Oriented Approach. Oxford: Wiley-Blackwell; 2009: 75–97

20 Österreichische Gesellschaft für Ultraschall in der Medizin (ÖGUM). http://www.oegum.at

21 Piepsz A. Radionuclide studies in paediatric nephrourology. Eur J Radiol 2002; 43(2): 146–153

22 Riccabona M. Cystography in infants and children: a critical appraisal of the many forms with special regard to voiding cystourethrography. Eur Radiol 2002; 12(12): 2910–2918

23 Riccabona M. Potential of modern sonographic techniques in paediatric uroradiology. Eur J Radiol 2002; 43(2): 110–121

24 Riccabona M, Lindbichler F, Sinzig M. Conventional imaging in paediatric uroradiology. Eur J Radiol 2002; 43(2): 100–109

25 Riccabona M, Sorantin E, Hausegger K. Imaging guided interventional procedures in paediatric uroradiology—a case based overview. Eur J Radiol 2002; 43(2): 167–179

26 Riccabona M, Simbrunner J, Ring E, Ruppert-Kohlmayr A, Ebner F, Fotter R. Feasibility of MR urography in neonates and infants with anomalies of the upper urinary tract. Eur Radiol 2002; 12(6): 1442–1450

27 Riccabona M. Imaging of renal tumours in infancy and childhood. Eur Radiol 2003; 13(Suppl 4): L116–L129

28 Riccabona M. Pediatric MRU—its potential and its role in the diagnostic work-up of upper urinary tract dilatation in infants and children. World J Urol 2004; 22(2): 79–87

29 Riccabona M, Ruppert-Kohlmayr A, Ring E, Maier C, Lusuardi L, Riccabona M. Potential impact of pediatric MR urography on the imaging algorithm in patients with a functional single kidney. AJR Am J Roentgenol 2004; 183(3): 795–800

30 Riccabona M. Vesicoureteral reflux. In: Carty H, Brunelle F, Stringer D, Kao SC, eds. Imaging Children. Vol. I. 2nd ed. Amsterdam: Elsevier Science Publishers; 2005: 671–690

31 Riccabona M. Urinary tract infection. In: Carty H, Brunelle F, Stringer D, Kao SC, eds. Imaging Children. Vol. I. 2nd ed. Amsterdam: Elsevier Science Publishers; 2005: 691–712

32 Riccabona M, Fritz GA, Schöllnast H, Schwarz T, Deutschmann MJ, Mache CJ. Hydronephrotic kidney: pediatric three-dimensional US for relative renal size assessment—initial experience. Radiology 2005; 236 (1): 276–283

33 Riccabona M. (Acute) renal failure in neonates, infants, and children – the role of ultrasound, with respect to other imaging options. Ultrasound Clin 2006; 1: 457–469

34 Riccabona M. Imaging of the neonatal genito-urinary tract. Eur J Radiol 2006; 60(2): 187–198

35 Riccabona M, Fotter R. Radiographic studies in children with kidney disorders: what to do and when. In: Hogg R, ed. Kidney Disorders in Children and Adolescents. Birmingham: Taylor & Francis; 2006: 15–34

36 Riccabona M, Schweintzger G, Leidig E, et al. Standarddokumentation der Sonografie des kindlichen Abdomens: Dokumentationsempfehlung für abdominelle Ultraschalluntersuchungen im Neugeborenen-, Kindes- und Jugendalter. Ultraschall Med 2006; 27: 504–505

37 Riccabona M. Lower urinary tract—the ureter and vesicoureteral reflux. In: Slovis TL, ed. Caffey's Pediatric Diagnostic Imaging. Vol 2, Part 13. 11th ed. Philadelphia: Mosby/Elsevier; 2007: 2315–2355

38 Riccabona M. Renal agenesis, dysplasia, hypoplasia and cystic diseases of the kidney. In: Fotter R, ed. Pediatric Uroradiology. 2nd ed. Berlin, Heidelberg & New York: Springer; 2008: 196

39 Riccabona M, Avni FE, Blickman JG, et al. Imaging recommendations in paediatric uroradiology: minutes of the ESPR workgroup session on urinary tract infection, fetal hydronephrosis, urinary tract ultrasonography and voiding cystourethrography, Barcelona, Spain, June 2007. Pediatr Radiol 2008; 38(2): 138–145

40 Riccabona M. Urinary tract imaging in infancy. Pediatr Radiol 2009; 39(Suppl 3): 436–445

41 Riccabona M, Avni FE, Blickman JG, et al. Imaging recommendations in paediatric uroradiology. Minutes of the ESPR uroradiology task force session on childhood obstructive uropathy, high-grade fetal hydronephrosis, childhood haematuria, and urolithiasis in childhood. ESPR Annual Congress, Edinburgh, UK, June 2008. Pediatr Radiol 2009; 39(8): 891–898

42 Riccabona M. Imaging of the paediatric urogenital tract. In: Puri P, Höllwarth M, eds. Pediatric Surgery—Diagnosis and Management. Heidelberg, London & New York: Springer; 2009: 809–824

43 Riccabona M, Avni FE. MR imaging of the paediatric abdomen. In: Gourtsoyiannis NC, ed. Clinical MRI of the Abdomen—Why, How, When. Berlin & Heidelberg: Springer; 2011: 639–676

44 Rohrschneider WK, Haufe S, Wiesel M, et al. Functional and morphologic evaluation of congenital urinary tract dilatation by using combined static-dynamic MR urography: findings in kidneys with a single collecting system. Radiology 2002; 224(3): 683–694

45 Schoellnast H, Lindbichler F, Riccabona M. Sonographic diagnosis of urethral anomalies in infants: value of perineal sonography. J Ultrasound Med 2004; 23(6): 769–776

46 Sorantin E, Fotter R, Aigner R, Ring E, Riccabona M. The sonographically thickened wall of the upper urinary tract system: correlation with other imaging methods. Pediatr Radiol 1997; 27(8): 667–671

47 Stein R, Beezt R, Thueroff JW, eds. Kinderurologie in Klinik und Praxis. Berlin & Heidelberg: Springer; 2011

48 Teele RL, Share JC. Transperineal sonography in children. AJR Am J Roentgenol 1997; 168(5): 1263–1267

5

6 Imaging of Pediatric Trauma

Marcus Hoermann

6.1 Introduction and General Considerations

Prerequisite for correctly recognizing/classifying fractures in growing skeleton: understanding of growth phenomena such as growth stimulation and inhibition, physiology of growing bone.

- Epiphyseal plate (growth plate, physis) responsible for longitudinal growth
- Enlarged cartilage cells mineralize at junction of metaphysis and growth plate, then transform into bone cells
- Growth in bone diameter controlled by perichondrium (surrounding growth plate)
- All three systems have own blood supply—metaphyseal and epiphyseal supply systems may be interconnected by perichondrial system

- Bone mineralizes from center on metaphyseal side toward periphery—both in individual bones and in axial system as a whole
- Growth plate wide open initially, becomes increasingly narrow until just before growth complete; followed by resting phase in which proliferation ceases
- Final closure of growth plate marked by fusion of metaphysis and epiphysis. Edges of epiphyseal plate appear indistinct at imaging. Growth plate closure proceeds centrally and medially from epiphyseal margin (epiphyseal blood supply)

6.2 Growth Disorders

Growth disorders can occur only while growth plates are still open—depend more on skeletal maturity at time of injury than on nature or severity of traumatizing force.

Growth disturbance may result from stimulation or inhibition of growth. Any manipulation such as reduction or surgery (including metal implant removal) may create growth stimulus. Growth stimulation—does not necessarily lengthen bone. Fractures before 10 years of age → tend to cause lengthening; after 10 years → shortening.

Stimulation

Growth stimulation has several possible causes:
- Hyperemia due to mechanical irritation from traumatizing force
- Remodeling (attempt to create stable bone quickly)
- Disturbances of callus formation

- Operative treatment
- Humoral, hormonal, local growth factors

Inhibition

Growth inhibition rare—may occur in severe injuries (destruction of growth plate cartilage = complete disruption of epiphyseal vascular system, e.g., due to extensive soft-tissue and crush injury).

Secondary inhibition in metaphyseal fractures: transient interruption of epiphyseal blood supply.

Partial inhibition due to fracture across growth plate—bar forms between metaphysis and epiphysis. Degree of growth disturbance depends on thickness of physeal bar.

Callus (Healing Fracture)

Manifestation of fracture healing = callus, important for healing and for estimating fracture age (e.g., in suspected child abuse).

Callus formation earlier and more abundant in younger children, much softer → mimics stability, lengthens time available for correction of deformity. Early (abundant) callus can establish diagnosis of fractures not visible initially.

Longer healing period, especially after open reduction and internal fixation → bone appears radiographically stable for exercise and weight bearing but still prone to refracture. Refracture may also follow inadequate immobilization time or tech- nique → radial and ulnar diaphyses that may refracture up to 6 months after cast removal (muscular atrophy more pronounced in children; clumsiness means greater injury risk; **Fig. 6.1**).

Nonunions in children—occur with unstable fractures and conservative treatment with failure of consolidation. Almost always result from insufficient stability/length of immobilization. Most nonunions in children will go on to form union.

Typical examples: complication of forearm greenstick fracture—proper consolidation does not occur due to axial malalignment → partial nonunion on side of complete fracture (**Fig. 6.2**). Nonunited fracture of humeral radial condyle (complicated pressure dynamics in radial part of elbow joint).

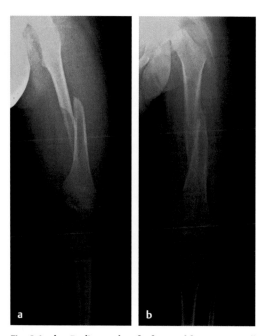

Fig. 6.1a, b Radiographs of a femoral fracture. Small child injured in motor vehicle accident.

a Survey radiograph shows displacement, axial malalignment, shortening, and external rotation of femur = transverse fracture of femur.

b Survey radiograph after cast removal. Prominent callus with remodeling causes temporary shortening of bone; should resolve spontaneously within 2 years.

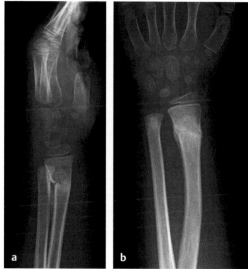

Fig. 6.2a, b Radial buckle fracture caused by a fall onto the hand. Lateral (**a**) and AP (**b**) radiographs after cast removal show definite fracture callus without deformity = buckle fracture.

6

Imaging of Fractures

See also Chapter 7.

Plain Radiographs in Two Planes

Mainstay of fracture diagnosis. Rules:
- Not all fractures have to be X-rayed. According to Lutz von Laer, radiographs needed only if they will influence treatment.
- Always include both neighboring joints in image.
- Stress radiographs and arthrograms are very rarely indicated in children.
- Increasing role of US (high-frequency linear probe); e.g., calvarial fracture, radial head dislocation (nursemaid's elbow), nondisplaced fracture of lateral humeral epicondyle, epiphyseal fracture or separation due to unossified epiphysis (in newborns and infants)

> With few exceptions, contralateral radiograph is obsolete.

Magnetic Resonance Imaging

Not first-line study for imaging limbs, but excellent second-line study for evaluating joints and tendons —has increasingly replaced arthroscopy.

Principal injuries in small children are ligament avulsions; ligament tears more common with aging. Can be clearly differentiated on radiographs → older children more often requiring joint evaluation by MRI.

Computed Tomography

Only for transitional fractures of radius or ankle joint or preoperative assessment of complex fractures.

Has other applications in child abuse; multiple injuries; soft-tissue, cranial, and spinal injuries.

Ultrasound

Time-consuming, but used increasingly for fractures (see above). Very good for evaluating associated soft-tissue injuries.

Follow-up Radiographs

Use judiciously. **Position check** at 4 days—alters treatment in only 20% of cases → use only for fractures prone to displacement (lateral humeral epicondyle, supracondylar fracture). X-ray 1 week after trauma only if swelling has completely subsided. Do additional position check in children > 12 years with diaphyseal fractures; later followups are pointless because fracture stable. Open reduction performed under general anesthesia and image intensifier/fluoroscopic control.
Check consolidation of:
- All fractures that were reduced
- Articular fractures
- All fractures expected to have consolidation problems
- Known axial malalignment

Image at 4 to 5 weeks. US can replace conventional radiographs for most follow-ups (axial malalignment, reliably distinguish between soft/hard callus).
Assess growth: clinically and by photographic documentation, not radiologically.

6.4   Nomenclature and Classification

Fracture classification during skeletal growth—complicated from diagnostic and therapeutic standpoints.

Special problems in children—bending fractures: buckle and greenstick fractures, shaft and epiphyseal fractures (Salter I–IV, Aitken I–III).

Epiphyseal injury (epiphysiolysis, **Fig. 6.3**). Classic classifications of **Salter-Harris** and **Aitken** (**Fig. 6.4**).

The **nomenclature system of the Li-La** ("Light and Laughter" for Sick Children, a non-profit organization for more effective, child-oriented pediatric health care) attempts to simplify and standardize classification of pediatric fractures; assigns fractures a numerical value that indicates a particular bone, a specific site in bone, articular involvement, fracture pattern, and degree of displacement (http://www.li-la.org).

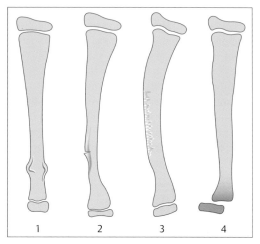

Fig. 6.3   Typical fractures in children. Buckle fracture (incomplete fracture) (1), greenstick fracture with cortical disruption on one side (incomplete fracture) (2), bending fracture (incomplete fracture) (3), and epiphysiolysis with or without epiphyseal displacement (4).

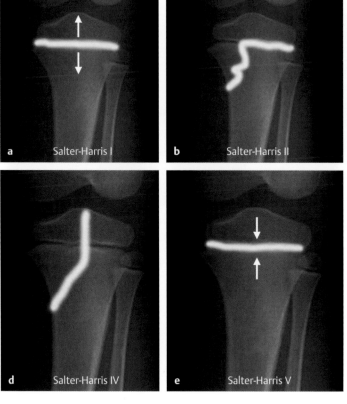

a   Salter-Harris I

b   Salter-Harris II

c   Salter-Harris III

d   Salter-Harris IV

e   Salter-Harris V

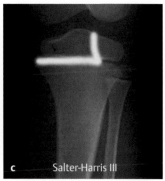

Fig. 6.4a–e   Salter-Harris classification of growth plate fractures.

a   Salter-Harris type I: transverse fracture through growth plate; width of growth plate is increased (direction of arrows).

b   Salter-Harris type II: runs through part of growth plate and continues along shaft.

c   Salter-Harris type III: runs through part of growth plate and continues into epiphysis.

d   Salter-Harris type IV: runs along shaft and epiphysis, crossing growth plate.

e   Salter-Harris type V: runs along growth plate, causing compression or crushing of plate (direction of arrows).

6

6.5   Frequency of Various Fractures in Children

Shaft fractures are 50 times more common than articular fractures. Most fractures involve metaphysis of upper limb. Shaft fractures also more common in upper limb; typical = forearm greenstick fracture. Common lower limb fractures = transverse femoral fracture and tibial torsion fracture.

Articular fractures are twice as common in upper limb as in lower limb. Typical fracture in upper limb = radial condyle fracture; in lower limb = fracture of medial malleolus. With open growth plates = fracture occurs not in weight-bearing zone but at joint margin (due to high flexibility). Fracture line in weight-bearing zone (transitional fracture) does not occur until adolescence, when growth plate is fused at its periphery.

Before 12 years of age, shaft fractures of upper limb more common than articular fractures, and ligament avulsions more common than midsubstance tears. Contusions and dislocations much rarer (exception: radial head dislocation at "sandbox" age; **Figs. 6.5, 6.6, 6.7, 6.8, 6.9, 6.10, 6.11, 6.12, 6.13**).

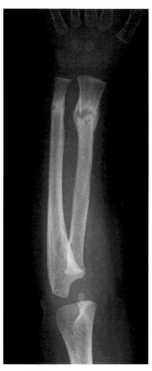

Fig. 6.5 Forearm fracture caused by fall onto hand. Survey radiograph after cast removal shows round "irritation callus." Note: irritation callus after treatment signals incomplete healing due to inadequate immobilization → high risk of refracture!

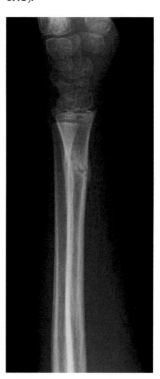

Fig. 6.6 Nonunion of arm fracture caused by fall onto hand during play. Survey radiograph. The nonunion has good prognosis for spontaneous healing.

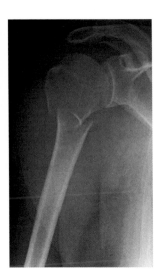

Fig. 6.7 Humeral fracture caused by fall from bicycle. Radiograph displays typical fracture of humeral shaft.

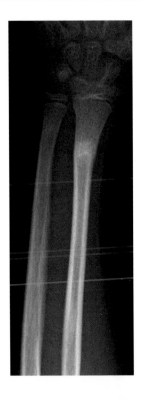

Fig. 6.8 Forearm fracture caused by fall onto hand. Radiograph shows buckle fracture without axial malalignment (common fracture in schoolchildren).

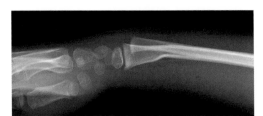

Fig. 6.9 Greenstick fracture caused by fall onto hand from playground equipment. Radiograph shows greenstick fracture with axial malalignment and cortical disruption on concave side.

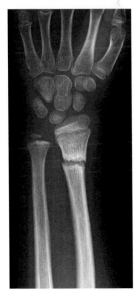

Fig. 6.10 Forearm fracture caused by fall from tree. Radiograph shows typical transverse fracture of radial shaft.

6

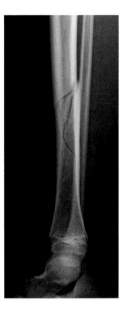

Fig. 6.11 Tibial fracture caused by one-legged jump onto uneven ground. Radiograph shows typical spiral fracture of tibial shaft.

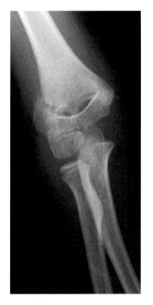

Fig. 6.12 Humeral fracture caused by diving into swimming pool. Radiograph shows fracture of radial condyle (if unclear, can usually be recognized in lateral view—if fracture line extends into growth plate). Note: growth plates start to close at about age 12 to 14. Comparison radiograph of opposite side is not indicated!

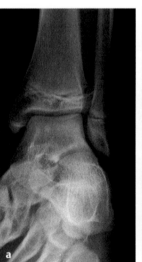
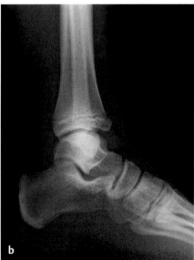
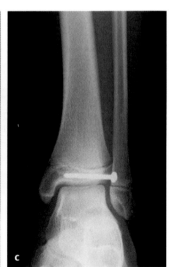

Fig. 6.13a–c Transitional fracture caused by skateboard injury. Survey radiographs in two planes.

a AP view = transitional fracture in adolescence occurs in weight-bearing zone due to incipient growth plate fusion.

b Lateral view = visible step-off in epiphysis is diagnostic.

c Treatment = screw fixation of epiphysis to prevent growth disturbance.

Cranial and Craniofacial Injuries

Injuries of skull and facial skeleton less common in children (except in child abuse), and imaging algorithm controversial.

Skull radiographs in two (or three) planes often ordered by trauma surgeons/pediatricians, but rejected by radiologists for several reasons: radiation risks, radiographs cannot exclude bleeding/contusion in absence of fracture, and fractures without neurologic symptoms have no treatment implications (**Figs. 6.14** and **6.15**).

Imaging algorithm: for head trauma (more differentiated in infants, see **Fig. 6.16**):

- Possible **indications for skull radiographs:** suspected impression fracture, child abuse, penetrating FB, subgaleal hematoma, third-party negligence, age 12 months or less.
- Multiple injuries, acute (moderately) severe head trauma/suspected basal skull fracture or midfacial fracture (only causes in children after severe motor vehicle accidents or fall from great height—much less common than in adults), acute neurologic symptoms → **CT**
- With protracted neurologic symptoms, follow-up → **MRI**
- **US** (using transtemporal approach): in first months of life detects subdural hemorrhage (SDH), epidural hemorrhage (EDH), intraventricular hemorrhage (IVH), intracerebral hemorrhage (ICH)
- Prompt/early detection of secondary CSF flow obstruction (see Sect. 4.2)

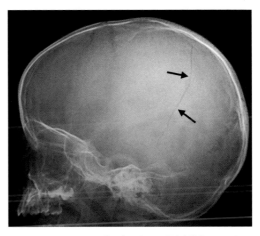

Fig. 6.14 Fracture of calvarium. Girl fell from swing, had no apparent neurologic abnormalities. Radiograph shows parietal lucent line (arrows) = skull fracture. Note: radiograph had no therapeutic implications.

Treatment: clinical observation—important for reasons that include possible lucid interval in children.

Findings:

- **US:** limited—reliable only during initial months (see Sect. 4.2)
- **CT:** ICH has same basic imaging features as in adults (**Fig. 6.17**). Not important to establish type (e.g., SDH or EDH), since same treatment (see also Sect. 6.10)

6

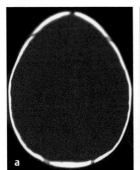
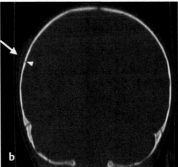
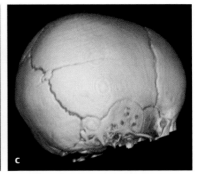

Fig. 6.15a–c Fracture of calvarium caused by falling from table. Unenhanced cranial CT with bone window. Axial reconstruction (**a**) with bone window shows no abnormalities. Coronal reconstruction (**b**) = subgaleal hematoma (arrow) and thin fracture line (arrowhead).

3D reconstruction (**c**) shows fracture line along axial reconstruction plane. No intracranial hemorrhage. Note: always review scout image to avoid missing a fracture that runs parallel to reconstructed image plane.

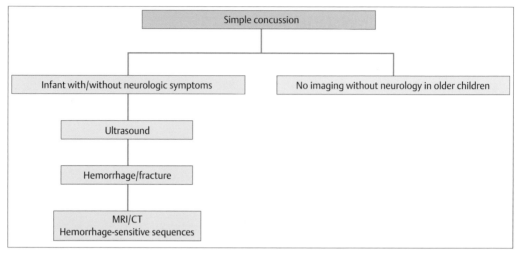

Fig. 6.16   Imaging algorithm for "simple" head trauma.

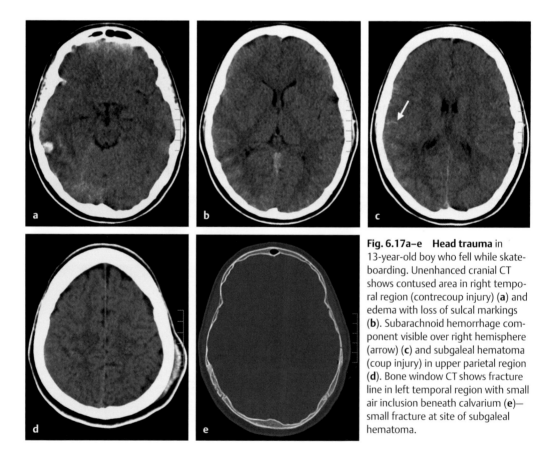

Fig. 6.17a–e   Head trauma in 13-year-old boy who fell while skateboarding. Unenhanced cranial CT shows contused area in right temporal region (contrecoup injury) (**a**) and edema with loss of sulcal markings (**b**). Subarachnoid hemorrhage component visible over right hemisphere (arrow) (**c**) and subgaleal hematoma (coup injury) in upper parietal region (**d**). Bone window CT shows fracture line in left temporal region with small air inclusion beneath calvarium (**e**)—small fracture at site of subgaleal hematoma.

Limitations in children: early stage of acute hemorrhage isodense to cortex → not visible on CT. Physiologically small extra-axial CSF spaces can mask hemorrhage. SDH may be isodense to CSF earlier than in adults

- **MRI** in head trauma—see Sect. 6.10

6.7   Spinal Injuries

Vertebral fractures in growing skeleton very rare. Thoracic spine most commonly affected, followed by lumbar spine. Cervical injuries least common. Exception: dens fracture (**Fig. 6.18**).

Due to high elasticity of pediatric skeleton, the most common spinal injuries are vertebral body compression fractures with anterior wedging and Chance fractures (spinal flexion injury).

Diagnosis: based on radiographs in two planes, anterior wedging of vertebral body in lateral projection (**Fig. 6.19**).

Differentiation from congenital deformity (Scheuermann disease) may be difficult. Diagnosis easy if anterior vertebral body height reduced by > 20%. With more subtle changes: determine ratio of anterior edge height to posterior edge height (abnormal if < 0.95 or > 3 segments), use scintigraphy (at least 48 hours after injury).

Presence of neurologic symptoms → evaluate by sectional imaging (CT for fracture investigation, MRI for cord symptoms and other neurology).

> **!** Caution: intraspinal/epidural hemorrhage!

Possible future options for functional MRI = fiber tracking and tensor diffusion imaging.

> Note: in preschool and school-age children, cervical spine often has physiologic step-off at C2-C3. Dens fractures easily missed on X-ray films → MRI or CT. Functional radiographs of cervical spine obsolete and deceiving → MRI better for ligament injuries.

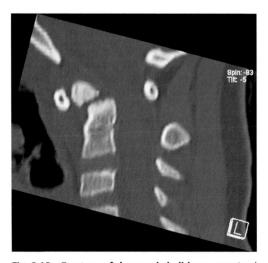

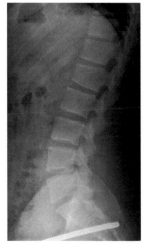

Fig. 6.18   Fracture of dens and skull base, sustained by back-seat child passenger in rear-end collision. Unenhanced cranial CT. Sagittal image reconstructed from low-dose CT shows displaced dens fracture (not visible on plain radiographs—cranial CT indicated for severe injury, also revealed basal skull fracture).

Fig. 6.19   Vertebral body compression fracture caused by fall during rollerblading. Lateral radiograph shows anterior wedging of L1 vertebral body (= compression fracture). Rest of spine appears normal, excluding congenital deformity.

6

6.8   Visceral Injuries and Children in Emergency Room

General: important to use child-appropriate algorithms in emergency room (ER) → develop, establish, and apply. Key concern is radiation safety (ALARA principle) = establish low-dose CT protocols, avoid unnecessary imaging (see Sect. 1.5). Note: differences in various countries based on local needs and jurisdiction.

Children more likely than adults to sustain craniofacial injuries in multiple trauma, also blunt abdominal injuries and vertebral injuries (seat belt) in motor-vehicle accidents. Thoracic injuries and injuries to long tubular bones less common because children's bones more pliable. Important aspects:

- **Different circulatory physiology in children:** blood vessels smaller, have greater capacity for vasoconstriction—bleeding may stop spontaneously, less frequent need for surgery → spleen and liver injuries more often amenable to conservative treatment

> ! Children may remain clinically stable for some time after serious injury, but may then decompensate very quickly.

- **Compensated shock in hemodynamically stable children:** hypoperfusion complex/hypovolemia syndrome—typical CT features (**Fig. 6.20**):
  - Inhomogeneous contrast enhancement of parenchymal organs, often with zones of complete ischemia
  - Small-caliber aorta and vena cava
  - Threadlike visceral branches from aorta
  - Hyperperfused adrenal glands and intestinal mucosa
  - Other unexplained free fluid

> ! Some children are still hemodynamically stable when typical CT signs of decompensation already present—poor prognosis warrants immediate treatment!

Emergency Room Management

Foremost principle = stabilize. Imaging evaluation of pediatric ER patients (**Fig. 6.21**) often starts with chest radiographs and **US** (**FAST** = focused abdominal sonography for trauma).

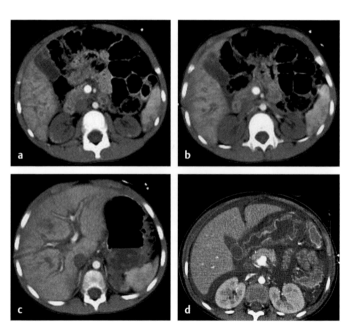

Fig. 6.20a–d Hypovolemia syndrome following motor-vehicle accident. Evaluated with CT protocol for multiple injuries. Axial scans show threadlike vessels with decreased blood flow to abdominal organs (here kidney—caution: not ruptured, although blood flow decreased), periportal fluid tracking, and adrenal hypervascularity (**a–c**). Axial CT in different patient (**d**) shows increased enhancement of intestinal mucosa. Typical features of hypovolemia syndrome.

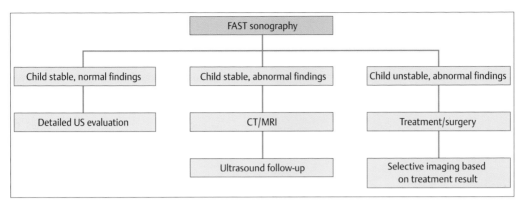

Fig. 6.21 Algorithm for pediatric patients in the emergency room.

But: FAST has not been adequately evaluated in children; significance of free fluid differs from adults. Sites of predilection for free fluid: perisplenic, perirenal, subhepatic, retroperitoneal (cul-de-sac) = evidence of parenchymal injury.

Nevertheless, use CT sparingly in children → use US whenever possible: parenchymal evaluation, free fluid—where, how, much, etc. US follow-up should be done by the same examiner if possible, but always by somebody experienced in pediatric US.

CT of multiple injuries: match protocol to child (age/weight); coverage should include skull, chest, abdomen, and whole spinal column (with image reconstructions in two planes). Spiral MDCT recommended. Also important to use soft-tissue and lung windows, obtain multiplanar reconstructions of skull (and facial skeleton) → pelvic radiograph not essential. Separate review of scout image helpful. Try to reduce number of phases—i.e., head = unenhanced scan, chest with cervical spine and upper abdomen (large vessels) = arterial phase, abdomen and pelvis = late parenchymal phase. Use delay triggering for arterial phase; some recommend split bolus technique. CT-cystography very unusual in childhood!

MRI = another option in stable patients—consider transport risk and logistical problems; special indications (cord injury, etc.; see Sect. 1.6).

Typical Patterns of Injury

Thoracic trauma: most common in multiple injuries due to motor vehicle accidents. Contusions (bleeding and edema in alveoli and interstitium) and lacerations (tissue tears). Rib fractures less common (higher elasticity). Thoracic injuries often missed or underestimated on X-ray films → evaluate by CT! Typical findings:

- Posterior location (posterior rib fractures, injuries close to spinal column)
- 50% curvilinear, 45% amorphous
- Combination of confluent patchy and nodular opacities
- Sparing of subpleural space; "hyperinflated" layer 1–2 mm wide between consolidation and adjacent chest wall

Pulmonary lacerations often associated with single/multiple pneumatoceles; may show air–fluid levels and hematoma—up to 4 months after trauma.

Blunt abdominal trauma: more common in boys, two age peaks: 6 to 8 years and 14 to 16 years. Thoracic cage more pliable = less protection for abdominal organs located at less protected sites.

- **Spleen** most commonly affected, sometimes (early posttraumatic period) cannot be evaluated with US → contrast-enhanced US, CT, or MRI (**Fig. 6.22**). Grading and appearance/findings same as in adults. Management much more conservative. Posttraumatic aneurysms and arteriovenous fistulas may occur
- **Pancreatic rupture** and cyst formation (pancreatic duct injury, **Fig. 6.23**) often caused by bicy-

6

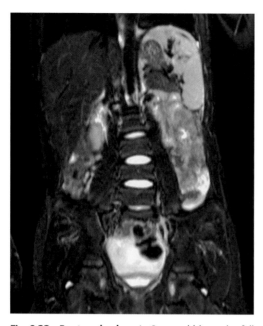

Fig. 6.22 Ruptured spleen in 8-year-old boy who fell from roof. Initial US scans = no detectable splenic lesion. Later scans showed increasing free fluid, ↓ general status → MRI (coronal, T2-weighted). Subcapsular splenic rupture has low T1- and T2-weighted signal intensity (old blood). Free fluid in lesser pelvis.

cle handlebar impact—only external signs are small bruises, but visceral injury common → always evaluate at least with detailed US and re-examine at 24 hours

- **Renal injury:** suggestive US signs—perirenal/subcapsular fluid, inhomogeneous perirenal tissue, free fluid in lesser pelvis

> (Power) Doppler important for early posttraumatic assessment of renal vascularity and hematoma detection. Avulsion of renal vascular pedicle = parenchyma initially appears normal; fresh hematoma = US appearance similar to renal parenchyma!

> **!** Caution: potential for bladder/ureteral injury.

CT—can also assess function (IVP very rarely indicated). Delayed scans (low dose) to check for bladder or ureteral injury only if highly supected. Grading same as in adults.

- **Seat belt injuries** in motor-vehicle accidents: spinal injury → CT
- **Hollow viscus injury:** associated injuries in 54%. Imaging detection difficult in early phase; air/free fluid not always present! Follow-up essential.

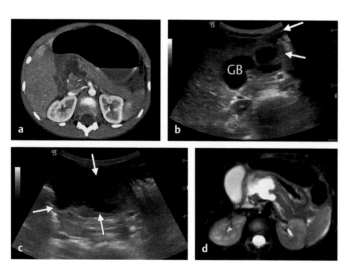

Fig. 6.23a–d Pancreatic trauma caused by fall from bicycle. CT, US, and MRI. Initial diagnosis on CT = pancreatic rupture (**a**). Subsequent US (**b, c**) shows expanding pseudo-cyst → MRI (**d**). Dilatation of pancreatic duct, enlargement of cyst. Outcome: full recovery with conservative treatment. GB, gallbladder.

6.9 Sports-Related Injuries and Chronic Trauma

Almost any injury in growth period is "sports-related injury." Typical sports-related injuries of ligaments, menisci, and cartilage are less common than generally assumed. Meniscal tears are very rare, commonly misinterpreted. Cruciate ligament tears also rare.

> Type I/II meniscal tears on MRI are usually normal finding in children!

More common fibulotalar ligament injury: open growth plates = usually bony avulsion, detectable on radiographs. < 12 years = ligament usually intact, > 12 years = ligament itself injured. With increasing growth plate closure → MRI in children with equivocal clinical findings.

Traumatic cartilage lesions = osteochondral fractures (flake fractures): detectable by MRI, full extent definable only by arthroscopy.

Patellar dislocation most common in young girls with hypoplastic, high-riding patella (patella alta). Diagnosed clinically. Radiographs serve only to exclude associated bony injury after reduction (osteochondral fracture → MRI/arthroscopy). Almost always associated with tear of medial retinaculum—does not require imaging.

6.10 Child Abuse

NAI = nonaccidental injury = battered child syndrome.

Radiology has significant role, especially in cases with subtle outward signs. The broad definition of "child abuse" is often surprising to parents and caregivers; explains high percentage of unreported cases.

Most commonly affected age group = children from birth to 3 years of age (55% < 1 year). Main perpetrators are parents and close relatives.

Signs and symptoms: Two main diagnostic groups:
- Soft-tissue and skeletal injuries = battered child syndrome
- CNS trauma due to shaking = shaken baby syndrome (often fatal or with neurologic deficit)

Imaging recommendations are broadly similar in most countries (check national guidelines if in doubt). Primary goal: noninvasive, minimal radiation burden to provide highest diagnostic yield at acceptable cost (**Figs. 6.24** and **6.25**).

Typical Fractures in Child Abuse

Metaphyseal fracture: caused by traumatizing force close to a joint—most commonly involves distal femur, proximal tibia, and fibula. Curvilinear transepiphyseal fracture (appearing on X-ray as thin lucent line along edge of metaphysis) = bucket-handle fracture (**Fig. 6.26**).

Diaphyseal fracture: most commonly affects femur, less commonly humerus and tibia. Transverse and spiral patterns common. Spiral fractures suggestive of abuse in children < 1 year; accidental diaphyseal fractures extremely rare < 2 years. Fractures of long tubular bones (especially humerus: oblique, spiral, or transverse fracture) in children < 3 years are suspicious for abuse. Finger and hand fractures suggestive of severe abuse.

> Exception: Toddler's fracture = accidental spiral tibial fracture in children just learning to walk.

Less impact on diaphysis—no fracture, only periosteal hematoma → not detectable on plain radiographs initially, only after incipient calcification (~ 10–14 days after trauma). Initial US can detect hematoma (bordering on bone).

Rib fractures: highly specific for child abuse, especially due to violent shaking → posterior rib fractures (never occur during cardiopulmonary resuscitation—pressure to anterior chest may fracture ribs in anterior axillary line). As a rule, rib fractures first detected in healing stage; presentation with fractures of different ages considered proof of child abuse. Oblique radiographs yield higher detection rate; some advocate low-dose chest CT.

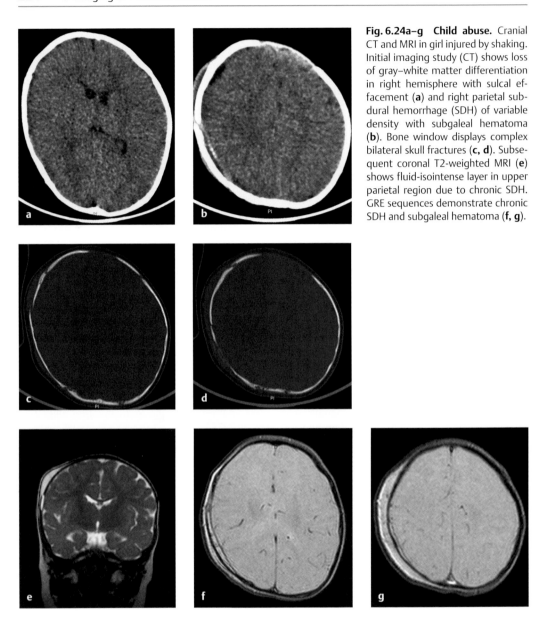

Fig. 6.24a–g Child abuse. Cranial CT and MRI in girl injured by shaking. Initial imaging study (CT) shows loss of gray–white matter differentiation in right hemisphere with sulcal effacement (**a**) and right parietal subdural hemorrhage (SDH) of variable density with subgaleal hematoma (**b**). Bone window displays complex bilateral skull fractures (**c, d**). Subsequent coronal T2-weighted MRI (**e**) shows fluid-isointense layer in upper parietal region due to chronic SDH. GRE sequences demonstrate chronic SDH and subgaleal hematoma (**f, g**).

Spinal injuries: rare, usually caused by shaking trauma = ligament tears, compression fractures, fractures, episural hematoma, and dislocations of facet joints.

Determination of Fracture Age

One of primary tasks in (pediatric) radiology is determination of fracture age. Metaphyseal injuries, complete fractures, and epiphyseal separations can be detected immediately after trauma; other injuries may be first identified in healing stage owing to associated callus. Estimation of fracture age is helpful in confirming abuse. Chronological guidelines are shown in **Table 6.1**.

Table 6.1 Chronological guidelines for estimating fracture age

Periosteal reaction	10–21 days
Indistinct fracture line (sclerosis)	10–14 days
Soft callus	14–21 days
Hard callus	21–90 days
Remodeling	3 months to several years

Specificity of Fractures in Child Abuse

High specificity: metaphyseal fractures, posterior rib and sternal fractures, clavicular fractures in infants, spinous process fractures, complex skull fractures, fractures of different ages.
Moderate specificity: bilateral fractures—also of different ages. Vertebral body fractures, digital fractures.

When Should Something Be Done?

Identification of child abuse—an interdisciplinary process, requires close cooperation of all physicians involved. Following situations considered suspicious for child abuse:
- Vague or contradictory history
- Long delay between injury and doctor visit
- Dehydrated and emaciated child (neglected appearance)
- Radiologic findings more serious than expected
- Known abuse of siblings
- Failure to thrive, (unexplained) scalds, burns

Radiologic survey by trained and experienced personnel should follow standard protocol (no "cloak and dagger" operations). With clinical suspicion late at night → admit child as inpatient, obtain photographic documentation if needed, and investigate next day.

Imaging Algorithm

In **children < 1 year of age:**
- Skeletal status including large joints (individual images, not "babygram"); good resolution—for detection of metaphyseal injuries

  - AP chest, lateral spine (may add AP view), oblique rib views if required
  - Long tubular bones = arms and legs, AP plus lateral (especially with apparent abnormalities)
- Skull in two planes, required in addition to CT (current neurology)
- Abdominal (and cranial) US; abdominal/pelvic radiographs if required
- CT/MRI of neurocranium (see below)

In **older children:**
- Any clinically suspicious area
- Commonly affected regions (fractures of different ages?)
- Skeletal scintigraphy
- AP chest radiograph
- CT/MRI—depending on (neurologic) presentation and availability
  - Role of whole body MRI yet undefined
  - Postmortem imaging rather alternative to nonforensic autopsy, may become more important in future (as already used in some countries)

Differential Diagnosis of Child Abuse

- Multiple fractures: osteogenesis imperfecta (characterized by marked osteopenia)
- Metaphyseal lesions: congenital syphilis
- Periosteal hemorrhage: scurvy
- Cortical hyperostosis: Caffey syndrome
- Other: osteomyelitis, analgesic syndrome (very rare)

Head Trauma in Child Abuse

High morbidity and mortality rates. Caused by shaking, blows to head, throwing against stable objects (**Fig. 6.25**).

Pediatric brain especially vulnerable—greater fluid content, brain immature and nonmyelinated, open cranial sutures → increased mobility.

6

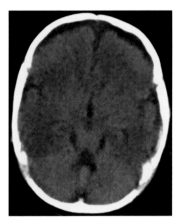

Fig. 6.25   Shaking trauma. Unenhanced CT scan after multiple shaking episodes shows enlarged subarachnoid spaces, loss of gray-white matter differentiation, and reversal of normal gray-white matter densities (reversal sign) with hyperattenuating cerebellum. Outcome: infant died from injuries.

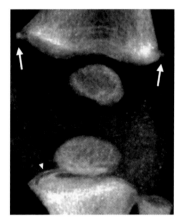

Fig. 6.26   Child abuse. Radiograph shows metaphyseal corner fragments (arrows), often visible only after callus formation, and transepiphyseal fracture (arrowhead). Fractures near joints typical manifestations of child abuse.

Effects of head trauma:

- Cerebral hemorrhage: usually SDH, EDH (near fracture site), occasionally SAH
- Retinal hemorrhage: characteristic of shaking trauma → always order an ophthalmologic examination in suspected child abuse
- Calvarial fractures: usually multiple, complex; bilateral and impression fractures
- Parenchymal lesions: usually dramatic; axonal damage (shearing injury) involving long tracts → paralysis; at gray-white matter junction → atrophy and loss of substance

- Brain edema: after hypoxia → ischemia, increased intracranial pressure, hyperemia, secondary (hemorrhagic) infarction, herniation, atrophy. Combination of brain edema and IVH/SAH is usually fatal

Imaging: X-rays and US limited → CT, or preferably MRI, can differentiate hematomas of different ages, CSF flow obstruction and herniation (**Fig. 6.26**).

> GRE and FLAIR sequences (MRI) better than SE sequences for detecting blood/blood breakdown products; potentially add DWI; always include susceptibility weighted sequence such as GRE or FFE.

6.11   Obstetric Trauma

Occurs in 1–2% of all births.

Diaphyseal fractures most common (in order of frequency: clavicle, humerus, femoral shaft).

Skull: impression fracture (greenstick fracture—periosteum intact).

Suspected obstetric trauma always requires detailed clinical examination (swelling, crepitation, hematoma, limited motion, pain on passive motion, pseudoparalysis, etc.).

Cervical plexus lesions and avulsions may be associated with significant nerve damage and protracted clinical course. Most severe trauma = cervical cord injury: complete cord lesion with paralysis—extremely rare.

Imaging: plain radiographs (soft-tissue swelling, joint space narrowing), targeted US (better for epiphysiolysis)—epiphyseal separations rare and difficult to detect (identify quickly and reduce at once to avoid growth disturbance).

Cervical cord injury and plexus injuries: bedside US (requires experienced examiner) supplemented by MRI including myelographic sequences—use high resolution and compare sides—coverage should extend to clavicle!

6.12   Intraocular Foreign Bodies

Intraocular FBs not uncommon, have variable consistency and opacity = rarely diagnosed on **radiographs** unless radiopaque objects.

Sectional imaging modalities much more sensitive—US can detect 95% of intraocular FBs (posttraumatic imaging limited by swelling, pain, and age-dependent tolerance for US examination). Treatment depends more on accurate localization than detection → CT (most commonly recommended in literature).

MRI = excellent alternative (radiation safety)—especially given reports that MRI can detect ferromagnetic FBs based on susceptibility artifacts (not always detectable by US or CT).

Case Study 6.1

History: Teenager injured in moped accident—admitted to ER with diffuse abdominal pain and small bruises. Rapid urine test positive for red cells.
Acute imaging modalities in this setting? Initial detailed US with serial examinations. Further investigation by spiral MDCT; possible late or delayed abdominal radiographs. Angiography occasionally used for potential interventional therapy (vascular injury—embolization, recanalization, etc.).

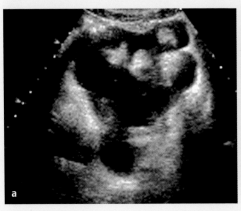 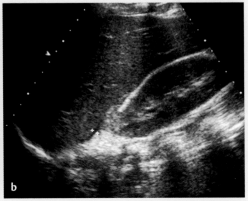

Fig. 6.27a–f

continued ▶

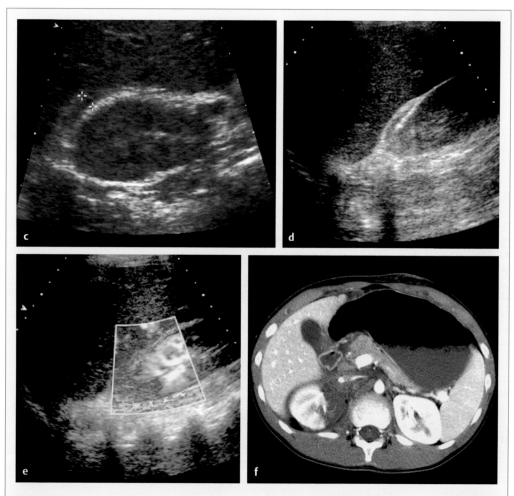

Fig. 6.27a–f

Available images: relevant early (**a–c**) and late (**d, e**) US scans, latter using power Doppler; also axial CT.
Findings: free intraperitoneal fluid in lower abdomen (**a**), thin fluid layer in Morison pouch (++) with slightly ill-defined outlines of upper pole of right kidney, which has somewhat atypical structure (**b** longitudinal scan, **c** transverse scan through right upper abdomen). Latter findings usually displayed better by high-resolution US (**d**), with power Doppler showing regional perfusion abnormality at upper pole (**e**). Note relatively poor B-mode visualization of renal laceration at this early posttraumatic stage! Abdominal contrast-enhanced spiral MDCT confirms finding (**f**).
Diagnosis: free intraperitoneal fluid due to renal laceration/rupture, with capsular tear, at upper pole of right kidney.
Additional tests: contrast-enhanced spiral MDCT if required (therapeutic implications? signs of other injuries? severe trauma/multiple injuries?), may include delayed images (contrast extravasation from renal pelvis?). (With kind permission of M. Riccabona, Graz, Austria.)

7 The Pediatric Musculoskeletal System

Peter Waibel, Kathrin Maurer

7.1 Normal Skeleton and Variants

Radiographic Morphology of Normal Bone Structure

X-rays almost completely attenuated by cortical (compact) bone. Cancellous (trabecular) bone faintly visible only at bone ends or when amount increased. Bony canals for nutrient vessels = sharply defined tubular defects with sclerotic margins.

Growth and Development

Developing fetus has cartilaginous skeleton at end of 2 months. Long bones have their primary ossification centers at midshaft. Secondary ossification centers are located in epiphyses. Neurocranium and viscerocranium formed mainly by membranous ossification. Bone growth is individualized process in every child. Age- and gender-specific bone lengths—comprehensive tables (Maresh 1955). Assessment of skeletal maturity based on longitudinal studies → atlases by Greulich and Pyle (1959) and Tanner et al. (1975)—determination of biological age, prediction of adult height.

Anatomic Variants

Anatomic variants can mimic proliferative and/or destructive lesions. If uncertainty exists—bone scintigraphy/MRI. Projection artifacts can simulate pathology, e.g., Mach band effect (= perceived accentuation of interfaces with abrupt change from dark to light → apparent fracture). Pseudosclerosis —caused by superimposed shadows and summation effects from bony structures.

Skull, Paranasal Sinuses

Formed by membranous ossification. Wormian bones = accessory bones, may have pathognomonic significance (e.g., osteogenesis imperfecta). Some named (e.g., Inca bone). Parietal foramina = areas of delayed ossification.

Hand and Wrist

- Sclerotic epiphyses = **"ivory epiphyses"** (distal phalanges and middle phalanx of fifth finger)
- **Cone-shaped epiphyses** = single/multiple, distal phalanx of thumb/middle phalanx of small finger (shortened, **Fig. 7.1**). Coning has pathologic significance when proximal phalanges/middle phalanx of third/fourth finger affected

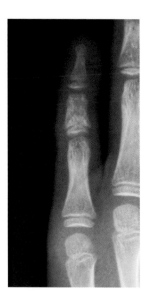

Fig. 7.1 Cone-shaped epiphyses. Radiograph of hand—fifth ray. Middle phalanx of fifth finger has cone-shaped epiphysis.

7

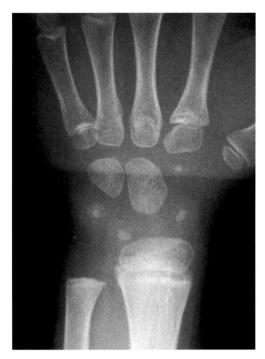

Fig. 7.2   Pseudoepiphyses. Hand radiograph for determining skeletal age in 10-year-old boy, incidentally shows partial pseudoepiphyses of second, third, and fifth metacarpals. Skeletal age dissociated: carpal 6 years, distal radioulnar 5 years.

- Accessory ossification centers: not uncommon, may appear in proximal second through fifth metacarpals and distal first metacarpal
- Pseudoepiphyses (**Fig. 7.2**)
- Carpal bones may ossify in irregular pattern due to multiple ossification centers. Approximately 25 accessory ossification centers known to occur in hand as normal variants
- Fusion = result of early embryonic segmentation disorder; lunate and triquetrum most commonly affected
- Sesamoid bones = formed by ossification of tendon attachments (first metacarpophalangeal joint—11th year in girls, 13th year in boys)

Forearm, Elbow, Shoulder

- Ulnar and radial styloid processes—often arise from separate ossification centers

Ulnar styloid process: difficult/sometimes impossible to distinguish from older fractures on ulnar side.

- Ossification centers in elbow joint—order of appearance follows timetable (capitellum → radial head → medial epicondyle → trochlea → olecranon → lateral epicondyle)

Accessory ossicles very rare, difficult to diagnose—virtually identical to intra-articular osteochondral fragments.

- Supracondylar process—bony remnant of supernumerary portion of pronator teres: do not mistake for osteochondroma (see **Fig. 7.65**)

! Tent-shaped epiphyseal plate of proximal humerus can mimic fracture line in certain projections.

Thorax

Frequent anomalies = bifid/double ribs, pseudarthrosis with adjacent ribs (**Fig. 7.3**). (3D)US may be an option to improve visualization of cartilaginous parts.

Pelvis, Femur

Typical male–female differences first appear during puberty. Accessory ossification centers most common at acetabular rim. Ossification of ischiopubic synchondrosis highly variable. Fusion on both sides may be complete by age 3 years. Up to half of all children over 6 years of age have bilateral swelling (**Fig. 7.4**) without pathologic significance. Ossification center for femoral head appears in fourth month of life; may have irregular, coarse granular appearance until second year of life (see **Meyer dysplasia**, p. 249). Diaphyseal periosteal reaction—adaptive response in infants and small children.

Incidental finding: well-circumscribed, elliptical osteolytic zones often found on back of femur = **fibrous cortical defect/nonossifying fibroma** (**Fig. 7.5**).

Multiple mineralization centers in distal femoral epiphyses, usually on medial side, most pronounced in preschoolers. Older children may have apparent defects in lateral border of femoral condyle due to irregular ossification (may resemble osteochondritis dissecans) (**Fig. 7.6**).

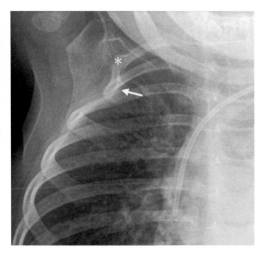

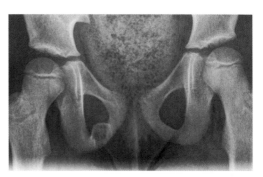

Fig. 7.4 Normal variants of ischiopubic synchondrosis. Pelvic radiograph of large, unilateral ischiopubic synchondrosis in a 6-year-old girl.

Fig. 7.3 Pseudarthrosis. Chest radiograph shows two-part first rib with pseudarthrosis (*) and neoarticulation with second rib (arrow).

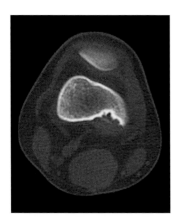

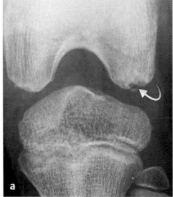

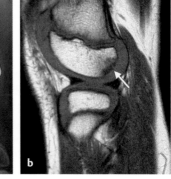

Fig. 7.5 Cortical defect. CT of distal femur shows irregular cortical defect with sclerotic margins of posteromedial femoral metaphysis.

Fig. 7.6a, b Tunnel view radiograph and sagittal MRI of knee.
a Atypical osseous defect in posterolateral femoral condyle of 10-year-old boy. Cause: delayed ossification.
b Unenhanced T1-weighted MRI shows hypointense tissue posterior to weight-bearing zone.

7

Knee, Tibia, Foot

- Patella: largest sesamoid bone in body, located in quadriceps tendon; different ossification centers and segmentation patterns (bipartite patella) are common
- Fabella: inconstant sesamoid bone in lateral head of gastrocnemius muscle

- Ossification centers for tibial tuberosity—extremely variable; diagnose aseptic necrosis only with associated soft-tissue swelling and clinical manifestations
- Cortical defects in tibia and fibula are common
- Separate ossification centers for medial malleolus—common, require differentiation from fracture fragments (**Fig. 7.7**)

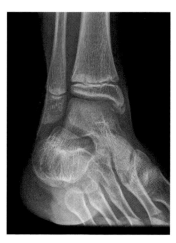

Fig. 7.7   Ossification variants in distal tibial epiphysis. AP radiograph of ankle joint shows multiple ossification centers in medial malleolus.

- Physiologic genua vara (bowlegs): normal bone structure in respect of child's age; tibiofemoral angle: infants = 17 degrees, first year = 9 degrees; mild varus < 11 degrees by third year. Normalizes by adolescence
- Foot: numerous accessory ossification centers/ sesamoids and cone-shaped epiphyses. Best known = **os tibiale externum (cornuate navicular** after growth is complete)

> Ossification of navicular bone is irregular, has physiologically late onset.

7.2   Regional Skeletal Malformations, Abnormalities of Bone Shape and Arrangement

Lower Limb

Proximal Femoral Focal Deficiency

PFFD has broad spectrum—from mild hypoplasia of femur and acetabulum to complete femoral aplasia. Often combined with ipsilateral changes such as fibular hemimelia, foot anomalies (pes equinovarus; **Fig. 7.8**).

Fibular Hemimelia

Isolated lesion/combined with PFFD. Ranges from mild hypoplasia to complete absence of fibula. Association with tibial shortening, postaxial aplasia of toes, patellar dysplasia, agenesis of anterior cruciate ligaments.

Tibial Hemimelia

Ranges from mild hypoplasia to complete absence of tibia (may appear as fibrous cord on MRI).

Tibial Pseudarthrosis

Spectrum from bowing to true pseudarthrosis (Crawford types I–IV). High incidence of neurofibromatosis type I in pronounced forms (**Fig. 7.9**)!

Tarsal Coalition

Failure of segmentation of primitive mesenchyme in developing foot. Important: differentiate from syndesmosis, synchondrosis, and synostosis. Most common forms: **talocalcaneal and calcaneonavicular coalition** (**Fig. 7.10**). Imaging depends on age and type of tissue → oblique radiographs can detect osseous calcaneonavicular coalition in adolescents; subtalar and fibrous coalitions best demonstrated by MRI.

Ball-and-Socket Talus

Usually sporadic occurrence.

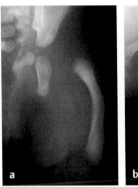

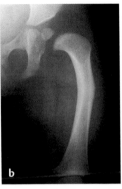

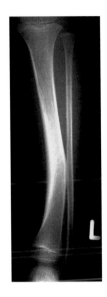

Fig. 7.9 Congenital tibial pseudarthrosis, Crawford type II. Radiograph of left lower leg shows varus angulation. Associated with increased fracture risk during first years of life.

Fig. 7.8a, b Proximal femoral focal deficiency. Thigh radiographs shows shortening and varus deviation of left proximal femur at birth (**a**) and 3 years later, after lengthening (**b**).

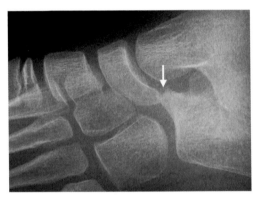

Fig. 7.10 Calcaneonavicular coalition. Radiograph of tarsal bones shows subtotal osseous fusion (arrow).

Anomalous Arrangement of Bones in Foot

- **Clubfoot** (pes equinovarus): common congenital anomaly, isolated/combined (intrauterine crowding?). Lateral radiograph of foot leads to parallel arrangement of talus and calcaneus (**Fig. 7.11**)
- **Pes planus** (flat foot): usually results from neuromuscular disease. Axis between talus and calcaneus > 60 degrees in lateral projection
- **Pes cavus** (high arch): extreme posterior angulation of calcaneus, plantar flexion of metatarsus

7

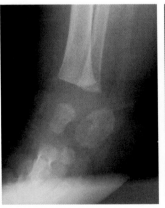

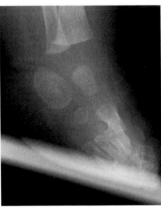

Fig. 7.11 Pes equinovarus (clubfoot). Radiographs of both feet. Lateral projection shows parallel arrangement of talus and calcaneus.

Upper Limb

Radioulnar Synostosis

Failure of longitudinal segmentation. Restricted range of pronation, no supination. Rare cases are syndromic/combined with hand anomalies.

Congenital Dislocation of Radial Head

Isolated/syndromic. Isolated dislocation usually autosomal dominant. Radial head small and elongated; unilateral/bilateral (**Fig. 7.12**).

Radial Aplasia

Ranges from hypoplastic thumb to complete absence of radius. Valgus and palmar deviation of hand due to muscular traction. Entire forearm shortened. Occasional absence of first ray and associated carpal bones. Bilateral in up to 50% of cases.

Possible associations: Fanconi anemia, TAR syndrome (thrombocytopenia with absent radius), Cornelia de Lange syndrome, VACTERL association, etc.

Ulnar Aplasia

Much rarer than radial aplasia. Most cases sporadic, 25% bilateral. Concomitant postaxial hand deformities (carpal, metacarpal, phalangeal). Elbow anomalies common (radiohumeral fusion).

Carpal Fusion

Most common between lunate and triquetral bones.

> **!** Caution: carpal fusion possible in rheumatoid arthritis.

Syndactyly

Fusion of adjacent fingers. May involve soft tissues alone or soft tissues and bone. Isolated/syndromic.

Symphalangism

Fusion of interphalangeal joints. Autosomal dominant inheritance.

Clinodactyly

Valgus/varus curvature of fingers, most commonly affecting distal fifth interphalangeal joint. Combined with shortening of middle phalanx (**brachymesophalanx**). Usually sporadic; may also be syndromic or posttraumatic.

Kirner Deformity

Palmar flexion of distal fifth phalanx with normal alignment of epiphysis (sporadic, may be inherited as autosomal dominant trait) (**Fig. 7.13**).

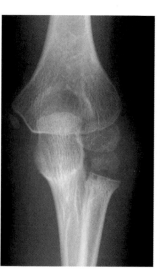 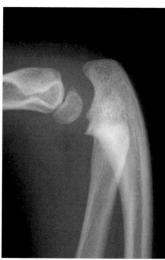

Fig. 7.12 Congenital dislocation of radial head. Elbow radiograph shows abnormal shape of radial head due to absence of articulation.

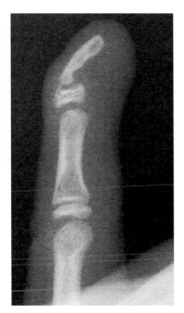

Fig. 7.13 Kirner deformity. Radiograph of small finger shows palmar flexion of distal fifth phalanx with normal alignment of epiphysis.

Regional Malformations

Congenital Annular Constrictions (Amniotic Bands)

Pathogenesis unclear. Theory: fetal body parts snared by loose amniotic and chorionic strands. Amputation possible in severe cases, hypoplasia in milder cases. High association with (soft-tissue) syndactyly (**Fig. 7.14**).

Arthrogryposis

Main radiologic sign = congenital contractures. Associated with other malformations (e.g., hip dysplasia, clubfoot). Arthrogryposis = descriptive diagnosis, not an etiology! Lower limbs predominantly affected. Muscles may be partially replaced by connective tissue.

Neurofibromatosis

Musculoskeletal changes correspond to mesodermal dysplasia. Most common spinal manifestation = scoliosis (see Sect. 7.4). Other features: leg length discrepancy, various forms of tibial pseudar-

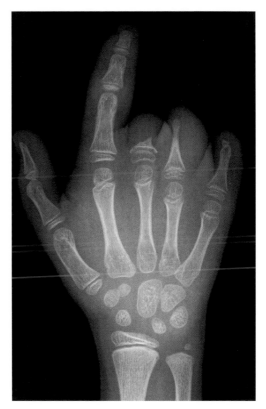

Fig. 7.14 Congenital annular constriction. Radiograph of right hand documents partial amputation of phalangeal segments combined with syndactyly.

throsis, multiple fibromas, and neurofibromas. Possible bone erosion, depending on site of involvement. See Sect. 4.1 for neuroradiologic aspects.

VACTERL/VATER Association

Musculoskeletal findings include vertebral anomalies, radial hypoplasia/aplasia, rib anomalies, hip dysplasia, tibial/fibular aplasia, vertical talus, PFFD. Other features described in Sect. 2.5 and Chapter 3.

Benign Bone Tumors, Tumorlike Changes

See also Sect. 8.6.

Approximately 50% of all bone neoplasms in children are benign, many have typical imaging features. Differentiation of benign from malignant

7

not always possible. Biologic aggressiveness can be roughly assessed with Lodwick classification. Projection radiographs should always be taken before any further (imaging) investigation.

Osteochondroma

Not true neoplasm, but developmental abnormality of metaphyseal bone. Bone forms cartilage-capped outgrowth with continuity of cancellous and cortical bone. May be sessile or pedunculated. Longitudinal axis always points away from joint. May occur anywhere, except on bone formed by membranous ossification (**Fig. 7.15**).

Osteochondroma may be secondary to irradiation. Multiple outgrowths have autosomal dominant inheritance.

Enchondroma

Typically occurs in shafts of short tubular hand bones. Appears as well-circumscribed round or spindle-shaped osteolytic area (Lodwick IA or IB), often with matrix calcifications.

Simple Bone Cyst

Fluid-filled cavity = lytic bone lesion with septation (Lodwick IA).
Sites of occurrence: metaphysis of long tubular bones; rare occurrence in pelvis/axial skeleton.

Usually detected incidentally or in association with fracture (**Fig. 7.16**).

Aneurysmal Bone Cyst

Eccentric osteolytic lesion that grows by expansion. May be primary or secondary.
Sites of occurrence: facial bones, vertebral elements, metaphyses of tubular bones.
CT/MRI: Fluid level due to sedimentation of blood breakdown products. May show signs of increased biologic activity—requires differentiation from telangiectatic osteosarcoma.

> Rare solid variant indistinguishable from an aggressive solid tumor.

Nonossifying Fibroma

Lodwick IA. Osteolytic lesion of large tubular bones in children. Corresponds biologically to persistent cortical defect (see Sect. 7.1).

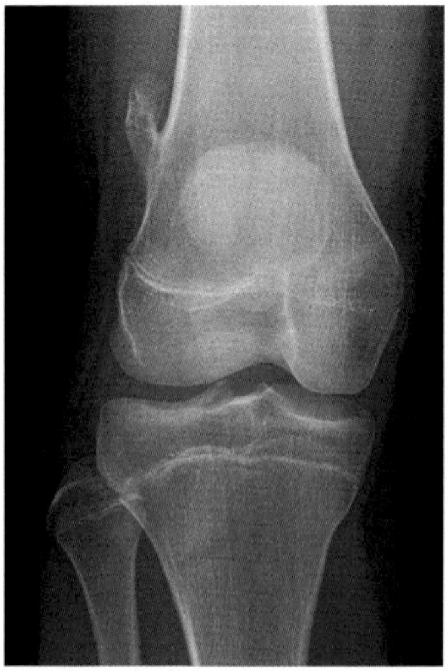

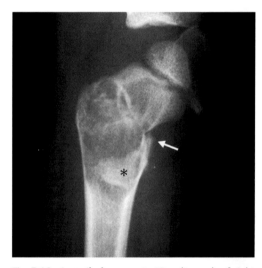

Fig. 7.15   Osteochondroma. AP radiograph of right knee shows pedunculated osteochondroma with typical growth direction toward diaphysis. DD: ossified tendon attachment.

Fig. 7.16   Juvenile bone cyst. AP radiograph of right hip shows fractured (arrow) juvenile bone cyst with "fallen fragment" sign (*).

Radiography: usually metaphyseal, eccentric, located on posterior circumference, associated cortical bulge, multilocular appearance.
MRI: hypointense to muscle on T1-weighted images, hypointense to fat on T2-weighted images (**Fig. 7.17**).

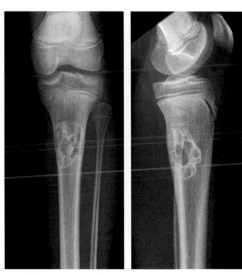

Fig. 7.17 Nonossifying fibroma. AP radiograph of proximal lower leg shows eccentric, multilobular osteolytic area with wide sclerotic rim.

Fibrous Dysplasia

May be mono-/polyostotic. More common in girls than boys. Not neoplasm in strict sense.
Radiography: sclerotic rim, dense center (ground-glass appearance) due to fibrous, partially calcified contents. Possible bone deformity.

Langerhans Cell Histiocytosis

Osteolytic lesions in tubular bones, usually diaphyseal, of variable aggressiveness (Lodwick I–II). Age 10 to 12 years. Typical sites of LCH occurrence besides femur: skull, mandible, pelvis, ribs, spinal column (vertebra plana).
MRI: nonspecific; whole-body MRI helpful in search for multiple lesions (many lesions "silent" on radionuclide scans; **Fig. 7.18**).

Chondroblastoma

See Sect. 8.6.

Osteoid Osteoma, Osteoblastoma

See Sect. 8.6.

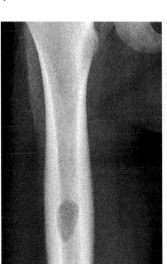

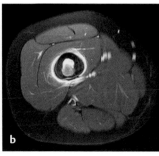

Fig. 7.18a, b   Unilocular Langerhans cell histiocytosis.
a Radiograph shows well-circumscribed osteolytic area in femoral shaft.
b Axial T1-weighted MRI (contrast-enhanced with fat suppression) shows intraosseous mass with inhomogeneous enhancement and periosseous soft-tissue reaction/periosteal enhancement.

7

7.3   Congenital Hip Dysplasia

Congenital hip dysplasia = developmental dysplasia of hip (DDH).

Developmental deficiency of pelvic acetabulum. Most severe form → hip dislocation.

Affects 2–5% of newborns in Central Europe, with female > male. Left > right. Hip dysplasia bilateral in 20 to 25% of cases.

Etiology and Risk Factors

Weakness of joint capsule and ligaments, promoted by estrogens. Mechanical factors—unfavorable limb position in utero.

Risk factors: positive family history (hip dysplasia in parents/siblings), breech delivery, intrauterine crowding (oligohydramnios—association with foot deformities/torticollis).

Clinical Findings

In newborns: asymmetry of gluteal folds, limitation of abduction, positive Ortolani sign. Later: delay in walking, leg length discrepancy, limping, limitation of motion. Late sequela: early onset of osteoarthritis.

Imaging

Ultrasound

Advantage = can define portions of hip joint preformed in cartilage—excellent for neonatal imaging. No radiation exposure.

Examination technique according to count: 5- to 12-MHz linear probe, lateral decubitus, hip flexed 20°, slight internal rotation (further details, e.g., at http://www.oegum.at).

Coronal scan through hip joint: key landmarks metaphyseal border, cartilaginous femoral head, greater trochanter, acetabulum, and gluteal muscles.

Standard US plane for taking measurements must include (**Figs. 7.19, 7.20, 7.21**):
- Inferior margin of ilium in acetabular fossa
- Straight, linear echo of ilium

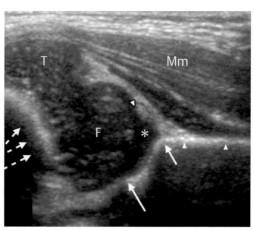

Fig. 7.19   Normal neonatal hip, Graf type I. Coronal US scan, side orientation deliberately reversed; right side of image = superior, left side of image = inferior. Correct plane for evaluating hip defined by thick inferior border of ilium at acetabular fossa (long arrow), straight contour of iliac wing (white arrowheads), bright acetabular labrum (arrowhead). Cartilaginous femoral head (F) and greater trochanter (T), metaphyseal border (short white arrows), gluteal muscles (Mm), superior bony rim of acetabulum (short arrow), cartilaginous rim of acetabulum (*).

- Acetabular labrum

Qualitative evaluation: bony and cartilaginous portion of roof, shape of bony promontory of superior bony acetabular rim, position of femoral head.

Quantitative evaluation: Measure angles formed by reference lines (**Fig. 7.20**).
- Baseline: parallel to ileal echo
- (acetabular) Bony roof line: tangent to inferior margin of ilium and bony promontory of superior bony rim of acetabulum
- Cartilage roof line: passes through tip of acetabular labrum and bony promontory of superior bony rim
- α = angle formed by baseline and bony roof line. β = angle formed by baseline and cartilaginous roof line

Dynamic examination: Cephalad pressure → (sub)luxation of femoral head? Caudad traction on femoral head → reduction? Essential whenever static US shows slightest abnormality!

Overall evaluation: Graf classification of infant hip (**Table 7.1**).

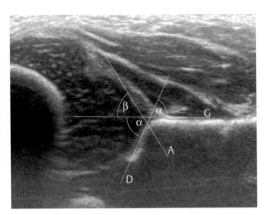

Fig. 7.20 Graf angle measurements in normal neonatal hip. Mature hip: α = 65°, β = 51°. Good bony contours, good femoral head coverage. Baseline (G), cartilage roof line (A), bony roof line (D), α angle (α), β angle (β).

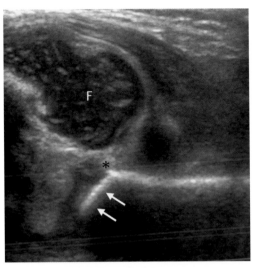

Fig. 7.21 Congenital hip dislocation, US on third day of life. Femoral head (F) displaced laterally upward, acetabulum (arrows) poorly formed, cartilaginous acetabular rim and labrum (*) displaced medially and downward into acetabular fossa.

Table 7.1 Graf classification of infant hips

Type	Superior bony rim of acetabulum	Bony roof contour	Cartilaginous acetabular roof	α angle	β angle
Type 1, mature hip joint	Angular/blunt	Good	Covers femoral head	≥ 60°	
Type 2a, physiologically immature before age 12 weeks	Round	Adequate	Covers femoral head	50–59°	
Type 2b, delay of ossification after age 12 weeks	Round	Deficient	Covers femoral head	50–59°	
Type 2c, critical range	Round to flat	Severely deficient	Still covers femoral head	43–49°	< 77°
Type D, decentering	Round to flat	Severely deficient	Displaced	43–49°	> 77°
Type 3, eccentric	Flat	Poor	Displaced upward	< 43°	
Type 4, eccentric	Flat	Poor	Displaced medially and downward		

7

Normal hip—α should be ≥ 60° by age 3 months at the latest! Angle measurements are meaningful only when correct plane is displayed!

Rosendahl method ("modified Graf classification")

Two steps: anatomical and functional assessment = hip morphology assessed by Graf method + Barlow maneuver testing for instability.

Classification: Hip morphology (= α angle) assessed in standard coronal view (Graf) with centered femoral head:

- If hip decentering, eccentric or dislocated hips (= Graf 2c, D, 3, 4)—femoral head relocated by mild traction + reassessment thereafter of hip morphology
- Irreducible hip—morphology assessed with dislocated femoral head

Note: even in anatomically normal hips, additional Barlow maneuver always performed to assess for coexisting instability.

Harcke method (US examination of hip): Dynamic sonography of neonatal and infant hip, patient in supine position; transducer positioned over lateral or posterior-lateral aspect of hip. Four steps:

1. Coronal neutral—similar to Graf standard plane. Femoral head visible posterior to triradiate cartilage = abnormal
2. Coronal flexion—same plane as above, hip in 90° flexion. Identification of triradiate cartilage. Barlow maneuver—femoral head moving over posterior lip of triradiate cartilage = instability
3. Transverse flexion—hip in 90° flexion, femoral head central to "U" produced by femoral metaphysis and ischium. Barlow maneuver—gap between head and acetabulum increases = instability
4. Transverse neutral—hip in neutral position; center of femoral head within acetabulum at level of triradiate cartilage

Definition of normal limits: femoral head in center of acetabulum at rest and with stress maneuvers.

Morin and Terjesen method: "femoral head coverage."

Assesses degree of lateralization of femoral head based on Harcke coronal flexion view; performed mostly in France.

Two lines drawn parallel to Graf baseline:

- One tangent to lateral part of femoral head
- One tangent to medial junction of head and acetabular fossa

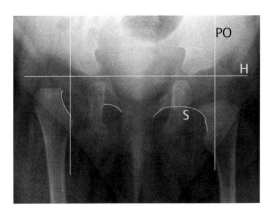

Fig. 7.22   Pelvic radiograph (5-month-old child with congenital dislocation of right hip and normal left hip). Neither femoral head displays ossification center at this time. Right femur displaced laterally and upward. The Perkins–Ombredanne line (PO) runs medial to femoral metaphysis, and obvious discontinuity noted in Shenton–Menard line (S). Acetabular roof poorly formed on right side, normal on left. H = Hilgenreiner line.

- Measure distance between medial and iliac lines + between medial and lateral lines
- Calculate ratio multiplied by 100 = percentage of femoral head covered by bony acetabulum

Modified Morin (= Terjesen method): Instead of iliac line—draw line through lateral bony rim of acetabulum parallel to long axis of transducer measuring "bony rim percentage," later named "femoral head coverage."

Anatomic landmarks: lateral part of femoral head, medial junction of head, acetabular fossa

Lower normal limits: boys = 47%, girls = 44%

Radiography

The radiographic criteria for DDH should be known, as pelvis often appears on radiographs taken for other indications. Femoral head position can only be estimated on films taken before capital femoral ossification center appears (months 3–6), evaluation performed more accurately when ossification center present.

Radiographic signs of **DDH** (**Fig. 7.22**): steep acetabular roof, small ossification center, superolateral displacement of femur, presence of pseudoacetabulum. Reference lines in pelvic radiograph:

- Hilgenreiner line: connects through superior border of triradiate cartilage

- Perkins–Ombredanne line: through superior cartilaginous rim, perpendicular to Hilgenreiner line; normal = capital femoral ossification center in inferomedial quadrant
- Shenton–Menard line: curved line formed by obturator foramen and medial border of femur; normal = no discontinuity
- Acetabular angle: between Hilgenreiner line and line tangent to acetabular roof

Magnetic Resonance Imaging

Indications = evaluate hips of children with irreducible dislocation, peri-/postoperative assessment, imaging in cast.

Differential Diagnosis

Hypoplasia of proximal femur = proximal focal femoral deficiency. Secondary hip dysplasia/dislocation in neurologic diseases due to abnormal muscle pull.

Treatment

Hip dysplasia: with stable, centered femoral head—treatment with flexion–abduction-external rotation harness or splint and regular US follow-ups.
Hip dislocation: femoral head first reduced, then stabilized with **retention orthosis** (e.g., flexion–abduction cast). Stabilized hip treated same as dysplasia. With later diagnosis: surgical intervention (e.g., corrective osteotomy).

Prognosis

Untreated cases → progressive deterioration and osteoarthritis due to unphysiologic muscle traction. Early diagnosis and appropriate treatment → excellent outcome.

Potential complication during treatment = aseptic necrosis of femoral head.

7.4   Spinal Column

Normal Anatomy

Vertebral elements formed by segmentation of mesenchyme around neural tube and notochord. "Notochord remnants" → posterior indentation of vertebral bodies (**Fig. 7.23**). Result = 32 to 34 elements in definitive spinal column. Notochord remnants → intervertebral disks. Cartilaginous precursor of vertebral segment contains chondral centers (two for each vertebral body and arch). Abnormal development/hypoplasia → hemivertebrae. Ossification centers start to appear in week 10 of gestation. Vertebral body centers finally unite in 10th year of life. Ossification centers of vertebral apophyses appear during puberty, require differentiation from anterior disk protrusions (**Fig. 7.24**).

Length proportions change dramatically: cervical spine ¼ of total spinal length at birth, decreasing to ⅕ to ⅙ in adults. Lumbar spine makes up ¼ to ⅓ of total spinal length.

Imaging displays 7 cervical, 12 thoracic, 5 lumbar, 5 sacral, and 4 to 5 coccygeal elements, with possible variations at each junction. C1 and C2 phy-

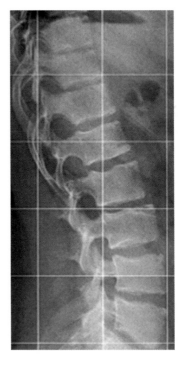

**Fig. 7.23
Notochord
remnants.**
Lateral radiograph of thoracolumbar junction shows posterior indentations in multiple superior vertebral margins, caused by remnants of regressed notochord.

7

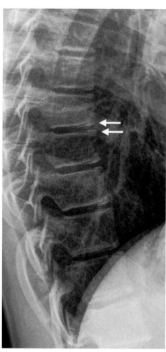

Fig. 7.24 Apophyseal rings of vertebral bodies (15-year-old boy). Lateral radiograph of thoracic spine shows partially ossified, still-unfused apophyseal rings (arrows).

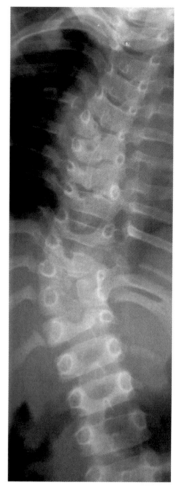

Fig. 7.25 Segmentation anomaly. Magnified view of AP chest radiograph in a newborn shows segmentation anomaly at T4–T6, characterized by failure of fusion of vertebral body ossification centers (cervical spine).

logenically distinct, arising from 5th and 6th occipital sclerotomes. Morphology of different vertebral elements changes significantly during lifetime. Neurocentral synchondroses visible until 6th year of life.

Notches visible in middle third of anterior and posterior vertebral margins on lateral radiographs: sinusoids/nutrient vessels. Vertebral body shape becomes less rounded and more rectangular with aging, while anterior notches disappear.

Cervical Spine

Arch of atlas (C1 vertebra) ossifies at age 9 to 12 months. Frequent ossification of atlanto-occipital membrane = arcuate foramen (marks course of vertebral artery).

Axis (C2 vertebra) has complex anatomy: dens and base each arise from two ossification centers; dentocentral synchondrosis fuses by 6 to 7 years. Sagittal alignment of cervical vertebral bodies varies with head position. Vertebral body offset appears at C2 to C4 (pseudosubluxation) due to more horizontal orientation of facet joints and increased elasticity. By school age, range of motion greatest at C5 to C6 level. Transverse process of C7 variable in size (may form cervical rib).

Thoracolumbar Spine

Vertebral body sizes increase from above downward to accommodate weight-bearing loads. Additional vertebrocostal joints present at thoracic level. Facet joints uniform except for L5: articular surface has coronal, oblique, or transverse orientation, frequent asymmetry.

Congenital Malformations: Segmentation Anomalies, Malformations in Dysraphism

Cervical Spine

Congenital partial ossification defects are not rare; most commonly involve arch elements. Usually detected incidentally (DD: destruction, infection). Hy-

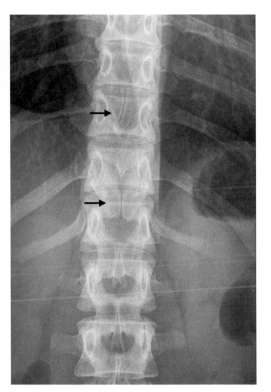

Fig. 7.26 Spina bifida occulta (17-year-old girl). AP radiograph of thoracolumbar junction reveals incomplete neural arch closure at T9 and T11 (arrow).

poplasia/aplasia of os odontoideum: present in many skeletal dysplasias (e.g., Morquio syndrome). Separate os odontoideum known to occur; post-traumatic etiology difficult to prove.

Delayed ossification considered normal variant.

Segmentation anomalies due to abnormal horizontal/vertical connections between embryonic cartilage rudiments, with subsequent ossification (designations: **cervical vertebrae, butterfly vertebrae**, fusions). **Klippel–Feil syndrome** = applied when cervical spine involved. In strict sense, this term also applies to short neck and elevated scapula (Sprengel anomaly).

Thoracolumbar Spine

Segmentation anomalies also occur in thoracolumbar spine. Not unusual to find circumscribed anomaly, also common in VACTERL children (**Fig. 7.25**).

Normal variants include indentation in posterior third of vertebral endplates, presumably related to notochord regression (**Fig. 7.23**).

Spina bifida vera = congenital vertebral arch defect with interposed spinal canal tissues (e.g., lipomeningocele). **Spina bifida occulta** = pure osseous defect, considered normal variant (common sites: C7, T11, L4–L5; see also Sect. 4.1) (**Fig. 7.26**).

Diastematomyelia: sagittal division of spinal canal by fibrous/cartilaginous/bony septum with circumscribed increase in interpedicular distance. May split spinal cord, depending on level, and prevent cord ascension.

Spinal Anomalies in Skeletal Dysplasias

See also Chapter 9.

Vertebral bodies: changes analogous to those in long tubular bones, but of lesser magnitude. **Achondroplasia:** decreased interpedicular distances, vertical shortening. Generalized **platyspondyly** in Morquio syndrome. Increased sagittal length in Kniest syndrome. Irregular vertebral body shape in **spondyloepiphyseal dysplasias. Mucopolysaccharidosis:** hook-like deformity of anterior vertebral margins due to protrusion of disk material. Generalized bone changes superimposed over vertebral changes. Some syndromes affect only spinal column and ribs = **spondylocostal dysostoses.**

Trauma

Conventional radiographs: lateral (supine, cross-table) and AP views. AP radiograph of dens often unrewarding in emergency settings (cervical collar in place). CT/MRI may be justified depending on clinical status/consciousness and with high trauma risk. See Chapter 6 for more details.

Important Measurements

Prevertebral soft tissues: useful to C3 level; < 5 mm after age 2 years, 3 mm after age 13 years. C1 to C2 distance ≤ 5 mm.

Craniocervical Trauma

Occipitocervical joints have near-horizontal orientation as result of embryonic development. Stability provided by strong ligaments (anterior and posterior atlanto-occipital ligaments, tectorial membrane). But child's head heavy in relation to body weight = condylar fractures may be combined with occipitocervical dissociation. Atlas and axis fractures account for up to 20% of vertebral fractures in children. Jefferson fracture (C1) = axial compression injury (**Fig. 7.27**). Dens fractures are most common.

Diagnosis is difficult due to synchondrosis. Atlantoaxial rotatory fixation/subluxation due to

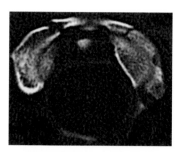

Fig. 7.27 Jefferson fracture. Axial CT of cervical spine displays multipart fracture of C1 arch.

trauma or infection: head flexion and lateral tilt plus rotation to opposite side. DD: Chiari I malformations, tumors of posterior cranial fossa, congenital anomalies of cervical spine.

Hyperflexion trauma to lower cervical spine often has no radiographic signs—known history of significant trauma plus persistent pain → MRI of discoligamentous structures. For biomechanical reasons, hyperflexion trauma is combined with posterior column injury!

Thoracolumbar Trauma

Radiographs in two planes with lateral cross-table view.

Difficult to demonstrate cervicothoracic and thoracolumbar junctions, especially in emergencies.

Important: shifts > 2 mm are pathologic; as well as circumscribed increase in paraspinal soft tissues. Aside from simple compression fractures (< 50% height reduction)—further investigation requires CT. Neurologic symptoms warrant MRI.

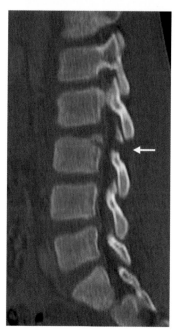

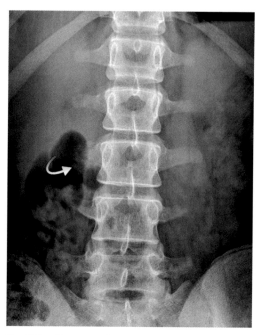

Fig. 7.28 Flexion-distraction fracture (Chance fracture). Sagittal reformatted CT image of lumbar spine shows approximately transverse fracture line through middle and posterior columns of L3 vertebra (arrow).

Fig. 7.29 Fracture of transverse processes. AP radiograph of lumbar spine shows healing fracture of right costal process of L3, manifested by callus reaction (→).

Severe compression fractures and burst fractures—unstable, result from large axial force on flexed spine. Distraction injury (seat-belt injury) = Chance fracture is typical (horizontal fracture line extending into vertebral arch—difficult to detect with axial CT alone; **Fig. 7.28**). Important: look for associated visceral/spinal injuries. Spinous process/transverse process/costal process fractures = isolated injury: concomitant injury is to soft tissues, not spinal canal (**Fig. 7.29**). Spondylolysis = fracture through pars interarticularis (usually of L5), usually caused by chronic repetitive stress, rarely by acute hyperextension.

Infections

Discitis

Most patients < 3 years of age (blood circulation through disk). Affected children refuse to walk, have back pain, usually no fever. Laboratory findings often nonspecific. Within 2 to 3 weeks of symptom onset: narrowing of disk space (**Fig. 7.30**). If uncertainty exists → MRI. No more than one-third of patients have positive blood cultures (usually *Staphylococcus aureus*). Cases may progress to vertebral fusion or complete disk recovery.

Spondylodiscitis, Vertebral Osteomyelitis

Results from hematogenous spread of typical organisms (*Staphylococcus aureus*, salmonella, brucella, etc.). Fever and positive blood cultures common. Rapidly destructive changes with disk space narrowing, followed later by reactive changes.

Tuberculous Spondylitis

Often affects > 2 vertebral elements. Process starts anteroinferiorly, spreads along anterior longitudinal ligament. Intervertebral disk involvement is late event. Predominantly destructive changes. Paraspinal abscess formation may precede bone involvement.

Neoplasms

See also Chapter 8.

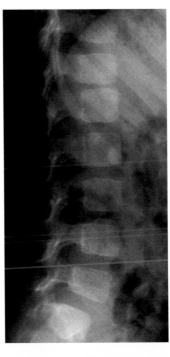

Fig. 7.30 Discitis (4-year-old girl). Lateral radiograph of lumbar spine shows uniform narrowing of infected T12–L1 disk space.

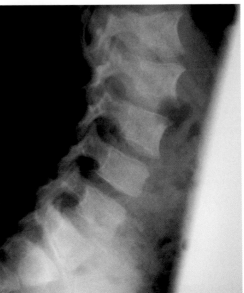

Fig. 7.31 Neurofibromatosis type I. Lateral radiograph of lumbar spine shows erosion of multiple lumbar vertebral bodies with anterior scalloping.

7

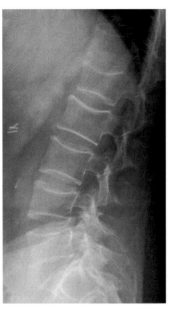

Fig. 7.32 Pathologic vertebral body fracture. Lateral radiograph shows multiple compression fractures at thoracolumbar junction as complication of high-dose steroid therapy.

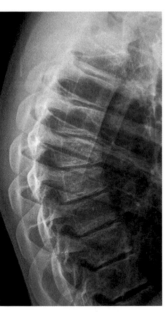

Fig. 7.33 Scheuermann disease. Lateral radiograph of thoracic spine shows pronounced kyphosis with vertebral body wedging, narrowing of several intervertebral disks, and multiple intratrabecular disk herniations at vertebral endplates.

Benign Lesions

Neurofibromatosis—may show multiple sites of vertebral involvement, with scalloping of vertebral margins (**Fig. 7.31**). Neurofibromas cause widening of intervertebral foramina.
Osteoid osteoma, osteoblastoma, and aneurysmatic bone cyst; two-thirds in vertebral arches. Expansile cystlike lesions. **Osteochondroma**—soli-

tary/multiple. Typical eccentric location in vertebral arch, may cause cord compression. **Vertebral hemangiomas** are rare. **LCH** → vertebra plana, vertebral arch rarely affected.

Malignant Neoplasms

Ewing sarcoma, lymphoma = aggressive-looking osteolytic areas.
Metastases—leukemias, neuroblastoma, sarcoma.
Compression fractures may result from diffuse metastatic involvement. DD: steroid therapy, osteogenesis imperfecta (**Fig. 7.32**).

Other Conditions: Scoliosis, Kyphosis

Adolescent Kyphosis (Scheuermann Disease)

Involves three or more vertebral bodies. Protrusion of disk material into vertebral endplates, associated vertebral height reduction, wedging of vertebrae, kyphosis. Typical site of occurrence: thoracolumbar junction (**Fig. 7.33**).

Scoliosis

Definition: present when lateral rotational curve(s) are > 10° based on Cobb measurements. Congenital scoliosis occurs in children with segmentation disorders; may be combined with spinal anomalies; possible VACTERL association (**Fig. 7.34**). Scoliosis common in Marfan syndrome, neurofibromatosis, congenital torticollis. Acquired forms in neurodegenerative disease, muscular dystrophy, cerebral palsy.

Most prevalent type = **idiopathic scoliosis**. Infantile form under age 3 years (left convex thoracic, M > F), juvenile at age 3 to 9 years, adolescent > 10 years (usually right convex thoracic; **Fig. 7.35**). Scoliosis with > 30% curve more common in girls (up to 7 : 1). Evaluated by conventional radiography, usually starting with iliac crest (**Risser sign** to assess growth potential). High association between scoliosis and congenital heart defects.

Intervertebral Disk Anomalies

Abnormalities of disk structure with degeneration and herniation into vertebral endplates and submarginal herniation beneath ring apophyses—

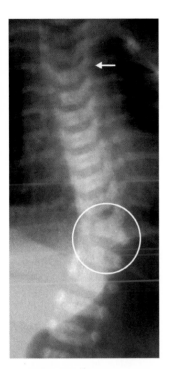

Fig. 7.34 VACTERL syndrome in newborn. AP radiograph of thoracic and lumbar spine shows complex segmentation and fusion anomaly at thoracolumbar junction leading to left convex scoliosis (circled). Esophageal atresia (arrow).

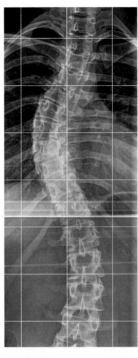

Fig. 7.35 Scoliosis. AP spine radiograph shows idiopathic adolescent scoliosis with rightward convexity and torsion. Normal vertebral body shapes.

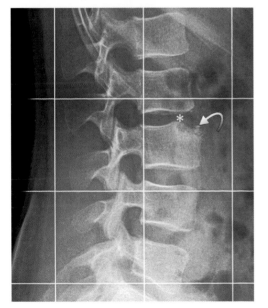

Fig. 7.36 Structural abnormality of spinal column. Lateral radiograph of lumbar spine shows monosegmental structural abnormality with submarginal herniation of intervertebral disk tissue (curved arrow).

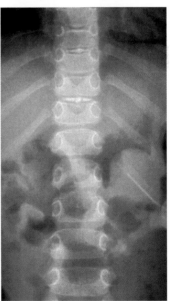

Fig. 7.37 Disk calcification. Multiple disk calcifications detected incidentally in plain abdominal radiograph.

symptomatic or incidental finding (**Fig. 7.36**). Possible abortive Scheuermann disease; rarely, residua of less aggressive spondylodiscitis.

Disk calcifications are rare in children. Incidence uncertain (asymptomatic). Etiology uncertain; often disappear spontaneously (**Fig. 7.37**).

7

7.5   Osteochondrosis and Aseptic Necrosis

Perthes Disease

General: idiopathic aseptic necrosis of femoral head. Incidence 1 : 1200 in children < 15 years old, 4 : 1 male preponderance, in Europe. Onset of disease between 3rd and 12th years of life, 10–20% bilateral, usually asymmetric.

Course: self-limiting, runs 3- to 4-year course. Ischemia → fragmentation → revascularization → reossification. Late sequel: 50% incidence of osteoarthritis after age 50 years.

Clinical features: persistent leg pain (hip pain often projected to knee), limp, limitation of hip motion, absence of trauma history.

Imaging:
- **Radiography:** AP pelvic radiograph and axial hip view—femoral epiphysis flattened, sclerotic, and fragmented (**Fig. 7.38a, b**). Radiographic Waldenström stages:
  - **Initial stage:** joint space widening, anterolateral flattening of femoral head, sclerosis of epiphysis

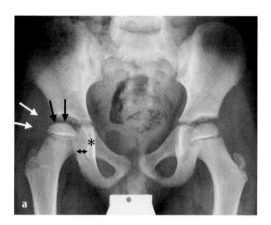
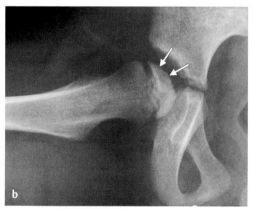
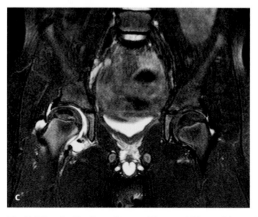
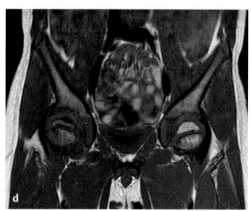

Fig. 7.38a–d   Perthes disease (5-year-old boy with persistent right hip pain).

a, b AP pelvic radiograph (**a**), axial projection of right hip (**b**). Right capital femoral epiphysis reduced in height and flattened anterolaterally (black arrows). Right joint space (double arrow) and acetabular teardrop figure (*) markedly widened. Fat lines displaced (white arrows).

c, d MRI of pelvis—coronal T2-weighted image (**c**) and coronal T1-weighted image (**d**). Necrotic portions of capital femoral epiphysis show decreased signal intensity in both sequences. Joint effusion.

- **Fragmentation stage:** subchondral fracture, inhomogeneous density and fragmentation of epiphysis, metaphyseal pseudocysts
- **Reparative stage:** resorption of fragments, remodeling of femoral head, broadening of metaphysis
- **Healed stage:** short broad femoral neck, cylindrical femoral head, incongruent articular surfaces, coxa vara with high position of greater trochanter
- In less severe cases with favorable course, hip joint may return to normal.

- **US:** moderately useful—findings can mimic transient synovitis. Recurrent/persistent hip effusion, irregularity of femoral epiphysis
- **MRI:** can provide early diagnosis in patients with equivocal radiographic findings: absence of enhancement in early arterial phase (dynamic perfusion sequence), joint effusion, synovitis. Typical pattern = hypointense epiphyseal marrow center in T1- and T2-weighted images (**Fig. 7.38c, d**). Later imaging can assess prognosis based on location and extent of hypoperfused areas, revascularization. MRI in healed stage can give accurate preoperative assessment of joint status (perfusion imaging may be used).
- **Bone scintigraphy:** can supply early diagnosis. Disadvantage = radiation exposure. Ischemia = decreased tracer uptake; revascularization = increased tracer uptake

Classification:
- **Catterall classification:** based on extent of affected portions of epiphysis
- **Salter–Thompson classification:** based on extent of subchondral fracture
- **Herring classification:** based on integrity of lateral pillar

Treatment: rest, nonsteroidal anti-inflammatory drugs (NSAIDs). 50% of cases have spontaneous recovery with good outcome. Incongruity of hip joint can be treated surgically.

DD:
- **Transient synovitis of hip:** acute, self-limiting synovitis with joint effusion, usually follows mild viral infection, no osseous changes; imaging consists of US (effusion) + plain film
- **Juvenile osteonecrosis:** aseptic necrosis of femoral head with known cause such as sickle-cell anemia, steroid therapy, or previous trauma—in

early stages only depictable by MRI or scintigraphy
- **Meyer dysplasia:** developmental disorder of femoral epiphysis, bilateral, asymptomatic, no perfusion deficit, no change of medullary signal intensity on MRI, diagnosis by MRI and plain film

Other Forms of Aseptic Necrosis

Osgood–Schlatter Disease

Aseptic necrosis of tibial tuberosity.
Imaging:
- **Radiography:** swelling of pretibial soft tissues, obliteration of infrapatellar fat pad, thickening of patellar tendon; fragmentation of tibial tuberosity (considered pathologic only in symptomatic patients with soft-tissue swelling) (**Fig. 7.39**)
- **US:** increased vascularity and hyperperfusion of aponeurosis

> No indication for MRI!

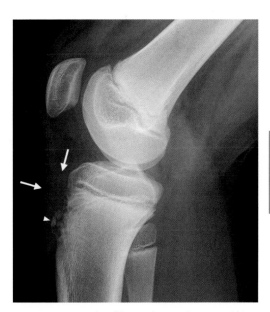

Fig. 7.39 Osgood–Schlatter disease (13-year-old boy with right knee pain). Lateral radiograph of right knee shows fragmentation of tibial tuberosity apophysis (arrowhead), obliteration of infrapatellar fat pad (long arrow), and swelling of pretibial soft tissues (short arrow).

7

Sinding–Larsen–Johansson disease

Aseptic necrosis of patellar apex.

Köhler Disease

Aseptic necrosis of navicular bone.
  Imaging:
- **Radiography:** sclerosis and fragmentation of navicular. Pathologic only in symptomatic patients with associated soft-tissue swelling, otherwise normal—even with side-to-side difference
- **DD on MRI:** abnormal medullary signal in Köhler disease

Osteochondritis dissecans

Definition: aseptic necrosis of subchondral articular bone. Common sites of occurrence: medial femoral condyle, talar dome, capitellum.
Cause: recurrent microtrauma. Typical age = adolescence.

Clinical features: persistent pain, aggravated by weight-bearing. With intra-articular loose body— intermittent catching of joint.
Imaging:
- **Radiography:** subchondral lucency with embedded bone fragment or elliptical defect with sclerotic margins. Detachment of fragment → intra-articular loose body (**Fig. 7.40a, b**)
- **MRI:** more sensitive than radiographs in early stage and for detecting intra-articular loose bodies; useful for evaluating articular cartilage (**Fig. 7.40c**). Later imaging can assess fragment viability and stability. Evidence of instability— size > 1 cm, fluid around fragment, cystic changes > 5 mm in adjacent bone

DD: normal irregular ossification of distal femoral epiphysis—asymptomatic, most common in lateral condyle, posterior location. Osteochondral fracture.
Treatment: may resolve spontaneously. (CT-guided) transchondral drilling (to induce revascularization).

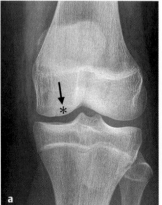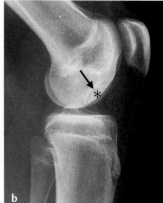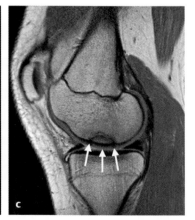

Fig. 7.40a–c   Osteochondritis dissecans (14-year-old girl with persistent left knee pain).

a AP radiograph of left knee.
b Lateral radiograph shows subchondral lucent line (arrow) with embedded bone fragment (*) at typical site in lateral portion of medial femoral condyle.

c MRI of left knee joint. Sagittal proton-weighted image shows intact cartilage (arrows) over bone fragment.

7.6   Osteomyelitis

Acute Osteomyelitis

General: usually hematogenous in children, rarely due to perforating injury/contiguous spread.

Causative organisms: staphylococci, occasional inoculation of *Haemophilus influenzae* or *Streptococcus pneumoniae*. With perforating injuries: *Pseudomonas aeruginosa*. In sickle-cell anemia: *Salmonella* species.

Sites of occurrence: metaphysis of long tubular bones—slow blood flow in sinusoids of metaphysis promotes bacterial colonization.

Spread: < 18 months: vessels pass through epiphyseal plate into epiphysis, promote rapid spread into joint—**septic osteoarthritis**. > 18 months: epiphyseal plate forms barrier. Spread occurs in medullary cavity, beneath periosteum, in surrounding soft tissues. Loose periosteal attachment in children allows extensive abscess formation.

Course: bacterial invasion → inflammatory reaction → rise of intramedullary pressure → subperiosteal/intramedullary spread → abscess formation → thrombosis → bone necrosis → subperiosteal new bone formation ("involucrum"—dead bone surrounded by newly formed bone).

Clinical features: pseudoparalysis in infants, often little systemic reaction. Older children—severe pain, swelling, redness, fever, systemic toxicity.

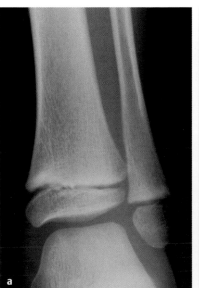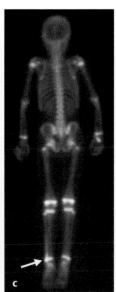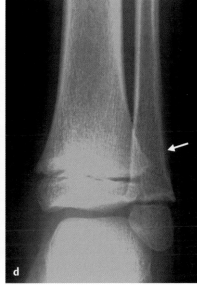

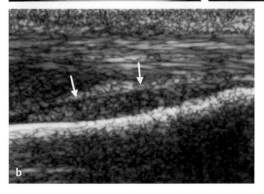

Fig. 7.41a–d   Acute osteomyelitis of left fibula.
a Initial AP radiograph of left ankle joint appears normal.
b Sagittal US scan of left distal fibula. Subperiosteal abscess (arrows).
c Bone scintigraphy shows increased uptake on lateral side of left ankle joint (arrow).
d Radiograph 10 days later shows faint periosteal reaction on distal fibula (arrow).

7

Imaging:

- **Radiographs:** often negative initially (**Fig. 7.41a**). May show swelling of deep soft tissues during first 3 days, displacement/obliteration of deep fat planes. Bone changes detectable by about 1 to 2 weeks = osteolysis of metaphysis (**Fig. 7.42a**) and periosteal reaction (**Fig. 7.41 d**)
- **US:** subperiosteal abscess (**Fig. 7.41b**) often detectable within 48 hours. Osteoarthritis—joint effusion with debris (**Fig. 7.43**). US-guided needle aspiration = diagnosis plus identification of causative organism, also therapeutic (for decompression in pyarthrosis)
- **MRI:** positive in first 24 to 48 hours, high sensitivity. Indication = initial workup of equivocal cases (DD: soft-tissue infection, osteomyelitis), poor response to antibiotic therapy, extensive abscess formation, preoperative. Whole-body MRI (with DWI) may be useful for multifocal osteomyelitis

  MRI findings: bone-marrow edema = hypointense on T1-weighted images, hyperintense on T2-weighted/STIR images. Marked enhancement of bone marrow and periosteum (inflammatory reaction; **Fig. 7.42b, c**). Soft-tissue edema = T2-hyperintense. Abscess = peripheral enhancement; necrosis = absence of enhancement

- **Scintigraphy:** positive within 24 to 72 hours (**Fig. 7.41c**)

Findings: increased tracer uptake in angiographic, blood-pool, and late phase. With infarction/abscess = central absence of tracer uptake. Advantage = detection of multifocal osteomyelitis (common in newborns). Disadvantages = radiation exposure, symmetrical involvement difficult to detect due to high physiologic tracer uptake in epiphyseal plate

- **CT:** not recommended! Increased bone marrow attenuation in early phase, occasional fat–fluid levels, gas inclusions, abscess formation. Later: osteolytic areas, periosteal new bone formation

Treatment: antibiotic therapy. With early use, radiographs often detect no bony changes by 14 days = complete recovery. Extensive (particularly intraosseous) abscess formation requires surgical intervention.

Late sequelae: result from damage to growth plate = growth disturbance, premature epiphyseal closure, deformity (40% of newborns with osteomyelitis).

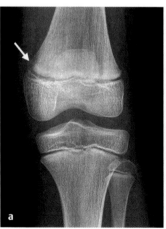
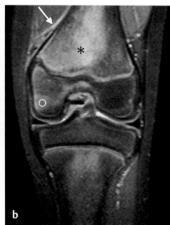
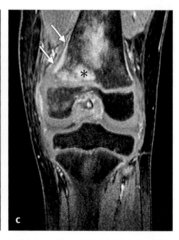

Fig. 7.42a–c   Acute osteomyelitis of right femur in (8-year-old boy with 4-day history of severe right knee pain).

a AP radiograph of right knee shows osteolysis of medial femoral metaphysis bordering on epiphyseal plate (arrow).

b, c Coronal MRI, TRIM sequence (**b**), coronal VIBE (volumetric interpolated breath-hold examination) with contrast medium (**c**) show increased signal intensity in medial part of metaphysis (*) and in soft tissues bordering metaphysis (arrows). Bone-marrow edema in medial condyle (o).

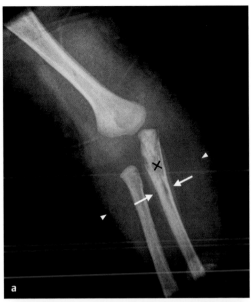

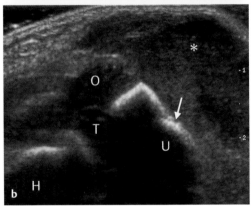

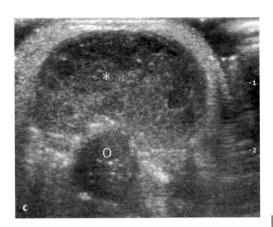

Fig. 7.43a–c   Acute osteoarthritis of right elbow (4-week old girl with 4-day history of slight fever, no malaise, and pseudoparalysis of right arm).
a   AP radiograph of right elbow shows extensive moth-eaten osteolytic area in proximal ulna (cross) with associated periosteal reaction (arrows). Marked soft-tissue swelling (arrowheads).
b, c   Posterior US scans of right elbow in sagittal (**b**) and axial planes (**c**) show large soft-tissue abscess (*) that communicates with elbow joint. Cortical disruption noted in proximal ulnar metaphysis (arrow). Olecranon (O), trochlea (T), distal humerus (H), proximal ulna (U).

Chronic Osteomyelitis

Chronic infection by organism of low virulence. Leads to osteolysis/reactive periosteal and medullary new bone formation = sclerosis.

Brodie Abscess

General: primary or may follow acute osteomyelitis. Well-encapsulated intraosseous fluid collection, occasionally with central bone sequestrum. Fluid usually sterile. Perifocal sclerosis.
Causative organism: *Staphylococcus aureus.*

Sites of predilection: tibia, femur—usually metaphyseal, occasionally diaphyseal.
Clinical features: recurring pain over period of months, swelling, local warmth.
Imaging:
- **Radiography:** circumscribed osteolytic area with sclerotic margins, occasionally periosteal reaction, bone sequestrum
- **CT/MRI:** osteolysis with peripheral enhancement; sequestra clearly visible on CT scans (**Fig. 7.44**)

7

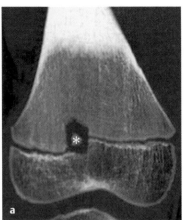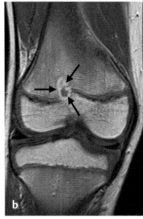

Fig. 7.44a, b   Brodie abscess of right knee. 9-year-old boy complained of knee pain for several weeks.
a Coronal reformatted CT shows osteolysis in distal femoral metaphysis with concomitant involvement of epiphyseal plate and adjacent epiphysis. Small bone sequestrum (*).
b Postcontrast coronal T1-weighted MRI shows enhancement of abscess membrane (arrows).

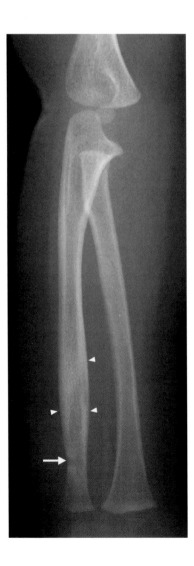

Sequestrum

Devitalized bone surrounded by inflammatory tissue in medullary space or cortex.

Fistula Formation

Bone marrow inflammation spreads through fistulous tract in cortex to surrounding soft tissues, sometimes to skin (**Fig. 7.45**).

Chronic Recurrent Multifocal Osteomyelitis

General: CRMO is an inflammatory bone disease of unclear etiology (immune response? occult viral/bacterial infection?). Lesions often symmetrical, asynchronous, most often involve metaphysis of tibia and distal femur, also clavicle. Self-limiting course. Presents clinically with pain and swelling.

◄ **Fig. 7.45   Chronic osteomyelitis with fistula formation.** AP radiograph of right forearm shows increased sclerosis and periosteal new bone formation in distal third of ulna (arrowheads). Fistulous tract in ulnar direction (arrow), marked soft-tissue swelling.

Imaging:

- **Radiography:** osteolysis and sclerosis with mild periosteal reaction and cortical thickening. Clavicle: hyperostosis in medial third (**Fig. 7.46**)
- **MRI:** changes as in bacterial osteomyelitis, but without abscess/fistula formation. If CRMO is suspected → whole-body MRI or scintigraphy to check for additional lesions. Accessible lesion selected for biopsy

DD: bacterial osteomyelitis, Ewing sarcoma, LCH, metastasis—biopsy required!

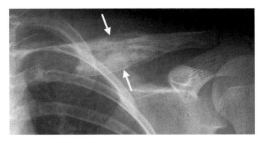

Fig. 7.46 Chronic recurrent osteomyelitis. Radiograph of left clavicle shows medial two-thirds affected by hyperostosis (arrows).

7.7 Diseases of Joints

Arthritis

General imaging aspects:

- Initial studies: **US** and **radiography**. Later: **US** (joint effusion, capsular thickening and pannus formation, increased vascularity). Option of US-guided percutaneous aspiration/injection
- **MRI:** most informative study (multiplanar capability, high soft-tissue contrast, vascular anatomy, best for imaging cartilage, connective tissue, synovium). Can also supply functional information (diffusion imaging, contrast-enhanced sequences)
- **CT** in selected cases (osseous changes near joints)

Juvenile Idiopathic Arthritis and Subtypes

General: Juvenile idiopathic arthritis (JIA) has onset before age 16 years. Runs course of at least 6 weeks. Important to exclude other causes (**Tables 7.2** and **7.3**).

Systemic arthritis (Still syndrome): up to 20% of cases, especially before age 5 years. Extra-articular symptoms include fever (**Table 7.3**). Chronic joint destruction, usually polyarticular, in up to 50% of cases. Sites of predilection: knee, wrist, ankle joint, cervical spine, hips.

Oligoarticular arthritis: most common form of JIA. Less than 5 joints affected at preschool age; knee and ankle joint most commonly involved, 50% with knee involvement only. Positive antinuclear antibodies (ANAs). Girls: high risk for uveitis. Up to 50% of cases develop extensive involvement, with more than five joints (**Figs. 7.47** and **7.48**).

Table 7.2 Joint diseases: radiologic signs of juvenile idiopathic arthritis (JIA)

Early signs	Late signs	Systemic signs
Joint effusion	Joint space narrowing	Serositis
Soft-tissue swelling	Joint incongruity	Generalized lymphadenopathy
Periarticular or diffuse parasternal	Bony erosions (caution: early sign in seropositive or systemic JIA)	Hepatosplenomegaly, activation of macrophages
Periostitis, tendinitis	Growth disturbance	Interstitial lung disease
	Ankylosis	Growth retardation
	Hypertrophic bursitis	Amyloidosis
	Synovial cysts	Rheumatoid vasculitis
	Compression fractures	Lymphedema

7

Table 7.3   Joint diseases: imitators of juvenile idiopathic arthritis (excerpt)

Radiology	Differential diagnosis
Joint effusion	Infectious arthritis, hemophilic arthropathy, transient synovitis, connective tissue disease, spondylarthropathy
Soft-tissue swelling	Infectious arthritis, hemophilic arthropathy, sarcoidosis
Osteoporosis	Leukemia, juvenile osteoporosis, connective tissue disease
Joint space narrowing	Hemophilic arthropathy, traumatic dislocation, infectious arthritis, idiopathic chondrolysis
Ankylosis	Spondylarthropathy, infectious arthritis, traumatic arthritis
Erosions	Hemophilic arthropathy, spondylarthropathy, infectious arthritis, carpal osteolysis, synovial osteochondromatosis
Periostitis	Trauma (including child abuse), osteomyelitis, osteoid osteoma, leukemia
Growth disturbances	
Epiphyseal overgrowth	Hemophilic arthropathy, spondylarthropathy, infectious arthritis, trauma, Perthes disease, skeletal dysplasia, Turner syndrome
Growth arrest	Turner syndrome, infections
Dysplastic changes	Mucopolysaccharidosis, mucolipidosis, camptodactyly arthropathy

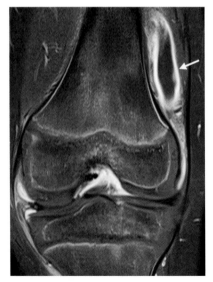

Fig. 7.47   MRI in oligoarthritis. Oligoarthritis with synovitis of left knee joint—early form. Normal cartilaginous/bone structure. Postcontrast coronal T1-weighted image with fat suppression = intense synovial enhancement (arrow).

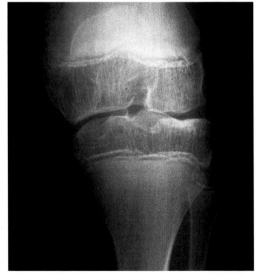

Fig. 7.48   Oligoarthritis. Oligoarthritis of left knee joint—late form. Radiograph shows joint space narrowing, cartilage destruction, subchondral erosion, and irregular joint contours.

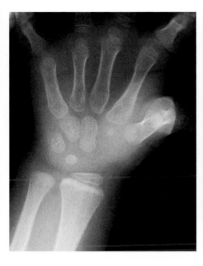
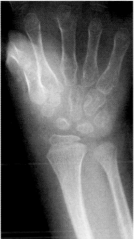

Fig. 7.49   **Juvenile idiopathic arthritis: polyarthritis.** Asymmetric form of polyarthritis involving right hand. Radiographs show cartilage loss with carpal joint space narrowing, erosion of hamate bone, and significant advancement of bone maturation relative to left side.

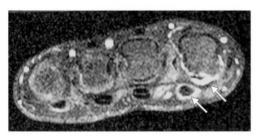

Fig. 7.50   **Juvenile idiopathic arthritis: enthesitis-associated arthritis.** Axial T1-weighted MRI with Gd and fat suppression shows synovial enhancement in the second DIP joint and flexor tendon sheath (arrows).

Polyarticular form: involves more than five joints in first 6 months. RF-negative (RF = rheumatoid factor): polyarthritis in early childhood. Typical presentation of RF-positive cases: adolescent girl with symmetrical involvement of small joints (**Fig. 7.49**). **Enthesitis-associated arthritis:** includes juvenile ankylosing spondylitis and arthritis associated with chronic inflammatory bowel disease. Often affects boys > 8 years of age. Human leukocyte antigen (HLA)-positive family history. Combination of arthritis and enthesitis = high index of suspicion. Arthritis associated with chronic bowel disease may have activity that parallels or is separate from course of bowel disease (**Figs. 7.50** and **7.51**). **Psoriatic arthritis:** affects midschool-age children. Arthritis may develop years before cutaneous manifestations. Asymmetric arthritis of knees, ankle

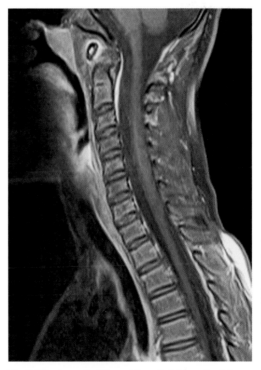

Fig. 7.51   **Juvenile idiopathic arthritis: enthesitis-associated arthritis.** Sagittal T1-weighted MRI of cervical spine with Gd and fat suppression shows homogeneous synovial enhancement in atlantoaxial joint = early form of spondylarthritis.

7

joints, hands (proximal interphalangeal joint/distal interphalangeal joint of one ray).

Infectious Arthritis

General: pathogenesis based on direct microbial invasion or postinfectious toxic process.

Most cases easily diagnosed from spinal column and pelvis. Hip, knee, and shoulder joint most commonly affected. Main causative organisms: *Staphylococcus aureus*, group B streptococci in newborns.
Primary imaging study: usually US, possibly MRI.

Transient Synovitis of the Hip

See also Sect. 7.5.
General: most common self-limiting joint disease in children. Affects boys more often than girls, age group = third to eighth year. Usually preceded by infectious disease, often minor. Acute onset of pain, limp.
Imaging: US (joint effusion). Radiographs normal except for narrowing of joint space and muscular asymmetry (**Fig. 7.52**).

> Diagnosed by exclusion—if symptoms persist > 14 days, investigate further (Perthes disease? JIA?).

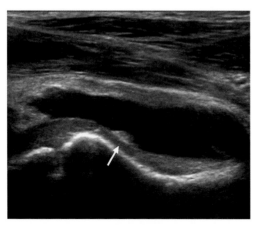

Fig. 7.52   Transient synovitis of hip (6-year-old boy). US of left hip shows approximately echo-free effusion in anterior recess of left hip joint. Aside from slightly enlarged villus (arrow), synovium appears normal.

Hemophilic Arthropathy

General: hemophilia, X-linked recessive, absence of factor VIII or IX.

Hemarthrosis in 90% of cases (knee, elbow, ankle). Joint swelling and subchondral resorption much greater than in JIA (typical findings in knee: widened intercondylar notch, squared-off patella; **Fig. 7.53**).
Imaging studies: usually US. MRI used for special investigations. CT rarely used.

Popliteal Cysts

General: most common fluid collection in enlarged semimembranosus bursa in children: one-third in patients < 15 years old. Unlike adults, usually not associated with knee effusion. Strong tendency for spontaneous resolution; (secondary) infection rare.
Imaging: US, possibly MRI.

> May extent into lower leg. Pseudotumor may result from pronounced reactive changes in synovial membrane.

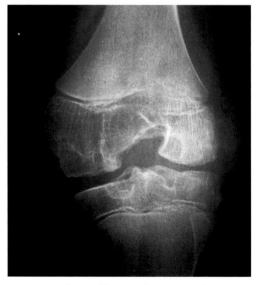

Fig. 7.53   Advanced hemophilic arthropathy of knee joint. AP radiograph of left knee shows cartilage destruction and subchondral bone destruction due to pannus formation. Typical finding: significant widening of intercondylar notch due to cruciate ligament involvement.

7.8   Changes in Soft Tissues

Calcifications, Ossifications, Foreign Bodies

General: calcifications after trauma or infection. Neoplastic: **pilomatrixoma** (**Fig. 7.54**), epidermoid cyst, lipoma. **Osteoma cutis** in disorders of parathyroid hormone metabolism. FBs not visible externally are common.
Imaging: US, possibly radiographs (incidental finding). US = primary tool for diagnosing nonmetallic FBs.

Myositis ossificans

General: benign ectopic bone deposition in soft tissues, usually muscle. Trauma history elicited in just two-thirds of cases. Etiology uncertain.
Imaging: radiography, CT. Typical roentgen signs usually present. US unrewarding.

> **!** Usually mimics malignancy on MRI (intense, irregular enhancement!). Lesions often look aggressive on radiographs, especially in early phase.

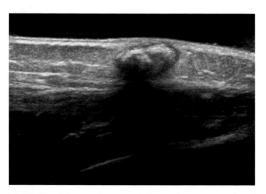

Fig. 7.54   Pilomatrixoma. High-resolution US with gel standoff shows clustered calcifications of varying sizes with hypoechoic rims in subcutaneous tissue.

Inflammatory Muscle Diseases

Juvenile Dermatomyositis

General: most common form of idiopathic inflammatory myopathy, manifested between 5 and 14 years of age.
Imaging: MRI—most sensitive modality, though nonspecific (DD: trauma, infection). Soft-tissue calcifications form in up to 70% of patients.

Pyomyositis

General: localized primary/hematogenous muscle infection (DD: trauma, tumor, hematoma). Main causative organism is staphylococcus, often not identified. Pelvic and lower limb muscles are principally affected (**Fig. 7.55**).
Imaging: US is not reliable with involvement of deep structures. MRI provides rapid and effective diagnosis; may show associated osteomyelitis (DD: osteomyelitis with associated myositis).

Fibrodysplasia Ossificans Progressiva

General: genetic disease, usually based on spontaneous mutation, or may have autosomal dominant inheritance. Typical finding: macrodactyly of both big toes. Children develop painful swellings with progressive ossification of muscles and connective tissue. Process usually starts at neck and shoulders and spreads to chest wall and below.
Imaging: masses hyperintense on T2-weighted MRI. Radiographs show macrodactyly of big toes. Diagnosis established radiologically by coexistence of progressive soft-tissue swellings and macrodactyly of big toes.

> **!** Biopsy contraindicated—may accelerate lesion growth!

7

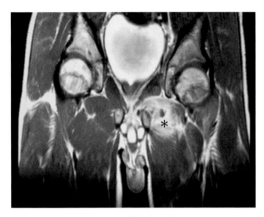

Fig. 7.55 Pyomyositis of left obturator externus muscle. Coronal T1-weighted MRI with Gd and fat suppression shows intense enhancement of muscle with small central abscess (*).

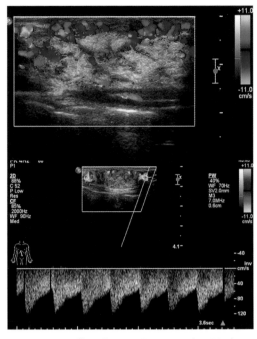

Fig. 7.56 Capillary hemangioma. Duplex US shows hypoechoic and echogenic components of subcutaneous mass with copious blood flow. Doppler spectrum shows diastolic hyperemia.

Neuromuscular Diseases

General: etiologically diverse group of diseases leading to degeneration of muscle tissue. Variable degree of atrophy and fatty replacement. Changes may be distinctive in early stages, become nonspecific in later stages (see also Chapter 9).
Imaging: often unproductive. US used to describe affected muscle (groups) and especially before biopsy to direct adequate tissue sampling (without too much fat or fibrous tissue).

Vascular Malformations

Current nomenclature (Mulliken and Glowacki) based on biologic activity and endothelial characteristics. Main groups: hemangiomas (rapid growth, gradual involution) and vascular malformations (dysplastic vessels without cellular proliferation).

Hemangiomas

General: usually visible only in first months of life. Typical raspberry-like surface appearance. Cutaneous and subcutaneous spread, rarely with visceral involvement (liver!). Most hemangiomas are subcutaneous. Orbital lesions may cause amblyopia.
Imaging: US with color duplex US, MRI = option for large lesions that may require treatment (**Fig. 7.56**). Characteristic findings:

- **US:** solid hypoechoic to echogenic mass
- **CDS (color Doppler US):** multiple vascular sections
- **Doppler spectra:** combination of arterial and venous waveforms, depending on flow rates and vascular resistance
- **MRI:** homogeneous, intensely enhancing mass; individual vessels cannot be identified

Vascular Malformations

Lesion growth proportional to body growth, except in cases with increasing/rapid blood flow. Designated according to main histologic component.

Venous Malformations

General: most common type of vascular malformations. Formerly called **cavernous hemangiomas**. Spread by infiltrating muscles and/or joints, occasionally bone. Intertwining vessels with low venous flow and no shunting of blood. Extension into joint = risk of hemarthrosis (**Fig. 7.57**).

Imaging:

- **US** with **CDS (color duplex US):** tortuous veins at atypical site
- **MRI:** veins of different calibers, appearing in multiple sections due to tortuosity. High T2-weighted signal intensity, intense enhancement after contrast administration
- **Venography:** available as pretreatment study (e.g., for FL-guided sclerotherapy)

Lymphatic Malformations

General: cystic malformation of heterotopic lymphatic tissue without drainage.

Imaging:

- **US:** microcystic, macrocystic and mixed-cystic malformation
- **CDS:** slight vascularity of solid elements/septa. Intralesional hemorrhage = internal echoes (may form sediment layer). Option of US-guided sclerotherapy
- **MRI:** (multi)cystic mass with low T1 and high T2 intensity. Fluid level due to intralesional hemorrhage/infection (**Fig. 7.58**)

Arteriovenous Malformations

General: high flow velocity! Hypertrophy of affected limb. When in liver → increased circulating blood volume → risk of heart failure!

Imaging: US—shows arterial flow in distended veins, defines feeding and draining vessel. Shunt usually very short (**Fig. 7.59**). CT angiography or MRA can give conspicuous survey view.

Capillary Malformations

Thickening of skin and subcutaneous tissue. Circumscribed vessels cannot be visualized.

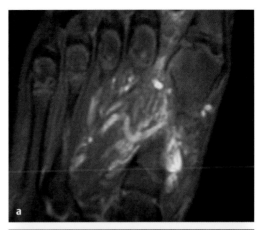

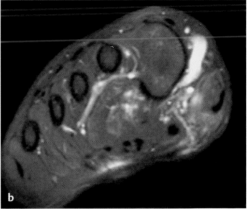

Fig. 7.57a, b Venous malformation. T1-weighted MRI with Gd enhancement and fat suppression. Axial (**a**) and coronal (**b**) images show multiple tortuous vessels located mainly in muscles of left forefoot.

Complex Lesions

General: mesenchymal mixed tumors with various components. Histological examination often necessary for classification. Manifestations and features defined by location and histology.

Klippel–Trenaunay syndrome = capillary lymphatic malformation with hypertrophy of affected limb. Defined by absence of deep veins, persistence of embryonic lateral marginal vein.

Imaging: US/CDS findings are often confusing. MRV is preferred.

7

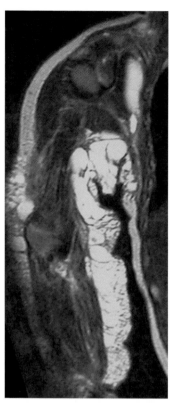

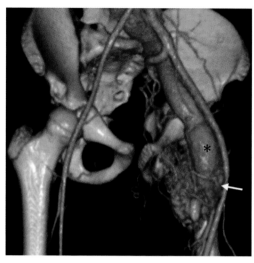

Fig. 7.59   Arteriovenous malformation in left groin. Preinterventional CTA (before coiling) shows short arteriovenous connection (arrow) feeding greatly expanded segments of left external and common iliac veins (*) along with multiple deep inguinal collateral veins communicating with territory of external iliac vein.

Fig. 7.58   Lymphatic malformation in right arm of newborn. Coronal T2-weighted MRI of right arm shows multiple subcutaneous and intramuscular masses, predominantly microcystic, with grotesque enlargement of arm and hand.

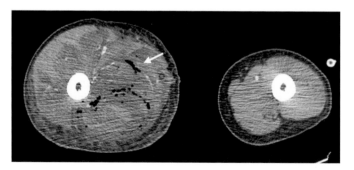

Fig. 7.60   Necrotizing fasciitis of thigh. Axial postcontrast CT scans of thigh show massive swelling of thigh muscles accompanied by epifascial gas (arrow).

Other Soft-Tissue Abnormalities

Cellulitis, Phlegmons, Soft-Tissue Abscesses, Fasciitis

Cellulitis, phlegmons: diffuse inflammation of skin and subcutaneous tissue, usually caused by bacterial infection. US shows diffuse, somewhat irregular increased echogenicity of tissue in early stage. Further progression → "fox-hole"-like fluid collections, circumscribed phlegmons.

Necrotizing fasciitis = involvement of deep structures, especially fascial planes, with detectable gas collections. Rare but life-threatening—most common in immunocompromised patients (**Fig. 7.60**).

Soft-tissue abscesses: may follow injuries, injections, or spread from abscessed lymph nodes. Imaging methods of choice = US and CDS; may be used to direct needle aspiration.

Lymphadenopathy

US = best for subcutaneous lymph nodes. Deeper lymph nodes = CT/MRI.

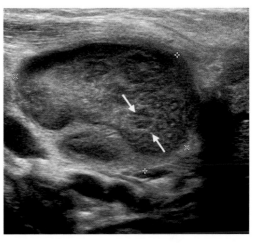

Fig. 7.61   Lymph node anatomy. High-resolution soft-tissue US of neck shows enlarged lymph nodes with typical hilar structure and enlarged secondary follicles (arrows).

Normal lymph nodes usually have elliptical shape (submental: spherical) (**Fig. 7.61**). Classification systems may be anatomical or clinically oriented (lymph node levels) (**Fig. 7.62**).

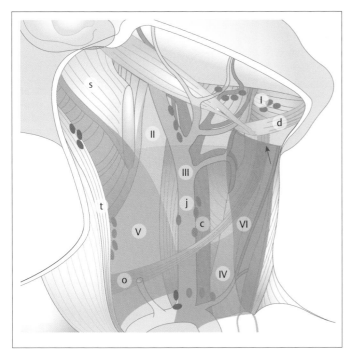

Fig. 7.62   Diagrammatic representation of lymph node levels in neck. Lymph node levels indicated by roman numerals, anatomic landmarks by lower-case letters. Carotid artery (c), internal jugular vein (j), omohyoid muscle (o), trapezius muscle (t), sternocleidomastoid muscle (s), digastric muscle (d). (Adapted from Saleh et al. 2008.)

7

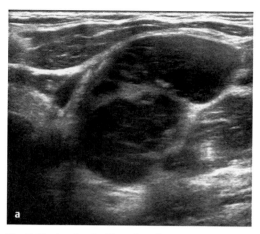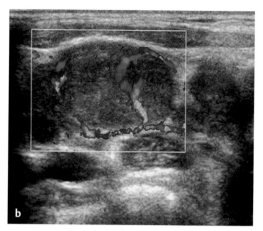

Fig. 7.63a, b   Cervical lymph node involvement by Hodgkin disease. High-resolution soft-tissue US of neck shows enlarged lymph node with loss of typical hilar structure (**a**). CDS = irregular perfusion (**b**).

All lymph node groups manifest similar findings and changes—cervical lymph nodes shown as example (approximately half of all lymph nodes in neck!). "Normal" cervical lymph nodes have maximum short-axis diameter of 10 mm (exception: jugulodigastric nodes range to 15 mm).

! Absence of enlargement does not exclude disease!

Benign and malignant lymph nodes overlap in US morphology. Following criteria, especially when combined, suspicious for malignancy: spherical shape (rather than elliptical), absent/displaced hilum, irregular outlines, necrosis, irregular flow pattern on CDS (**Fig. 7.63**).

Reactive lymph node changes by far the most common: uniform enlargement, decreased echogenicity, hyperemia of central hilar vessels.

Not uncommon to find rounded intraparotid nodes.

Peracute bacterial inflammations mostly unilateral, may form abscesses. (Power) Doppler can detect liquefaction (**Fig. 7.64**). CT/MRI useful for suspected retropharyngeal abscess.

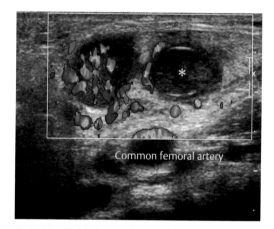

Fig. 7.64   Right inguinal lymphadenopathy. Duplex US of left groin shows two acutely inflamed and enlarged right inguinal lymph nodes. The more medial node contains central abscess (*).

Quiz Case 7.1

History: 6-year-old girl fell on her elbow.

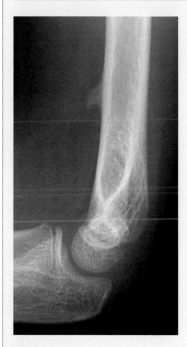

Questions	Correct answers
What images would be appropriate?	Radiographs in two planes of affected joint, (only one relevant image reproduced above). Note: no routine initial film of opposite side for comparison indicated
What images are available?	Lateral radiograph of elbow
Findings?	Bony protuberance located on anterior side of distal humeral shaft, points distally
Diagnosis?	Supracondylar process
DD?	Osteochondromas would be located in metaphysis and would point toward shaft

Fig. 7.65

7

Quiz Case 7.2

History: 8-year-old boy with palpable abnormalities on both femurs.

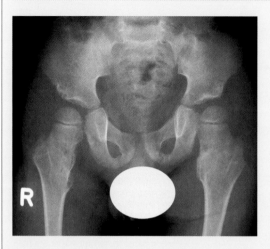

Fig. 7.66

Questions	Correct answers
What images would be appropriate?	Pelvic survey radiograph that covers thighs
What images are available?	Pelvic survey radiograph
Findings?	Asymmetric, lobulated bone masses protruding from proximal femurs and pelvis
Diagnosis?	Multiple sessile osteochondromas of both femurs (= metaphyseal bone dysplasia)
Can imaging contribute to treatment?	Follow-up of growth

Quiz Case 7.3

History: multiple bony-hard tumors in chest.

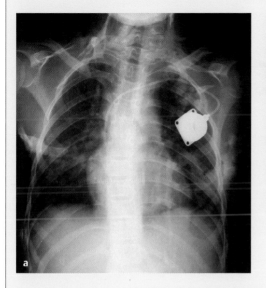

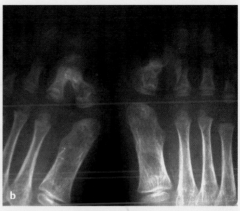

Fig. 7.67a, b

Questions	Correct answers
What images would be appropriate?	Radiographs, US, MRI, CT
What images are available?	Chest radiograph (Fig. **a**), radiograph of medial forefeet (Fig. **b**)
Findings?	Multiple ossifications of varying shape in thoracic and cervical soft tissues, some intramuscular. Bilateral widening and shortening of big toes
Diagnosis?	Fibrodysplasia ossificans progressiva
DD?	With normal big toes: dystrophic calcifications, ossifications, calcinosis cutis, parasitic infection

7

Bibliography

1 Barnard LB, McCOY SM. The supra condyloid process of the humerus. J Bone Joint Surg Am 1946; 28(4): 845–850

2 Fishman SJ, Mulliken JB. Vascular anomalies. A primer for pediatricians. Pediatr Clin North Am 1998; 45(6): 1455–1477

3 Graf R. Hip Sonography: Diagnosis and Management of Infant Hip Dysplasia. Berlin, Heidelberg: Springer; 2006

4 Greulich WW, Pyle SI. A Radiographic Atlas and Skeletal Development of the Hand and Wrist, 2nd ed. Stanford, CA: Stanford University Press; 1959

5 Jaramillo D, Laor T. Pediatric musculoskeletal MRI: basic principles to optimize success. Pediatr Radiol 2008; 38(4): 379–391

6 Jaramillo D. What is the optimal imaging of osteonecrosis, Perthes, and bone infarcts? Pediatr Radiol 2009; 39(Suppl 2): S216–S219

7 Jurik AG. Chronic recurrent multifocal osteomyelitis. Semin Musculoskelet Radiol 2004; 8(3): 243–253

8 Keats TE. An Atlas of Normal Roentgen Variants that May Simulate Disease. St. Louis: Mosby; 2001

9 Kuhn JP, Slovis TL, Haller JO. Caffey's Pediatric Diagnostic Imaging. Philadelphia: Mosby; 2004

Quiz Case 7.4

History: 11-year-old girl with acute right-sided calf pain.

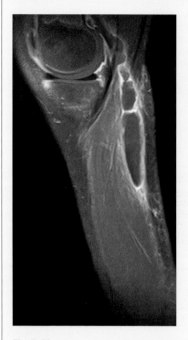

Questions	Correct answers
What images would be appropriate?	Radiographs, US, MRI, possibly venography
What images are available?	MRI of proximal lower leg (fat-suppressed T1, sagittal, postcontrast)
Findings?	Septated liquid intramuscular mass in gastrocnemius muscle with enhancing septa; no joint effusion
Diagnosis?	Popliteal cyst with inflammatory changes, extending far between crural muscles
DD?	Cystic synovialoma, partially organized hematoma, postnecrotic abscess

Fig. 7.68

10 Maresh MM. Linear growth of long bones of extremities from infancy through adolescence; continuing studies. AMA Am J Dis Child 1955; 89(6): 735–742

11 Paltiel HJ, Burrows PE, Kozakewich HP, Zurakowski D, Mulliken JB. Soft-tissue vascular anomalies: utility of US for diagnosis. Radiology 2000; 214(3): 747–754

12 Pyle SI, Waterhouse AM, Greulich WW. A Radiographic Standard of Reference for the Growing Hand and Wrist. Cleveland, OH: Case Western Reserve University Press; 1971

13 Restrepo R, Oneto J, Lopez K, Kukreja K. Head and neck lymph nodes in children: the spectrum from normal to abnormal. Pediatr Radiol 2009; 39(8): 836–846

14 Rosendahl K, Toma P. Ultrasound in the diagnosis of developmental dysplasia of the hip in newborns. The European approach. A review of methods, accuracy and clinical validity. Eur Radiol 2007; 17(8): 1960–1967

15 Saigal G, Azouz EM, Abdenour G. Imaging of osteomyelitis with special reference to children. Semin Musculoskelet Radiol 2004; 8(3): 255–265

16 Saleh A, Mathys C, Mödder U. Staging von Kopf-Hals-Tumoren mit bildgebended Verfahren. Teil II: N- und M-Staging. Radiologie up2date 2008; 1

17 Tanner JM, Whitehouse RH, Marshall WA, et al. Assessement of Skeletal Maturity and Prediction of Adult Height (TW2 Method). London: Academic Press; 1975

8 Pediatric Oncoradiology

8.1 General Introduction and Basic Principles

Michael Riccabona

Goals of Oncologic Imaging

- Evaluation/detection of tumors suspected clinically/detected incidentally
- Tumor description, quantification, localization: tumor size, local findings (invasive/localized, capsule, vascular invasion, necrosis, local metastasis), acute/impending dangers (e.g., hemorrhage, elevated-pressure hydrocephalus, tracheal compression, etc.)
- Tumor characterization: identification of entity if possible (tentative diagnosis—almost never replaces histology!). Clinically important benign–malignant differentiation—often possible
- Staging: local and systemic (distant metastases), if malignant
- Preoperative imaging: relation to surrounding structures (vessels, adjacent organs, urinary tract, bowel, bile ducts, etc. = assess operability/visualize surgical risks)
- Postoperative assessment: residual tumor, surgical changes, complications
- Follow-up: response to (chemo)therapy? recurrence? complications?
- Treatment-associated secondary changes (avascular necrosis, etc.)
- Long-term monitoring: late/secondary changes, organ growth, late recurrence/metastasis, etc.

Imaging Options

- **US:** initial investigation and follow-up of abdomen and small parts/soft tissues, especially lymph nodes. Preoperative US is adequate for some (benign/intermediate) tumors such as teratoma, mesoblastic nephroma, etc. Contrast-enhanced US (ce-US) may also provide tumor char-

acterization (especially in liver—same criteria as in adults). 3D US improves tumor volumetry
- **Plain radiographs:** essential for bone tumors (two planes), otherwise of limited importance (e.g., relevant pulmonary metastasis, initial detection of certain intrathoracic tumors, tumor calcification, bone infiltration/metastasis)
- **FL:** still used occasionally for GI/bladder tumors, but largely replaced by MRI and CT. May have role in biopsy and intervention (e.g., embolization therapy, percutaneous decompression and drainage, complicated venous access, etc.) or treatment (e.g., tumor-associated intussusception and reduction, etc.)
- **MRI:** "workhorse" of pediatric oncoradiology in all body regions—except for evaluating very small pulmonary lesions (mostly metastases) and bone architecture (DD of certain bone tumors). T1-, T2- and contrast-enhanced T1-weighted sequences (always in three planes), at least one with fat saturation; tumor volumetry. Preoperative MRA (or MRU) and 3D acquisitions sometimes helpful (include them in initial protocol?). Increasing utilization of chemical shift imaging (in-phase and out-of-phase), dynamic perfusion sequences and DWI (characterization, therapeutic response, etc.), whole-body MRI (staging, etc.). Potentially, MR spectroscopy if available and/or required (see Sect. 1.6)
- **CT:** if MRI not available or contraindicated. Always used for small pulmonary lesions, bone structural evaluation

Specific, individualized planning recommended. Assess need for precontrast scans, postcontrast phase of interest, possible need for CTA, and coverage extent (may acquire 1 phase with shorter range)—respect ALARA criteria (see Sect. 1.5). In abdominal cases, always precede CT by detailed US! Use child-appropriate age-adapted CT protocols! Note requirements of specific oncologic study protocols.

- **Scintigraphy:** skeletal scintigraphy (staging, DD of bone tumors), special tests (e.g., meta-iodo-benzyl guanidine [MIBG] for neuroblastoma, rarely gallium scans for liver tumors, etc.)
- **PET (-CT/MRI):** increasingly important for certain entities (lymphoma, recurrence, etc.).

Tumor localization: criteria helpful for localizing to specific organ: mobility (e.g., with respirations) relative shift, vascular supply, crescent sign (**Fig. 8.1**).

Tumor investigations are replete with pitfalls, "mimics" common. Tumor exclusion, while often desired, is not possible in some settings! Note requirements of specific oncologic study protocols.

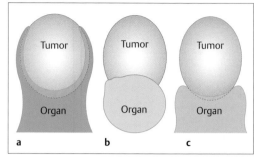

Fig. 8.1a, b   Localizing tumors and determining their origin. Morphologic criteria for determining tumor origin, useful in all imaging modalities (especially for large tumors of parenchymal organs with little or no infiltration, destruction, or spread outside the organ). Tumor originating from organ may appear to emerge from organ (**a**), separating parenchymal edges. Tumor originating outside organ may abut adjacent organ without altering its shape (**b**), or may cause visible impression (**c**).

8.2   ## Tumors of the Brain, Orbit, and Spine

Gabriele Hahn

Brain Tumors

General: supratentorial brain tumors more common than infratentorial tumors in children under 3 years old. Infratentorial tumors predominate from 4th to 10th year. Infra- and supratentorial tumors show equal distribution thereafter.

Most common brain tumors in **first year of life = teratoma, suprasellar astrocytoma, ependymoma, choroid plexus tumor, rhabdoid tumor**. Other less common types also encountered.

Imaging: MRI—mainstay for diagnosis and preoperative imaging. CT and US not sufficient for treatment planning. Standard MRI sequences for brain tumors: T1-, T2-weighted, and FLAIR sequences, preferably in axial planes, slice thickness < 5 mm; almost cover entire head. Add sagittal and coronal images to better define extent and delineate from surrounding brain. T1-weighted sequences after contrast administration—generally acquired in three planes. Tumors characterized and classified based on location, delineation, signal intensity, mass effects, and contrast enhancement.

Infratentorial Brain Tumors

Most common intra-axial tumors of posterior cranial fossa: mebulloblastomas (WHO IV, in fourth ventricle, T2 isointense to gray matter), astrocytomas (WHO I, in cerebellar hemispheres, T2 hyperintense), ependymomas (WHO III, spread along CSF pathways, T2 isointense to gray matter) (**Table 8.1**).

- Mebulloblastoma and ependymoma: usually inhomogeneous, variable contrast enhancement, may spread along CSF pathways (**Fig. 8.2**)
- Astrocytoma: mixed nodular or irregular enhancement pattern with cystic components (Case Study 8.1, **Fig. 8.9**)
- Brainstem tumors: differentiated by location (medulla oblongata, pons, mesencephalon) and spread (focal = < 50% cross-section, diffuse = > 50% cross-section). Most common histology: astrocytoma. Less common: ganglioglioma, etc. **Pontine glioma** with typical MRI features (= expanded pons, T1 hypointense, T2 hyperintense, indistinct margins, usually no disruption of blood–brain barrier [BBB]) does not require histologic confirmation (**Fig. 8.3**)

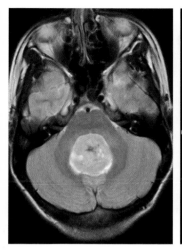

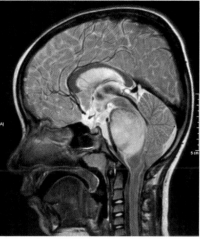

Fig. 8.2 **Infratentorial mebulloblastoma.** Axial T2-weighted MRI shows inhomogeneous tumor in fourth ventricle, predominantly isointense to cortex, with narrow rim of hyperintense CSF. Note absence of perifocal edema in adjacent pons and cerebellum.

Fig. 8.3 **Pontine glioma.** Sagittal T2-weighted MRI shows large hyperintense tumor in pons causing complete compression of fourth ventricle.

Fig. 8.2   **Fig. 8.3**

DD: of intraparenchymal infratentorial mass: **abscess, ADEM, MS, cavernoma.**

- Abscess—marked diffusion abnormality at lesion center, linear or irregular BBB disruption at periphery (= contrast enhancement)
- Cavernoma (acutely symptomatic)—hemorrhagic areas and perifocal edema in all MR sequences → may be indistinguishable from other tumor with intralesional hemorrhage

> Detection of hemosiderin/blood very specific in T2*-weighted sequences owing to susceptibility artifacts.

Extra-axial infratentorial tumors: dermoid/epidermoid, schwannoma, meningioma, skull-base tumor. Differentiation of extra-axial from intra-axial tumors essential for preoperative planning.

> Epidermoid can be positively identified with FLAIR and diffusion-weighted sequences (FLAIR = hyperintense; diffusion-weighted sequences = diffusion abnormality). MR morphology very different from arachnoid cyst, for example.

Supratentorial Brain Tumors

Best classified by their location: sellar/suprasellar, in cerebral hemispheres, in ventricular system, in pineal region, in calvarium/meninges.

Table 8.1 Differential diagnosis of infratentorial brain tumors

Type of tumor	T1	T2	FLAIR	Contrast enhancement	Other criteria
Mebulloblastoma	↓	←	↑	Inhomogeneous	In 4th ventricle, may spread along CSF pathways
Ependymoma	↓ ←	↑ ←	↑	Inhomogeneous	In 4th ventricle, may spread along CSF pathways
Pilocytic astrocytoma	↓ ←	↑	↑	Marked, nodular, or bandlike/irregular pattern	Intracerebellar, possible cysts
Brainstem tumor	↓	↑	↑	Absent or moderate	

Arrows = signal intensity relative to gray matter.

8

Sellar/Suprasellar Brain Tumors

Most common suprasellar tumor entities = **craniopharyngioma, astrocytoma, pituitary adenoma, germ cell tumor, Rathke pouch cyst, LCH.**

- Craniopharyngioma—arises from remnants of craniopharyngeal duct, has typical morphology (predominantly multicystic with few if any solid elements). Cysts with peripheral hypointense calcifications hypo-, iso-, or hyperintense in T1-weighted sequences, almost always show cyst wall enhancement after contrast administration (**Fig. 8.4**)
- Suprasellar astrocytomas—arise from optic chiasm/hypothalamus, usually occur in setting of neurofibromatosis type I (NF I; see also Sect. 4.1). T1 hypointense, T2 hyperintense, usually show inhomogeneous enhancement
- Suprasellar germ cell tumors—characteristics similar to LCH and lymphocytic hypophysitis. Typical clinical presentation = diabetes insipidus. MRI shows thickening and enhancement of infundibulum

Brain Tumors of the Cerebral Hemispheres

Most common hemispheric tumor = astrocytoma. Also **teratomas** in newborns. Other tumors in young children: **ependymoma, ganglioglioma, oligodendroglioma, PNET, DNET**—important in DD.

- Astrocytoma—typically located deep in hemisphere, may also occur in white matter or cortex. T1 hypointense, T2 hyperintense, well-defined margins. Portions of tumor may show marked enhancement, may contain cystic areas.

- DNET—benign brain tumor, occurs mainly in cortex. Patients usually present clinically with partial complex seizures. MR morphology highly variable. T2 hyperintense, may contain cystic areas, rarely shows enhancement

Brain Tumors in the Ventricular System

Most common: **choroid plexus papilloma** and **carcinoma.** Choroid plexus carcinomas differ from papillomas in presence of necrosis, tissue inhomogeneity, parenchymal invasion, and inhomogeneous enhancement (papilloma = homogeneous) (**Fig. 8.5**). Both tumors may spread along intracranial and intraspinal CSF pathways.

Brain Tumors of the Pineal Region

Important in pediatric age group: **germ cell tumor, pineoblastoma, pineocytoma, teratoma, glioma, simple cysts.** Germ cell tumors (germinoma, teratoma, other rarer types) most common. In most cases, CSF spread already present at time of diagnosis.

MRI: round, inhomogeneous in T1- and T2-weighted sequences; inhomogeneous enhancement pattern.

Different pineal tumors can rarely be differentiated by their MR morphology.

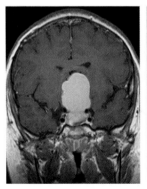

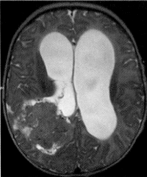

Fig. 8.4   **Fig. 8.5**

Fig. 8.4   Craniopharyngioma. Coronal T1-weighted MRI after contrast administration shows very hyperintense intra- and suprasellar median mass extending into third ventricle and into foramen of Monro on each side. Distinct linear enhancement seen at tumor periphery.

Fig. 8.5   Choroid plexus carcinoma. Axial T2-weighted MRI shows irregular intraventricular mass, isointense to cortex, in right lateral ventricle (LV). Parenchymal invasion in right hemisphere associated with hyperintense regional edema. Hydrocephalus with dilatation of LVs due to excessive CSF production by choroid plexus carcinoma.

Brain Tumors of the Calvarium and Meninges

Tumors arising from cranial coverings very rare in children: **meningioma, cartilaginous and bone tumors** (chondrosarcoma, osteosarcoma, Ewing sarcoma). Neuroblastoma often metastasizes to cranial bone.

Neurocutaneous Syndromes

See also Sect. 4.1. Neurocutaneous syndromes (phakomatoses) = congenital malformations predominantly affecting structures of ectodermal origin. Four classic diseases:

- **NF I (von Recklinghausen disease)**
- **Tuberous sclerosis (Bourneville–Pringle disease)**
- **Retinocerebellar angiomatosis (von Hippel–Lindau disease)**
- **Encephalotrigeminal angiomatosis (Sturge–Weber syndrome)**

Today, about 30 additional diseases are included under the heading of neurocutaneous syndromes (but diagnosed only sporadically).

Neurofibromatosis Type I

NF I = most common autosomal dominant CNS disease. Incidence of **optic glioma** in children = 15%

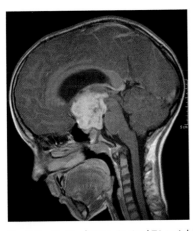

Fig. 8.6 Optic glioma. Sagittal T1-weighted MRI after contrast administration shows inhomogeneous, enhancing suprasellar tumor extending into third ventricle and prepontine area. Optic chiasm glioma compressing pituitary from above sella in child with (known) neurofibromatosis type I.

(highly variable MRI signal characteristics and contrast enhancement, **Fig. 8.6**). Other specific changes: focal signal changes in brain parenchyma (high T2-weighted and FLAIR signal intensity— caused by **atypical myelination** with vacuolization) in brainstem, cerebellar white matter, globus pallidus, corpus callosum, and **extracranial plexiform neurofibromas**. This atypical myelination develops after 1 year of age and resolves by age 20. Differentiation from astrocytoma at typical sites may be difficult (criteria: mass lesion, contrast enhancement).

> Brainstem gliomas and astrocytomas at other sites usually imply better prognosis for patients with NF I.

Tuberous Sclerosis

Large range of phenotypic variability in affected patients, with highly variable intracranial manifestations. Characteristic lesions = **subependymal hamartomas, (sub)cortical tubers, linear white matter lesions, giant cell astrocytoma at foramen of Monro.** Changes most conspicuous in still unmyelinated brain (white matter = T1 hypointense, T2 hyperintense in small infant). With progressive myelination, lesions become isointense to white matter → seen most clearly in FLAIR sequences (tuberomas, white matter lesions).

Sturge–Weber Syndrome

Pathognomonic features: facial angiomatosis (not always present), **cortical calcifications, pial angiomatosis, enlargement of choroid plexus** with **anomalous venous drainage**.

Pial angiomatosis visible only in postcontrast MRI, appearing as linear enhancement along brain surface. Underlying cortex atrophies only with increasing age. Typical cortical calcifications not yet present in small children.

Von Hippel–Lindau Disease

Typical features = multiple **hemangioblastomas**— cerebellar, in brainstem, hemispheric, and in spinal cord. Typical appearance = very vascular nodule in wall of fluid-filled cyst, may be completely solid. Solid components enhance intensely after contrast administration.

8

Rarely symptomatic and rarely diagnosed in children. Associated with other changes and extracranial tumors (e.g., pheochromocytoma, renal cell carcinoma, etc.).

Intraorbital metastatic neuroblastoma → permeative bone destruction, T1 hypointense, T2 hyperintense in fat-saturated sequences, homogeneous enhancement pattern.

Orbital Tumors

General: extraocular orbital mass = metastatic neuroblastoma, RMS, LCH, encephalocele, malformative tumors (dermoid, epidermoid, hemangioma, cavernoma, lymphangioma, colloid cysts; **Fig. 8.7**). Intraocular tumors = retinoblastoma, Coats disease, persistent hyperplastic primary vitreous, infections (Case Study 8.2, **Fig. 8.10**).
Imaging: mainly US and MRI in children. For US capabilities, see Sect. 4.2. MRI employs fat-suppressed T2- and T1-weighted sequences before and after contrast, using coronal imaging and high resolution (another option: isotropic 3D acquisition).

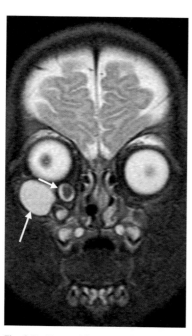

Fig. 8.7   Dermoid. Coronal fat-suppressed T2-weighted MRI shows two circumscribed dermoid tumors of right orbit, one hyperintense throughout (longer arrow) and other with hypointense center (shorter arrow).

Spinal Tumors

Spinal tumors are rare in children—most grow slowly, present with nonspecific early symptoms (e.g., back pain).
Imaging: MRI—key role in diagnosis and classification. Important for treatment planning = can differentiate intra- and extramedullary tumors (intramedullary mass = expands cord; extramedullary tumor = narrows CSF space and compresses cord, depending on size). Imaging strategy = T1- and T2-weighted sequences in all planes, contrast administration.

> Spinal intramedullary tumors are difficult to distinguish from focal demyelination (e.g., in MS or ADEM).

Intramedullary Tumors

Astrocytoma more common in children than **ependymoma**. Other rare tumors = ganglioglioma, gangliocytoma, germinoma, PNET, etc.

Criteria and appearance on spinal MRI: cord expansion, T1 hypointensity, variable T2 hyperintensity—the higher the malignancy and cellularity, the less free water content → T2 signal ↓, as in all other (brain) tumors. Cysts and necrotic zones demarcated after contrast administration. Two most common entities show moderate enhancement (ependymoma = sharper margins than astrocytoma).

> Nonneoplastic intramedullary syrinx may appear above and below tumor.

Extramedullary Intraspinal Tumors

Intradural tumors—most are drop metastases from brain tumors along subarachnoid space (medulloblastoma, ependymoma, glioblastoma, germ cell tumor, choroid plexus tumor, pineal tumor) or primary intramedullary tumors. Consist of individual nodules or patchy subarachnoid masses encasing cord—often detectable only after contrast administration (**Fig. 8.8**).

Extradural tumors—may originate from vertebral body, may be benign (aneurysmatic bone cyst, giant cell tumor, osteoblastoma) or malignant (osteosarcoma, Ewing sarcoma, LCH). Very rare: meningeal tumors (meningioma) and spinal nerve tumors (schwannoma, neurofibroma).

> Paraspinal tumors that invade spinal canal secondarily through neuroforamina (mainly neuroblastoma, occasionally lymphoma or PNET) important in pediatric age group (Case Study 8.3, **Fig. 8.11**).

Congenital spinal tumors—include teratomas, lipomas, dermoids, epidermoids, and hamartomas. Often associated with spinal malformation (e.g., MMC, etc.) and possible secondary tethered cord (see also Sect. 4.1). Initial imaging study in small infants = spinal US, owing to incomplete ossification of spinal column (see also Sect. 4.2). MRI can be added for treatment planning, also used in older children.

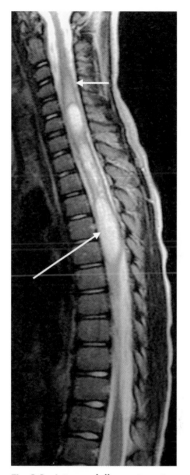

Fig. 8.8 Intramedullary astrocytoma.
Sagittal T2-weighted MRI of spine shows elongated, hyperintense intramedullary mass (long arrow) with associated cord expansion. Perimedullary CSF space significantly narrowed at cervical and thoracic levels. With hyperintense neoplasm, it is not possible to distinguish tumor from tumor-associated myelopathy at or above (short arrow) intramedullary tumor level.

8

Case Study 8.1

Clinical findings: 5-year-old girl with 3-week history of increasing retching and vomiting. Headache, papilledema.
Imaging options: MRI (possibly CT).

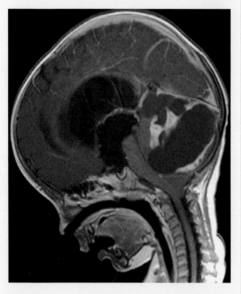

Fig. 8.9

Available image: cranial MRI, sagittal T1 after Gd.
Findings: infratentorial mass with cystic components almost isointense to CSF and with enhancing peripheral irregular components. Obstructive hydrocephalus due to aqueductal compression and foramen magnum herniation.
Diagnosis: infratentorial pilocytic astrocytoma.
DD: hemangioblastoma.

Case Study 8.2

Clinical findings: visual deterioration on left side.
Imaging options in the orbit: US, MRI.

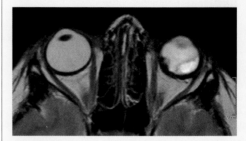

Fig. 8.10

Available image: axial T2 MRI of orbit.
Findings: left eye smaller than right, hyperintense retinal detachment in left eye due to protein-rich exudate.
Diagnosis: Coats disease.
DD: retinoblastoma, infection (*Toxicaris canii*, aspergillus), persistent hyperplastic primary vitreous.

Case Study 8.3

Clinical findings: progressing cord lesion.
Imaging options: MRI.

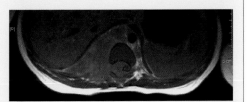

Fig. 8.11

Available image: axial T1 spinal MRI after contrast administration.
Findings: weakly enhancing retrocrural and transforaminal tumor extending into spinal canal. Cord completely encased by tumor and displaced to left side. Infiltration of back muscles, mainly on right side.
Diagnosis: neuroblastoma.

Bibliography

1 Barkovich AJ. Pediatric neuroimaging. Philadelphia: Lippincott Williams & Wilkins; 2005
2 Barkovich AJ, Moore KR, Grant E, et al. Diagnostic Imaging: Pediatric Neuroradiology. Salt Lake City: AMIRSYS; 2007

8.3 Neuroblastoma, Adrenal Masses, and Thoracic Tumors

Marcus Hoermann, Michael Riccabona

Neuroblastoma

General: after Wilms tumor, second most common abdominal tumor in children; second or third most common tumor after leukemia and CNS tumors; 7% are older than 15 years at diagnosis, responsible for childhood death in 15%. Many children with neuroblastoma die within 2 years; >90% of cases diagnosed in children under 5 years of age, 30 to 50% are diagnosed in first month of life.

Etiology: like benign ganglioneuroma and ganglioneuroblastoma, derived from ganglion cells of embryonic neural crest anywhere along sympathetic trunk.

Sites of occurrence: often retroperitoneal; adrenal glands (35%), along abdominal sympathetic trunk (30–35%), mediastinum (20%). Occasionally arise from organ of Zuckerkandl. May also form in pelvis or cervical sympathetic trunk (1–5%). Sporadic cases are metastatic from unknown primary tumor.

Screening, Clinical Features, and Diagnosis

Screening: under discussion; based on vanillylmandelic and homovanillic acid urine test in 6-month-old children.

Diagnosis: usually detected incidentally by US (or chest radiography) done for other indications (trauma, different disease). Confirmed by clinical examination and laboratory blood and urine analysis. Bone marrow involvement assessed by bone marrow biopsy.

Imaging: US, scintigraphy, CT, MRI—diagnosis, staging, etc. (see Sect. 8.1 and **Figs. 8.12, 8.13, 8.14**). Staging criteria (**Table 8.2**): local effects—displacement, invasive growth. Relationship to vessels—renal hilum, celiac trunk, portal vein, spread across midline, neuroforamen/intraspinal involvement, lymph nodes, metastases.

8

Table 8.2   International Neuroblastoma Staging System (INSS)

Stage	Definition
1	Localized tumor with complete gross excision, with or without microscopic residual disease; ipsilateral lymph nodes negative for tumor microscopically; nodes adherent to primary tumor and resected with it may be positive
2A	Localized tumor with incomplete gross excision; representative ipsilateral lymph nodes negative for tumor microscopically
2B	Localized tumor with or without complete gross excision, with ipsilateral nonadherent lymph nodes positive for tumor; enlarged contralateral lymph nodes negative microscopically
3	Unresectable unilateral tumor infiltrating across midline, with or without regional lymph node involvement; *or* localized unilateral tumor with contralateral regional lymph node involvement; *or* midline tumor with bilateral extension by infiltration (unresectable) or by lymph node involvement
4	Any primary tumor with dissemination to distant lymph nodes, bone, bone marrow, liver, skin, or other sites, except as defined for stage 4S
4S	Small localized tumor in children < 12 months (as defined for stage 1, 2A, or 2B); involvement limited to skin, liver, or bone marrow

Clinical presentation: depends on site of tumor/metastases, paraneoplastic syndrome. Three main manifestations:
- **Localized tumor:** about 40% paraspinal; 5 to 15% show intraforaminal growth → neurologic symptoms due to root irritation and cord compression: motor weakness, sensory deficit, pain. Cervical spine involvement → Horner triad, dysphagia, stridor. Renin-mediated hypertension due to renovascular compromise
- **Paraneoplastic syndrome:** two main symptoms:
  - watery diarrhea, resistant to treatment, with failure to thrive (secretion of vasoactive peptides)—resolves immediately after tumor excision
  - opsoclonus–myoclonus syndrome (Kinsbourne syndrome) in 2 to 4%—rapid eye movement; ataxia, uncontrolled muscle movements.

- **Metastatic disease:** 50% of patients already have locoregional spread (lymph node in close proximity to primary tumor) or distant metastases (cortex of bones, bone marrow, liver, distant lymph nodes) at time of diagnosis (**Figs. 8.13** and **8.14**). Unexplained tendency to metastasize to orbital bone causing local ecchymosis ("raccoon eyes"; see Sect. 8.2). Cutaneous metastases—shiny blue skin nodules, may be earliest clinical sign. DD: hemangioma

> These manifestations should not be mistaken for child abuse.

- **4S disease:** seen in just 5% of small primary tumors, but associated with metastasis to liver, skin, and bone marrow

> (Primary) tumors may regress spontaneously.

▪▪ Case Study 8.4 ▪▪▪▪

History: 4-year-old boy with palpable abdominal mass on right side.
Suitable modalities: US, MRI, CT.

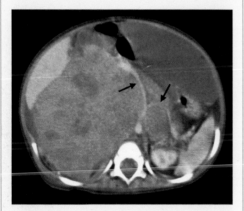

Fig. 8.12

Available image: axial multislice spiral CT (MSCT) with intravenous nonionic contrast medium.
Findings: giant, inhomogeneously enhancing mass arising from right adrenal bed, extending across midline, encasing and displacing visceral vascular branches (arrows) of abdominal aorta.
Diagnosis: high-risk neuroblastoma.

▪▪ Case Study 8.5 ▪▪▪▪

History: 4-year-old boy with palpable abdominal mass on right side. Staging of patient in **Fig. 8.12.**
Suitable modalities: US, MRI, CT.

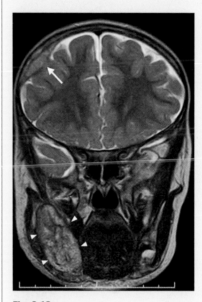

Fig. 8.13

Available image: coronal T2 MRI, TSE sequence.
Findings: inhomogeneous, well-circumscribed expansion of right mandible (arrowheads) and right parietal mass (arrow).
Diagnosis: bone metastases.

8

━━━ **Case Study 8.6** ━━━

History: 4-year-old boy with palpable abdominal mass on right side. Staging of patient in **Figs. 8.12** and **8.13**.
Suitable modalities: US, MRI, CT.

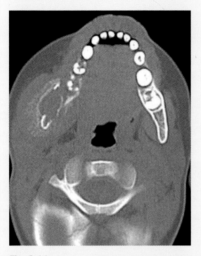

Fig. 8.14

Available image: axial MSCT with bone window.
Findings: lesion in expanded right mandible. Marked bone destruction with visible soft-tissue component and calcified tumor matrix.
Diagnosis: bone metastases.

━━━ **Case Study 8.7** ━━━

History: 2-year-old girl with large mass above right kidney detected by US.
Other imaging options: MRI, CT, scintigraphy.

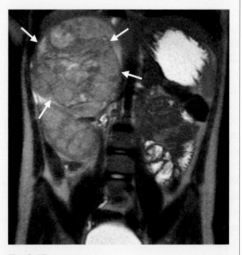

Fig. 8.15

Available image: coronal T2-weighted sequence on MRI.
Findings: inhomogeneous tumor with sharp margins, partially lobulated, with fluid-equivalent areas in right adrenal bed (→). Tumor displacing kidney.
Diagnosis: neuroblastoma.

Staging

Depending on whether patients are in a study cohort, either system below may be used.

International Neuroblastoma Staging System (INSS), 1993 revision, commonly used in United States, defines stages based on radiologic and scintigraphic findings, lymph node involvement, bone marrow involvement, resectability, macro- and microscopic postoperative features (**Table 8.2**).

International Neuroblastoma Risk Group (INRG)—newer staging system classifies tumors as having high, intermediate, or low pretreatment risk. Most commonly used in Europe for newer study cohorts.

- High risk: tumor with metastases at diagnosis (excludes pediatric 4S tumors) and all N-myc-amplifying tumors, regardless of age
- INRG stage I: localized disease without local invasion
- INRG stage II: locally invasive disease
- Stages M and MS: tumor with distant metastasis or 4S tumor

Other prognostic factors: biology and histopathology = favorable or unfavorable depending on neuroblastic differentiation, schwannian stromal content, age at diagnosis. Biologic criteria = N-myc amplification, diploidy in DNA index. Genetic defects = deletions on short arm of chromosomes 1, 11, 17.

Fetal Neuroblastoma

Neuroblastoma with teratoma = neoplasm most commonly diagnosed in utero. Has more favorable prognosis. Presents as mass in adrenal region. Most common DD: adrenal hemorrhage, extrapulmonary sequestrum, mesoblastic nephroma. Greater use of fetal MRI → increasing rates of detection and postnatal treatment (**Fig. 8.15**).

Imaging: initial study = US, which shows heterogeneous mass, predominantly hypoechoic, often with linear or stippled echogenic calcifications (little acoustic shadowing if small!). Tumor grows by expansion, may encase blood vessels—CDS important adjunct to B-mode. Hepatic metastasis more common than direct invasion of liver—can be clearly differentiated with US (see Sect. 8.1).

Detailed evaluation/staging: MRI or CT, especially if MRI unavailable (multidetector CT = MSCT; see **Figs. 8.12** and **8.14**). Always administer contrast. MRI superior for spinal involvement and bone marrow infiltration—but primary tumor does not have typical signal characteristics (**Fig. 8.16**). CT better for detecting rare pulmonary metastases and tumor calcifications.

Scintigraphy: ^{123}I-MIBG scanning—essential search tool for primary tumors and metastases. Another option: ^{99m}Tc-methylene diphosphonate scintigraphy.

Evaluating treatment response: scintigraphy is superior to MRI at present. Postoperative US and MRI (MSCT)—local evaluation of operative site. Often difficult to distinguish residual tumor from scar.

Other Pediatric Adrenal Tumors and Entities Important in Differential Diagnosis

Other adrenal tumors in pediatric age group: pheochromocytoma (rare, usually suspected clinically, sometimes bilateral, associated with von Hippel-Lindau, multiple endocrine neoplasia syndrome; **Fig. 8.18**), teratoma, adrenal carcinoma (rare, aggressive; **Fig. 8.17**), adrenal cysts, inflammations (Tb), adrenal hyperplasia, and adrenal hemorrhage (see Chapter 9).

▬▬	**Case Study 8.8**	▬▬

History: tumor detected at prenatal US.
Other postnatal imaging options: US, MRI, CT, scintigraphy.

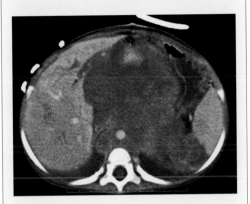

Fig. 8.16

Available image: contrast-enhanced axial MSCT.
Findings: giant, well-circumscribed, inhomogeneous mass on midline (= crossing midline) with both solid and liquid components. The mass has encased aorta and IVC without obstructing blood flow. Concomitant ascites, bilateral pleural effusions.
Diagnosis: high-risk neuroblastoma.

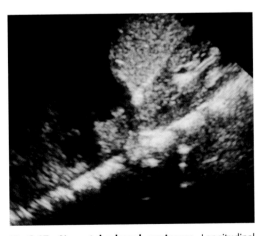

Fig. 8.17 Neonatal adrenal carcinoma. Longitudinal US scan through right adrenal gland and diaphragm shows aggressive adrenal tumor that has invaded chest. Note reactive pleural effusion and massive destruction by this extremely aggressive adrenal carcinoma in an infant.

8

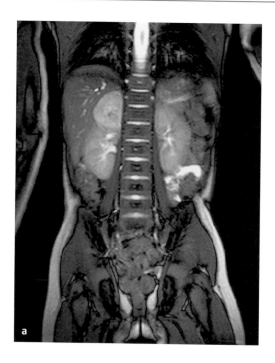

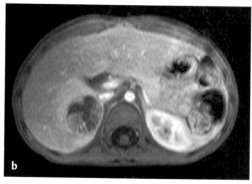

Fig. 8.18a, b   Pediatric pheochromocytoma.
a Coronal MRI (SSFP sequence) in 3-year-old girl with unexplained hypertension, urinary catecholamines ↑ ↑ ↑. MRI confirms right adrenal mass detected by US.
b Axial T1-weighted MRI after contrast administration shows almost spoked-wheel enhancement pattern in right adrenal tumor (pheochromocytoma).

Important Thoracic Tumors in Children

Lung Tumors—General

General: rare in children and adolescents; most distant metastases from age-specific primary tumors. Two-thirds of primary lung tumors are malignant.

Primary malignant lung tumors in order of frequency: carcinoid, bronchogenic carcinoma, mucoepidermoid carcinoma, pleuropulmonary blastoma (PPB).

Secondary blastomas: Wilms tumor, osteosarcoma, Ewing sarcoma, hepatoblastoma, neuroblastoma, RMS, germ cell tumor, malignant hematologic systemic disease (leukemia, lymphoma) (**Table 8.3**).

Clinical and radiologic features: usually nonspecific, with signs similar to pneumonia (with costophrenic angle effusion) or airway obstruction (hyperinflation) → delay in diagnosis → increased morbidity.

Imaging:

- **Chest radiograph:** initial imaging study of choice. Lateral view can be added to aid direct (tumor) detection or look for indirect signs of pathology (hyperinflation, consolidation, hypoventilation, effusion, etc.)

- **CT:** for further investigation, highest sensitivity. Gives accurate morphologic assessment; often yields biologic information and aids benign–malignant differentiation. Contrast should be administered for mediastinal evaluation and benign–malignant differentiation. Thin-slice acquisition allows multiplanar reconstructions and 3D reformations for virtual bronchoscopy. Multislice CT is helpful for diagnosis, surgical planning, and posttreatment follow-up. Sedation reduces motion artifacts in children < 4 years old (general anesthesia rarely necessary due to short examination time). Older children usually comply with breath-hold commands. Emphasize ALARA principle in oncologic patients (probable need for many repeat CT scans). Low-dose protocols come preinstalled on new CT systems, which should be modified on-site for individual needs (see Chapter 1).

- **US:** often can "see" tumor or chest wall invasion if situated in accessible space; usually inadequate for detailed evaluation of intrapulmonary masses.

Table 8.3 Relative frequency of lung tumors in children

Tumor	Frequency (%)
Carcinoid	33
Bronchogenic carcinoma	28
Mucoepidermoid carcinoma	9
Pleuropulmonary blastoma (**Fig. 8.20**)	8
Leiomyosarcoma	6
Rhabdomyosarcoma	5
Fibrosarcoma	4
Adenoid cystic carcinoma	2
Hemangiopericytoma	1
Teratoma (**Fig. 8.19**)	< 1
Plasmacytoma	< 1
Myxosarcoma	< 1

- **MRI:** valuable for chest wall invasion. MRI evaluation of intrapulmonary tumors currently under investigation, used increasingly at many centers
- **PET/CT (^{18}F-FDG):** promising method for staging and distinguishing tumors from others

Primary Malignant Lung Tumors

See **Table 8.3**.

Endobronchial Tumors

- **Adenoma:** most common primary malignant tumor. Three entities: bronchial carcinoid (80%), adenoid cystic carcinoma, and mucoepidermoid carcinoma
- **Carcinoids:** derived from Kulchitsky epithelial cells (APUD system [amine precursor uptake and decarboxylation]); may secrete neuroendocrine peptides. Carcinoid syndrome associated with hepatic metastases
- **Bronchial carcinoid:** polypoid endoluminal tumor causing complete obstruction of affected bronchi → pneumonia, atelectasis, hyperinflation, bronchiectasis may develop as late sequelae. Rich blood supply = frequent hemoptysis

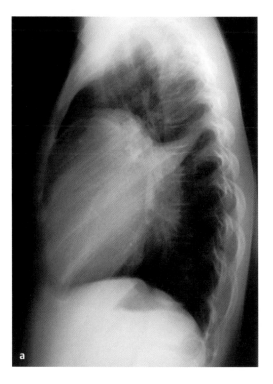

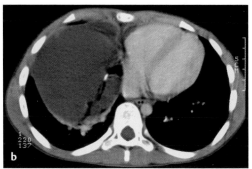

Fig. 8.19a, b Thoracic teratoma (with kind permission of G. Staatz, Mainz, Germany).
a Lateral radiograph displays large intrathoracic mass of soft-tissue density (*histology*: teratoma). Lateral chest radiograph useful for tumor localization, detection, or exclusion of effusion, and initial DD.
b Axial contrast-enhanced CT shows small calcification and peripheral elements of fat attenuation in cystic mass—virtually pathognomonic for teratoma.

8

▬▬▬ **Case Study 8.9** ▬▬▬

History: 5-year-old girl with respiratory distress, mild fever, diminished basal breath sounds, and dyspnea.
Suitable modalities: radiograph, US, CT, MRI.

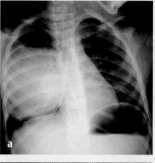 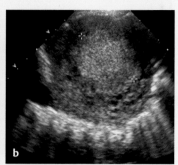

Fig. 8.20a–c

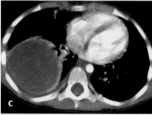

Available images: chest radiographs, US, contrast-enhanced CT.
Findings:

a   Radiograph: intrathoracic mass of soft-tissue density on right side, extending from chest wall to pulmonary hilum.
b   Initial further investigation by thoracic US: complex, partially solid soft-tissue mass (++) extending to hilum and chest wall, no evidence of pneumonia, minimal concomitant effusion.
c   CT confirmed findings, showed capsulelike rim of peripheral enhancement—no specific tissue diagnosis.
Diagnosis: lung tumor. *Histology*: pulmonary blastoma/PPB.
DD: other pediatric lung tumors, complicated echinococcal cyst.

! Proceed carefully during bronchoscopy!

- **Mucoepidermoid tumors:** develop only occasionally in bronchial epithelium
- **Adenoid cystic carcinoma:** slow-growing malignant tumor, predominantly submucous. Propensity for local recurrence

Treatment of endobronchial tumors: complete resection. Some malignancies may also require chemotherapy and radiation.

Pleuropulmonary Blastoma

Occurs almost exclusively before 6 years of age. Classified with "mesenchymal neoplasms" in WHO classification of lung tumors. Peripheral-/pleural-based tumor without chest wall invasion. More common on right side, with associated effusion, occasional pneumothorax. Rare type I, early form (16%)—often appears as multiseptated cyst with proliferation of stromal and mesenchymal cells. Typically diagnosed in first 2 years of life. Metastasizes chiefly to brain, bone, or liver. Often confused with congenital bronchogenic cysts/CCAM. Often

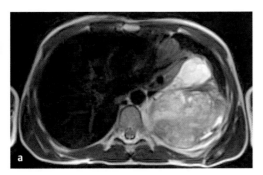

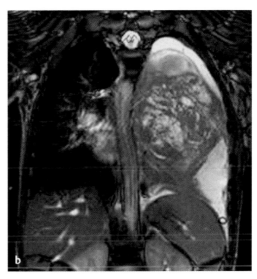

Fig. 8.21a, b   MRI of thoracic tumor (PNET). Axial T2-weighted TSE sequence (**a**) and coronal SSFP sequence (**b**) demonstrate large, complex intrathoracic mass (*histology*: PNET). (With kind permission of G. Staatz, Mainz, Germany.)

misinterpreted as "cystic RMS," arising from congenital cysts or CCAM, or cystic mesenchymal hamartoma.

Type I PPB may progress to more aggressive, mixed cystic-solid form (type II) or purely solid form (type III) with increasing tumor grade.

DD: with cystic forms—congenital pulmonary cyst, congenital lobar emphysema.

Cranial MRI important for staging and follow-up—high recurrence rate. Treatment = surgical removal and neoadjuvant chemotherapy.

> Thoracic uni-/multilocular lesion in children < 2 years of age = PPB until proven otherwise. Imaging cannot positively distinguish type I or IV CCAM from type I PPB.

Bronchogenic Carcinoma

Aggressive tumor with early metastasis, low survival rate (~ 7 months). Often presents with typical pulmonary symptoms, metastasis-associated complaints (bone pain, weight loss). May develop in setting of CCAM—similar to RMS?

Malignant Mesenchymal Lung Tumors

Sporadic occurrence: leiomyosarcoma (6%, most common), bronchopulmonary fibrosarcoma, RMS, malignant mesenchymoma, pulmonary hemangiopericytoma. RMS and malignant mesenchymoma may occur in congenital malformations (pulmonary cyst, CCAM). High-grade malignancy, but good prognosis with surgery and chemotherapy.

Metastases

In order of frequency: Wilms tumor, osteosarcoma/Ewing sarcoma/rhabdomyosarcoma, leukemia, lymphoma, hepatocellular carcinoma, hepatoblastoma, neuroblastoma, germ cell tumor. Hematogenous/lymphogenous spread or direct extension. Solitary or multiple lesions.

Imaging: CT/chest radiograph/MRI—rounded, well-circumscribed nodules, usually in periphery of lung, with predilection for basal lung zones. Reticular pattern, consolidation, or small nodular density in lymphoma, leukemia, neuroblastoma. Intrapulmonary degenerative foci typical of Wilms tumor, Hodgkin disease, osteosarcoma (frequent calcification).

8

Primary Benign Lung Tumors

- **Pulmonary plasma cell granuloma** (synonyms: inflammatory pseudotumor, myofibroblastic tumor, pulmonary fibroxanthoma, pulmonary endothelioma, pulmonary histiocytoma): most common in children < 10 years old. Nodular tumors range 0.5 to > 30 cm in diameter; isolated calcifications—predominantly affect right lung and upper lobe, may be accompanied by effusion
- **Hamartoma:** similar to adult tumors—peripheral nodular lesions with popcornlike appearance, calcifications, fatty elements. Very often associated with syndromes (Cowden syndrome, pulmonary hamartoma syndrome, etc.). Equivocal findings should be investigated, e.g., by fine-needle biopsy. Growing lesions should be resected
- **Leiomyoma:** occurs in children with AIDS/immunocompromise. Association with Ebstein-Barr virus. Usually shows endobronchial growth
- **Mucous gland adenoma, laryngotracheal papillomatosis, schwannoma:** extremely rare
- **Hemangioma/vascular malformation:** extremely rare; low-flow lymphangioma most common

Other Thoracic Tumors and Differential Diagnosis

- Mediastinal tumors: see Chapter 2
- Bone tumors of thoracic skeleton: see Sect. 8.6
- Sequestrum and other pulmonary changes: see Chapter 2

Bibliography

1 Burnei G, Draghici I, Gavriliu S, et al. The assessment of primitive or metastatic malignant pulmonary tumors in children. Chirurgia 2013; 108(3): 351–359
2 Brisse HJ. Staging of common paediatric tumours. Pediatr Radiol 2009; 39(Suppl 3): 482–490
3 Cohen MC, Kaschula RO. Primary pulmonary tumors in childhood: a review of 31 years' experience and the literature. Pediatr Pulmonol 1992; 14(4): 222–232
4 De Bernardi B, Nicolas B, Boni L, et al; Italian Co-Operative Group for Neuroblastoma. Disseminated neuroblastoma in children older than one year at diagnosis: comparable results with three consecutive high-dose protocols adopted by the Italian Co-Operative Group for Neuroblastoma. J Clin Oncol 2003; 21(8): 1592–1601
5 Hancock BJ, Di Lorenzo M, Youssef S, Yazbeck S, Marcotte JE, Collin PP. Childhood primary pulmonary neoplasms. J Pediatr Surg 1993; 28(9): 1133–1136
6 Hiorns MP, Owens CM. Radiology of neuroblastoma in children. Eur Radiol 2001; 11(10): 2071–2081
7 Kubin K, Hörmann M, Riccabona M, Wiesbauer P, Puig S. Benign and malignant pulmonary tumors in childhood. [Article in German] Radiologe 2003; 43(12): 1095–1102
8 McHugh K. Renal and adrenal tumours in children. Cancer Imaging 2007; 7: 41–51
9 Maris JM, Hogarty MD, Bagatell R, Cohn SL. Neuroblastoma. Lancet 2007; 369(9579): 2106–2120
10 Pianca C, Pistamiglio P, Veneselli E, et al; De Bernardi B. Neuroblastoma with symptomatic spinal cord compression at diagnosis: treatment and results with 76 cases. J Clin Oncol 2001; 19(1): 183–190
11 Woodward PJ, Sohaey R, Kennedy A, Koeller KK. From the archives of the AFIP: a comprehensive review of fetal tumors with pathologic correlation. Radiographics 2005; 25(1): 215–242

8.4   Tumors of the Urogenital Tract

Jens-Peter Schenk

Nephroblastoma, Wilms Tumor

General

Nephroblastoma (Wilms tumor) = most common renal tumor in pediatric age group (< 15 years old). Typical age at onset = 2 to 4 years.

Associated with syndromes: Denys–Drash syndrome, WAGR (Wilms tumor, aniridia, genitourinary abnormalities) syndrome, Wiedemann–Beckwith syndrome (WBS), Perlman syndrome, aniridia, hemihypertrophy. With syndromic clinical picture → evaluate radiologic findings; increased likelihood of nephroblastoma.

In hemihypertrophy/WBS—benefit from screening US at intervals of 4 months or less for children under the age of 7 years.

Imaging: US: first imaging test for any clinically suspected tumor (e.g., asymptomatic upper abdominal swelling). Can detect or exclude tumor, localize tumor to kidneys as site of origin

Detailed US scan—can determine size, exclude other renal lesions, evaluate intra-abdominal tumor extent (local staging)

Calcification evaluation—pattern important for DD (see neuroblastoma/renal cell carcinoma)

Focused examination of renal vein and IVC (B-mode plus CDS)—vascular invasion (tumor thrombus)? – US supplemented with CDS often better than other modalities!

- **MRI:** can confirm US findings, measure tumor volume (using formula for ellipse). High soft-tissue contrast → detection of nephroblastomatosis lesions after IV contrast injection. Make final, comprehensive evaluation of MRI, US, and Doppler findings.
  Typical MRI investigation:
  – **Protocol:** survey = fat-saturated (fs) coronal images (TIRM, T2-TSE fs, STIR [short-tau inversion recovery]) and axial T2-weighted TSE (for typical tumor pseudocapsule, PCS involvement, hyperintense vascular invasion in hypointense IVC) (**Fig. 8.22**). Essential to obtain T1-weighted sequence after contrast (tumor extent relative to residual kidney, exclusion of multifocal tumors/nephroblastomatosis)
  – **Findings:** tumor hyperintense in T2-weighted sequences, hypointense in T1-weighted sequences; heterogeneous structure (hemorrhage, fat, necrosis, cysts)

Goal of imaging in SIOP/GPOH studies (SIOP = International Society of Pediatric Oncology, GPOH = Society for Pediatric Oncology and Hematology): high versus low probability that nephroblastoma is present, as preoperative chemotherapy justified for high-probability cases without biopsy confirmation.
Goal of imaging in COG studies (COG = Children Oncology Group—commonly used in North America): preoperative staging because of upfront surgery principle.
MRI and MRA have completely replaced angiography and IVP.

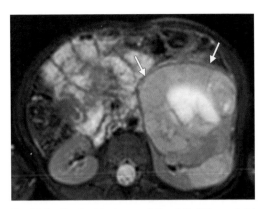

Fig. 8.22   Nephroblastoma of the left kidney. Axial T2-weighted TSE sequence shows typical appearance of inhomogeneous renal mass with hypointense pseudocapsule (arrows).

- **Abdominal CT:** use only if MRI is contraindicated/unavailable

Special considerations: venous vascular invasion in 5 to 10%; thrombus of viable tumor tissue may extent into right atrium (Case Study 8.11, **Fig. 8.28**). Bilateral nephroblastomas in 4 to 13%.

Staging with abdominal MRI or CT and chest radiographs in two planes. With pulmonary nodules, add thoracic CT scans. Skeletal metastases present in only about 3% of cases.

Staging of Nephroblastoma—By Extent

European staging system of SIOP (European International Society for Pediatric Oncology) and COG (Children Oncology Group) staging system consist of five stages based on surgical result, histologic extent, and radiologic findings. (Differences between the systems are to be taken out of therapy protocols.) Simplified staging system in **Table 8.4**.

Can subtypes be differentiated? Malignant tumors with moderate to high histologic grade cannot be differentiated by imaging. Predominantly cystic mass (little solid tissue) = **cystic nephroblastoma. Cystic partially differentiated nephroblastoma (CPDN)** = tumor with honeycomb texture throughout (no solid components), indistinguishable radiologically from multilocular cystic nephroma.

8

Table 8.4 Simplified staging system for nephroblastoma

Stage	Definition
I Complete excision	Tumor limited to kidney, complete excision
II Complete excision	Viable tumor tissue extends outside kidney, complete excision
III Residual tumor	Viable/regressive tumor tissue at surgical margin, tumor rupture, open biopsy, viable/regressive lymph node metastasis; tumor thrombi at surgical margins
IV	Metastases
V	Bilateral nephroblastomas

Most common sites of metastasis: abdominal = liver, retroperitoneal lymph nodes. Distant metastasis = mainly to lung.

DD: most important DD for all renal tumors = **neuroblastoma** (see Sect. 8.3). With upper-pole renal tumor of uncertain origin (renal, adrenal/retroperitoneal/sympathetic trunk) → MIBG scintigraphy.

Detection of Other Renal Tumors

Congenital Mesoblastic Nephroma

General: most common in first 3 months of life. SIOP classification: low risk. Metastases extremely rare.
Imaging: no pseudocapsule. Larger cysts occur in cellular subtype (patients > 3 months old).

Multilocular Cystic Nephroma

General: benign, occurs in small children or adult women. May occur segmentally—then difficult to differentiate from segmental cystic dyplasia/segmental multicystic dysplastic kidney.
Imaging: honeycomblike cystic mass with thin septa (US, MRI).

Metanephrogenic Adenoma

General: rare benign tumor. Usually detected incidentally.
Imaging: no specific imaging features or findings. Usually smaller than nephroblastoma.

Renal Clear Cell Sarcoma

General: cannot be differentiated from nephroblastoma. SIOP classification: high risk. Metastasizes to bone in 6% of cases, to brain in 12%. Not bilateral.
Imaging: same as nephroblastoma. Imaging should cover CNS and skeletal system (scintigraphy, whole-body MRI).

Rhabdoid Renal Tumor

General: extremely aggressive—SIOP classification: high risk. Synchronous and metachronous cerebral metastases. Early pulmonary metastasis (first year of life). Tumor often bordered by subcapsular hemorrhage.
Imaging: same as nephroblastoma. Imaging should cover CNS and skeletal system (scintigraphy, whole-body MRI).

Renal Cell Carcinoma

General: patients typically > 10 years old. Renal cell carcinoma more likely than nephroblastoma in patients > 15 years old.
Imaging: same as nephroblastoma. May have necrotic parts. Typically small cysts, usually smaller than nephroblastoma. Central calcification has been described.

Angiomyolipoma

General: associated with **tuberous sclerosis**. AML usually bilateral in these cases, may also occur in other organs (see also Sect. 4.1).
Imaging: same as nephroblastoma. Hyperechoic on US (fat and blood vessels). MRI (CT)—detects fat (fs sequence/chemical shift imaging, low attenuation) (Case Study 8.10, **Fig. 8.27**).

Some large AMLs (> 3–6 cm, cut-off value varies with institution) treated by prophylactic selective transaortic percutaneous embolization to prevent threatening acute hemorrhage.

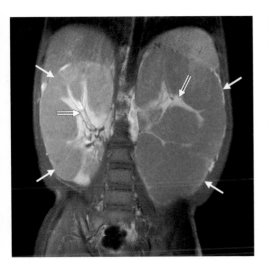

Fig. 8.23 Diffuse nephroblastomatosis. Coronal T1-weighted contrast-enhanced TSE image of both kidneys. Monstrous nephroblastomatosis (white arrows) appears as hypointense mass surrounding small amount of central, enhancing residual renal tissue (barely visible; barred arrows).

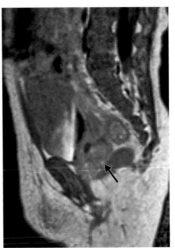

Fig. 8.24 Vaginal germ cell tumor. Sagittal T1-weighted isotropic SPACE sequence after Gd shows tumor (arrow) arising from posterior vaginal wall. Intravaginal tumor mass visible below cervix.

> May have atypical appearance in older children; may present as inhomogeneous mass due to intralesional hemorrhage.

Nephroblastomatosis

General: immature embryonic renal tissue, may degenerate. Differentiation from nephroblastoma sometimes difficult (may coexist).

Definition and types: multiple nodules in intralobar nephroblastomatosis.

Diffuse perilobar nephroblastomatosis—loss of corticomedullary differentiation, massive renal enlargement. MRI shows hypointense tissue layer along renal border (**Fig. 8.23**).

Imaging:
- **US:** may depict focal lesions of nodular disrupted cortical echogenicity and peripheral vascularization on aCDS; ce-US particularly helpful
- **MRI:** mandatory for follow-up under long-term chemotherapy to detect nephroblastoma nodules; ce-MRI superior to native sequences. Signal change in T2-weighted images can indicate change into fibrotic nephrogenic rests.
- **CT:** should be avoided because of radiation exposure. Small lesions difficult to differentiate

from small cysts. If ce-CT necessary, avoid too frequent follow-up, only use one phase and adapted protocol settings

> Modality of choice = MRI. If contrast-enhanced T1-weighted sequences show inhomogeneities and nodular masses with pseudocapsula, particularly with regression of nephroblastomatosis in response to chemotherapy → suspicion of nephroblastoma.

Rare Tumor Entities

Reninoma, ossifying renal tumor in children.

Uterine, Vaginal, and Bladder Tumors in Children and Adolescents

Vaginal and Uterine Tumors

General: usually present clinically with bloody discharge and visible bulge at vaginal introitus.

Most common tumor (usually diagnosed in first years of life) = **embryonic RMS.** Origin = anterior vaginal wall, level of anterior fornix/cervix, bladder.

Botryoid sarcoma protrudes from vaginal introitus (or when arising from the bladder—into bladder lumen).

8

Endodermal sinus tumor of vagina **(yolk sac carcinoma)** occurs in older girls. Origin = posterior vaginal wall. **Clear cell adenocarcinoma** usually occurs after menarche. **Vaginal germ cell tumor** (**Fig. 8.24**).

Imaging:

- **US:** initial imaging study, may use transvesical/transperineal or translabial approach. DD: hematocolpos.
- **MRI:** precise localization to site and organ. Sagittal T2- and T1-weighted postcontrast sequence, angled transverse sequence through vaginal/uterine long axis. May add coronal sequence (lateral vaginal wall) or isotropic 3D acquisition. High resolution with isotropic voxel and high matrix recommended. Watch for local infiltration of pelvic soft tissues (uterus, bladder, ureters, rectum). Endovaginal instillation of NaCl may be helpful
- Tumor can also be localized by **genitography** (vaginography–catheter technique). Combined with **VCUG** using dual-catheter technique

> Metastasis—to lung, liver, local, and retroperitoneal lymph nodes.

Bladder Tumors

General: RMS of bladder or urachus is most common. Occurs in first years of life. Infiltrates vagina, can originate from prostate.
Imaging:

- **US:** detection—mass, bladder wall thickening. Always scan with full bladder

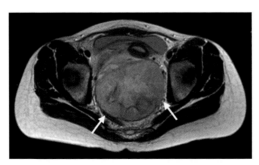

Fig. 8.25   Germ cell tumor of the right ovary. Axial T2-weighted TSE sequence shows slightly inhomogeneous, hyperintense retrovesical and parauterine mass (arrows) in lesser pelvis.

- **MRI:** in three planes, for confirmation and localization. Always use Gd and fat saturation
- **VCUG:** filling defects, urethral obstruction (on voiding)

Ovarian Tumors in Children and Adolescents

General: all age groups. Large ovarian tumors detectable by physical examination (palpable mass). May also be detected incidentally at US for abdominal pain.

Most common entity in children: (mixed) **germ cell tumors** (teratomas, dysgerminomas, endodermal sinus tumors, yolk sac tumors; **Fig. 8.25**). Very rare in children: epithelial ovarian tumors (cystadenoma, cystadenocarcinoma), stromal tumors.

> Always look for/exclude tumor in children with precocious puberty.

Imaging: general principles: differentiated cystic, mixed, and solid mass. Pain is often due to torsion. Tumor localization aided by targeted search for normal ovary.

- **US:** initial examination; watch for calcifications (teratoma, dysgerminoma), intracystic hemorrhage, free abdominal fluid, hepatic metastases, retroperitoneal lymph nodes. Also look for peritoneal dissemination and omental involvement ("caking")
- **Abdominal MRI:** evaluate invasiveness, intestinal and urinary tract obstruction, staging, operability

Special characteristics of teratomas: cystic tumor. Look for raised "teratoma nodule" projecting into cyst cavity (US, MRI; Case Study 8.12, **Fig. 8.29**). Important: exclude tumor in contralateral ovary

- **Abdominal radiograph:** rounded hypodensities with adjacent calcification
- **US:** regional increased echogenicity (fat, hairs). Acoustic shadowing from calcium, bone/teeth
- **MRI:** T1, fs, and chemical shift sequences

> Most important DD from primary ovarian tumor = adnexal/ovarian thickening due to lymphoma or leukemia. Ovarian torsion can mimic or mask tumor (Doppler sometimes helpful).

Testicular Tumors in Children and Adolescents

General: may present clinically as acute scrotum or painless swelling.

Typical tumor entities in prepubescent children: yolk sac tumor, teratoma, epidermoid cyst, mixed germ cell tumor, Leydig and Sertoli cell tumor, juvenile granulosa cell tumor, gonadoblastoma, RMS, metastatic leukemia, or lymphoma.

Paratesticular tumors in children: connective tissue tumor (leiomyoma, leiomyosarcoma, fibroma, fibrosarcoma, hemangioma, lipoma, liposarcoma), paratesticular RMS (17% of intrascrotal tumors in children, **Fig. 8.26**) in infants and teenagers.

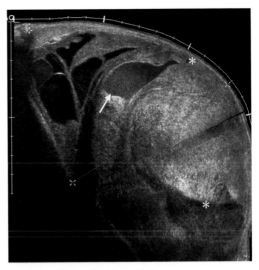

Fig. 8.26 Paratesticular rhabdomyosarcoma in the left scrotal compartment. Panoramic US scan of scrotum shows infiltrating mass with mostly homogeneous center (++) in left scrotal compartment with liquid pseudocystic areas (arrow).

Case Study 8.10

History and clinical presentation: seizures.
Effective imaging options: MRI, US (possibly CT).

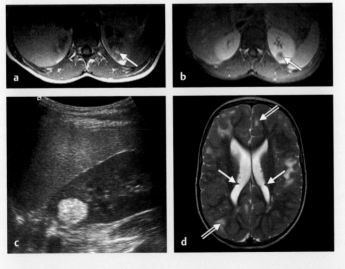

Fig. 8.27a–d
Available images: cranial MRI, US and MRI of kidneys.
a Axial T1-TSE of kidneys.
b Axial T1-TSE fs post-Gd of kidneys.
c Longitudinal US scan of left kidney.
d Cranial MRI, axial T2-TSE.

Findings: subependymal cerebral nodules (→) and hyperintense (sub)cortical tubers (=>). Inhomogeneous renal mass (→) with high T1 signal intensity and low signal intensity in T1 fs post-Gd (fat signal). US shows well-circumscribed globular hyperechoic mass.
Diagnosis: kidney AML in tuberous sclerosis.

8

Case Study 8.11

History and clinical presentation: fatigue, lethargy, palpable right abdominal mass.
Imaging options: US, MRI (possibly CT).

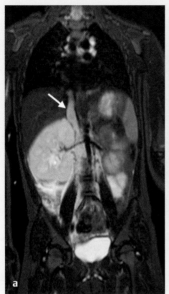

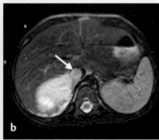

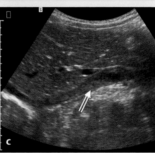

Fig. 8.28a–c

Available images: US and MRI.
a   abdomen MRI, coronal T2-
    TIRM.
b   abdomen MRI, axial T2-TSE
    fs.
c   Longitudinal US scan of vena
    cava from right side.

Findings: MRI shows hyperintense mass in axial T2-weighted TSE and coronal TIRM sequences and hyperintense mass almost completely filling IVC (→) originating from right renal tumor. US shows hyperechoic structure (=>) filling IVC lumen.
Diagnosis: tumor thrombus due to IVC invasion by nephroblastoma.

Imaging:
- **US including Doppler:** initial examination; findings more or less (non)specific:
  - Leydig cell tumor: hypoechoic focal lesion with partially ill-defined margins in testicular parenchyma
  - Teratoma: same as ovarian teratoma
  - Other tumors: mixed echogenicity, partly cystic, replace testicular tissue, may involve epididymis
- **MRI:** adjunct for lymph node staging

> Venous and lymphatic drainage along testicular vein.

DD: ectopic adrenal tissue in testis due to adreno-genital syndrome (US shows focal testicular hypo-echogenicity). Testicular swelling due to torsion, epididymal swelling due to epididymitis (acute scrotum).

Bibliography

1 Agarwal PK, Palmer JS. Testicular and paratesticular neoplasms in prepubertal males. J Urol 2006; 176(3): 875–881
2 Avni F, Riccabona M. MR imaging of the paediatric abdomen. In: Gourtsonyiannis N, ed. Clinical MRI of the Abdomen. Why, How, When. Berlin, Heidelberg, New York: Springer; 2009: 639–676
3 Brisse HJ, Smets AM, Kaste SC, Owens CM. Imaging in unilateral Wilms tumour. Pediatr Radiol 2008; 38(1): 18–29

Case Study 8.12

History and clinical presentation: several days of abdominal pain unrelated to menses, palpable mass in lower abdomen.
Imaging options: US, MRI (possibly CT).

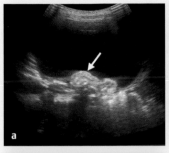

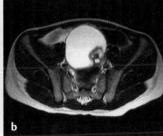

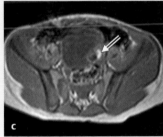

Fig. 8.29a–c
Available images: US, MRI.
a Longitudinal US scan of lower abdomen.
b abdomen MRI, axial T2-TSE.
c abdomen MRI, axial T1-fl2d.

Findings: cystic retrouterine mass (probably ovarian), solid mural component visible on US and MRI (→). US: shadowing echo. MRI: high signal intensity (T1 fl2d sequence) = cystic mass, solid mural component with fat and calcium (=>).
Diagnosis: ovarian teratoma.

4 Brisse HJ. Staging of common paediatric tumours. Pediatr Radiol 2009; 39(Suppl 3): 482–490

5 Choyke PL, Siegel MJ, Craft AW, Green DM, DeBaun MR. Screening for Wilms tumor in children with Beckwith-Wiedemann syndrome or idiopathic hemihypertrophy. Med Pediatr Oncol 1999; 32(3): 196–200

6 Fotter R. Pediatric Uroradiology. Berlin, Heidelberg, New York: Springer; 2001: 395–411

7 Furtwängler R, Schenk JP, Reinhard H, et al. Nephroblastom – Wilms-Tumor. Genetik, radiologische Diagnostik und Therapiekonzept – eine Übersicht. Onkologe 2005; 11: 1077–1089

8 Kuhn JP, Slovis TL, Haller JO. Caffeys Pediatric Diagnostic Imaging. 10th ed. Philadelphia: Mosby/Elsevier; 2003: 1958–1965

9 Lowe LH, Isuani BH, Heller RM, et al. Pediatric renal masses: Wilms tumor and beyond. Radiographics 2000; 20(6): 1585–1603

10 Olsen OE. Imaging of abdominal tumours: CT or MRI? Pediatr Radiol 2008; 38(Suppl 3):S452–S458

11 Owens CM, Brisse HJ, Olsen OE, Begent J, Smets AM. Bilateral disease and new trends in Wilms tumour. Pediatr Radiol 2008; 38(1): 30–39

12 Riccabona M. Imaging of renal tumours in infancy and childhood. Eur Radiol 2003; 13(Suppl 4): L116–L129

13 Rohrschneider WK, Weirich A, Rieden K, Darge K, Tröger J, Graf N. US, CT and MR imaging characteristics of nephroblastomatosis. Pediatr Radiol 1998; 28(6): 435–443

14 Schenk JP. Renal tumours, neuroblastoma and other suprarenal tumours. In: Troeger J, Seidensticker PR, eds. Paediatric Imaging Manual. Berlin, Heidelberg, New York: Springer; 2008: 97 p.

15 Schenk JP, Graf N, Günther P, et al. Role of MRI in the management of patients with nephroblastoma. Eur Radiol 2008; 18(4): 683–691

8

8.5   **Gastrointestinal Tumors and Tumors of Liver, Pancreas, Spleen, Bowel, and Mesentery**

Erich Sorantin, Michael Riccabona

Liver Tumors

Comprise about 0.5 to 6% of intra-abdominal neoplasms in children. **Malignant:** at age < 5 years hepatoblastoma (most common), metastasis (neuroblastoma, Wilms tumor); at age > 5 years hepatocellular carcinoma/adenoma, undifferentiated embryonic sarcoma, metastasis. **Benign:** epithelial lesion (focal nodular hyperplasia), epithelial tumors (adenoma), cyst and tumorlike mesenchymal lesion (cystic mesenchymal hamartoma), mesenchymal tumor (hemangioma, hemangioendothelioma, lipoma), teratoma.

Hepatoblastoma

General: most common tumor at age < 5 years. Median age 12 months; m : f = 2–3 : 1. Level of α1-fetoprotein ↑ in 90% of cases, 60% in hepatic right lobe. Distant metastasis in 10% of patients at initial diagnosis (lung, lymph nodes, ovaries, bone, CNS). Association with Beckwith–Wiedemann syndrome, familial adenomatous polyposis, glycogen storage diseases, Gardner syndrome, biliary atresia (BA).
Imaging:
- **Plain radiographs:** 55% calcifications
- **US:** variable echogenicity (necrosis, hemorrhage), usually well-circumscribed; possible vascular invasion and tumor thrombi in portal vein and hepatic veins (color duplex sonography [CDS]—hypervascular thrombus = DD from ordinary thrombosis)
- **CT:** tumor hypodense on unenhanced scans, rarely hyperdense; homogeneous or inhomogeneous depending on subtype; heterogeneous enhancement pattern
- **MRI:** morphology depends on histologic subtype and cellularity. Hemorrhagic areas: T1 hypointense, T2 hyperintense. Fibrous bands/septa = T1/T2 hypointense. Epithelial types show homogeneous Gd enhancement, mixed-cell tumors show inhomogeneous enhancement (**Fig. 8.30**)

Hepatocellular Carcinoma

General: most common liver tumor in patients > 5 years old. Metastasis rate: 50% at diagnosis.

Association with tyrosinemia, glycogen storage diseases, α1-antitrypsin deficiency, BA, Alagille syndrome, hemachromatosis, Wilson disease, galactosemia, viral hepatitis (B, C), alcohol-induced cirrhosis, aflatoxin (improper storage of grain, corn, peanuts).

Multifocal, (multi)nodular lesions or diffuse infiltration, possible capsule; calcifications less frequent than in hepatoblastoma. Difficult to detect in cirrhotic liver. Portal vein invasion in 44% of cases. Invasion of hepatic veins/IVC is rare (~4–6%), bile duct invasion even rarer. Diameter > 3 cm = central necrosis/hemorrhage.
Imaging:
- **US:** < 3 cm = 50% hypoechoic, posterior acoustic enhancement;   3–5 cm = hyperechoic/mixed; > 5 cm = peripheral hypoechoic halo. CDS for vascular invasion—ordinary thrombi without internal vessels!

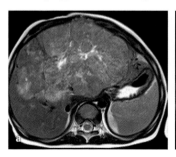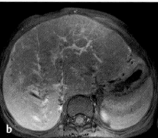

Fig. 8.30a, b   MRI in a 9-month-old boy.
a Axial T2-weighted image demonstrates giant, inhomogeneous liver tumor.
b T1-weighted image after Gd shows inhomogeneous tumor enhancement (hepatoblastoma).

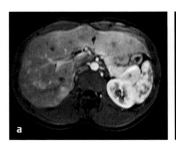
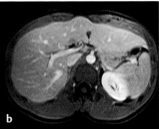

Fig. 8.31a, b Gd-enhanced T1-weighted MRI in young woman.
a Early phase—multiple nodular, ring-enhancing lesions with non-enhancing centers.
b Late phase—more homogeneous enhancement without focal abnormalities. Atypical focal nodular hypoplasia.

- **CT:** hypo- to isodense to liver on unenhanced scans. Encapsulated lesions have hypodense rim. Fatty metamorphosis (mainly in Asians) → hypodense areas. Arterial phase may show intense enhancement. Necrotic areas heterogeneous, capsule hypodense—difficult to distinguish in portal venous phase when capsule hyperdense (due to enhancement).
- **MRI:** variable appearance on unenhanced images = T1 hypointense, T2 hyperintense (hemorrhagic areas), fibrous capsule less intense in T1- and T2-weighted sequences. Inhomogeneous after Gd administration—depends on necrosis/hemorrhage/calcification.

Focal Nodular Hypoplasia

General: second most prevalent benign pediatric liver tumor, more common in girls. Needle biopsy: cannot distinguish FNH from well-differentiated hepatocellular adenoma/carcinoma → open biopsy and excision in doubtful cases/when large.

Association with Kasai surgery, oral contraceptive use (not causative, but growth-promoting).

Usually affects right lobe of liver, multiple in 20% of cases. Composed of hepatocytes, Kupffer cells, radial fibrous septa, and bile ducts (which do not communicate with biliary tract). Central scar contains AVM (contrast enhancement!). No capsule.
Imaging:
- **US:** well-circumscribed tumor, hypo-/isoechoic to liver. Central scar detectable in 20%—detection of arterial flow in scar diagnostic. Dynamic ce-US helpful
- **CT:** hypo-/isodense on unenhanced scans. Scar in 20%, calcifications in 1%. Marked arterial enhancement after contrast administration. Isodense to liver in portal venous phase. Scar

shows intense enhancement in late phase (up to 73%)
- **MRI:** iso-/hyperintense to liver, central scar hypointense on unenhanced T1-weighted images. Tumor shows slightly increased signal intensity on T2-weighted images, with hyperintense scar. Spoked-wheel enhancement pattern (= septa) after Gd. Scar shows late-phase enhancement in 80–100% of cases (**Fig. 8.31**)
- **Scintigraphy:** intense uptake in Kupffer cells; colloid = pathognomonic

Hepatic Adenoma

General: rare tumor, more common in females. Associated with glycogen storage disease, diabetes mellitus, anabolic steroids, oral contraceptives, prior chemotherapy (DD: regenerating nodules). Solitary in 80% of cases. More than four adenomas = adenomatosis. Hepatocytes contain fat. With larger tumor—necrosis and intralesional hemorrhage = symptomatic.
Imaging:
- **US:** nonspecific. Lipid-rich = hyperechoic with hypoechoic halo. Inhomogeneous with intratumoral hemorrhage. Hypo-/isoechoic = no halo. Prominent subcapsular vessels on CDS and central venous flow, mixed arterial–venous signals at periphery (differentiation from FNH—latter has arterial flow in scar)
- **CT:** noncontrast scans show well-circumscribed, hypodense tumor with hypodense capsule in 25% of cases, calcifications in 50%. Heterogeneous with intratumoral hemorrhage/fatty components. Variable enhancement on postcontrast scans; frequent transient (early) arterial enhancement and detection of subcapsular vessels. Tumor isodense to liver (masked) in late phase images

8

- **MRI:** heterogeneous on unenhanced images (necrosis, intratumoral hemorrhage, fat). Early arterial enhancement after Gd; isointense with detectable vascularity in late phase (see CT)
- **(Gallium) scintigraphy:** gallium uptake decreased, no colloid uptake (excludes Kupffer cells). Biliary tracers show early uptake that persists in late images

! Caution: high radiation exposure from gallium scintigraphy!

Infantile Hemangioma/Hemangioendothelioma

General: vasoproliferative anomaly with nonspecific clinical and imaging features. Common infantile hemangiomas develop in 10% of infants by age of 1 year, clinical course in actively proliferating = angiogenic phase, spontaneous regression leads to decreased size and complete disappearance. If hemangioma is fully developed at birth = congenital hemangioma, consisting of two types: RICH (rapidly involuting congenital hemangioma)—spontaneous and complete resolution before 14 months; NICH (noninvoluting congenital hemangioma).

Hemangioendothelioma = proliferates rapidly in first year of life, slowly regresses over next 5–8 years.

Multiple hepatic hemangiomas = hemangiomatosis. Hemangiomas in more than two organs = disseminated hemangiomatosis. Second most common liver tumor in children < 5 years old (12%; 85% < 6 years). Clinical manifestations appear after first month; f : m = 2 : 1.

Complications: rupture → hemorrhage, thrombocytopenic coagulopathy (Kasabach–Merrit syndrome), anemia, refractory cardiac decompensation with high shunt flow and steel phenomena, jaundice.
Imaging:
- **Plain radiographs:** hepatomegaly, tiny disseminated calcifications in 16% of cases
- **US:** variable echogenicity, often hyperechoic, usually well-circumscribed. Marked (peripheral) hypervascularity (CDS), possible shunt flow and hyperemia (DDS). Typical centripetal enhancement on ce-US (as in CT)
- **CT:** hypodense. Calcifications in up to 40% of tumors. After contrast administration, en-

hancement fills in from periphery (iris phenomenon, also known as iris diaphragm sign); central portions enhance in late phase (except with necrosis, thrombosis, or hemorrhage)
- **MRI:** hypointense to liver on unenhanced T1-weighted images. T2 hyperintense, large lesions inhomogeneous (hemorrhage). Enhancement pattern after Gd (dynamic scan) same as in CT (iris phenomenon)
- **Scintigraphy:** blood-pool scintigraphy pathognomonic—uptake initially low, then high

In all modalities—large shunt volume marked by prominent feeder arteries, and abrupt caliber change in abdominal aorta distal to celiac trunk.

Spleen

General: splenic tumors are extremely rare, usually benign. **Benign:** hemangioma/hamartoma/lymphangioma. Splenic cyst = congenital (epidermal origin = epidermoid, dermoid/transitional cell cysts) or acquired (posttraumatic, infectious—Echinococcus). DD: lymphangioma(s) (generalized = Gorham–Stout disease = generalized lymphangiectasis, chylothorax, bone lesions), old abscess. **Malignant:** angiomatous tumor (e.g., hemangiopericytoma/angiosarcoma), metastatic in systemic diseases (leukemia/lymphoma).
DD: infarction, hemorrhage/trauma, abscess, infiltrative (systemic) granulomatous disease.
Splenomegaly: in leukemia and lymphoma; in NHL with poorly defined hypoechoic areas (US). More diffuse with focal infiltration in Hodgkin disease (more common than in NHL).
Imaging:
- **US, CT, MRI:** US usually sufficient—especially for diagnosing cysts

Syndromic association, systemic cystic disease, etc.

Diffuse involvement—frequent spurious/negative findings. Contrast administration for focal involvement (always image late phases in all three modalities). Ce-US and (a)CDS are helpful. US-guided biopsy—option for equivocal focal lesion.
- **PET:** more sensitive for detecting organ involvement by systemic disease

Pancreas

Benign and malignant pancreatic tumors are rare in children. Frantz tumor = solid-cystic pseudopapillary tumor, pancreaticoblastoma, islet cell tumor, carcinomas even rarer (acinar cell carcinoma, ductal adenocarcinoma, inflammatory pseudotumor—e.g., in systemic granulomatous disease/HIV, tuberculosis, etc.).

Islet Cell Tumor

General: hormone-secreting tumor with benign and malignant variants. Common site of occurrence: head of pancreas.

Possible hormone production: B cells → insulin (= "insulinoma," most common form in children; DD: diffuse islet cell hyperplasia = nesidioblastosis); A cells → glucagon; G cells → gastrin; D cells → somatostatin; D1 cells → vasoactive intestinal peptide = VIP ("VIPoma," causes secretory diarrhea, hypokalemia, hypochlorhydria).

Associated with multiple endocrine neoplasia syndrome (= presence of other/different tumors with endocrine activity), gastrinoma in Zollinger–Ellison syndrome.

Imaging:
- **US:** round to oval mass, usually well-circumscribed (if large enough), hypoechoic, may have echogenic rim. Ce-US improves detection (early arterial enhancement, fading enhancement in later phases). Intraoperative US is helpful for localization
- **CT/MRI:** marked (early) arterial enhancement

Gastrointestinal Tumors

Tumors of Small Bowel

Usually **benign**, mostly polyps (polyposis syndrome; common manifestations = GI bleeding, intussusception). Others: vascular malformation (hemangioma), neurofibroma, telangiectasia, fibroma, (lipo)leiomyoma, gastrointestinal stromal tumor (GIST), lipoblastoma.

Malignant tumors other than (Burkitt) lymphoma are extremely rare. Malignant variants of benign tumors may occur (Peutz–Jeghers syndrome). Carcinoids: most common in appendix (better prognosis than ileal lesions).

Table 8.5 Polyposis syndromes in children

Polyps—hamartomas
Juvenile polyposis
Juvenile polyposis of infancy
Peutz–Jeghers syndrome
Cowden syndrome

Polyps—adenomas
Classic familial adenomatous polyposis
▪ Attenuated classic familial adenomatous polyposis
▪ Gardner syndrome
▪ Turcot syndrome

Peutz–Jeghers Syndrome

General: autosomal dominant polyposis syndrome (hamartous polyps and mucocutaneous pigmentary changes). Pigmented spots (face, lip, buccal mucosa, palm, sole of foot) in first 2 years of life—disappear in adolescence. Occurrence: 95% in small bowel → jejunum and ileum, occasionally the stomach (25%) and colon (30%). Other sites: nose, bladder, lung. Typical age at diagnosis = 11 years. Risk of adenocarcinoma (not from malignant transformation of hamartous polyps, but from coexisting adenomas!). These cases often have additional malignancies (stomach, ovary, lung, thyroid, breast, skin, pancreas, uterus, testis, multiple myeloma), with 93% overall risk of malignancy.

Imaging:
- **US:** detects intussusception (highest sensitivity and specificity), allows direct detection of intraluminal polyps (improved by orally administered small bowel fluid or—if in colon—saline enema for US). Bowel wall thickness > 1 cm and associated lymph node > 1 cm = suspicious for Burkitt lymphoma
- **Small bowel follow through:** mural contrast voids and filling defects. Burkitt lymphoma—opacified small bowel lumen with thickened walls
- **CT/MRI:** second-line studies → staging and evaluation of extraluminal components

8

Tumors of Large Bowel

General: large bowel tumors are extremely rare in children. Mostly juvenile/hamartous–adenomatous polyps (**Table 8.5**). Colon carcinoma 20 times more common in Crohn disease than in normal population. Ulcerative colitis = premalignant disease (see Sect. 3.4). DD: inflammation, intestinal duplication.

Imaging:

- **US:** nonspecific, same as with small bowel polyps. Improved by hydrocolon (= NaCl instillation for US examination). Can detect intussusception; very thick, hypoechoic colon wall

> **!** Caution: Burkitt lymphoma.

- **Contrast enema/small bowel double contrast, UGI series:** former gold standards; endoscopy always used today
- **CT/MRI:** virtual endoscopy, staging (lymph nodes, extraluminal component, etc.) for malignancy and DD (Crohn disease, etc.)

Juvenile Polyps

Present with painless rectal bleeding between 6th and 10th years of life. Colocolic intussusception rare. Frequency declines from anus to cecum (75–85% in rectosigmoid). No malignant potential.

Juvenile Polyposis Coli, Juvenile Polyposis of Infancy

Autosomal dominant inheritance. Hamartous polyps with malignant potential. Occur frequently in sigmoid colon and rectum. Five to 10 polyps necessary for diagnosis.

Juvenile polyposis of infancy = aggressive variant. Presents in first months of life with intussusception, malabsorption, and diarrhea.

Gastric Tumors

Benign Tumors

General: polyps → association with polyposis syndromes, benign lymphoid hyperplasia (in children with immunoglobulin diseases), mesenchymal tumors—mainly in adolescents: leiomyoma, (neuro)-fibroma, hemangioma, lipoma, teratoma (m > f, common in first year of life), carcinoid.

Carnie triad: multiple gastric leiomyomas, pulmonary hamartoma, neuroblastoma.
Imaging: lymphoid hyperplasia = widening of antral folds > 5 mm (US/FL/CT/MRI). Intramural tumors—mass effect, possible small bowel intussusception. Teratoma → calcifications, fatty/cystic components (MR/CT/US/radiography).

Malignant Tumors

Gastric carcinoma → associated with familial polyposis; rarely leiomyosarcoma, lymphoma.
Imaging: same as for adults.

Gastrointestinal Stromal Tumor

General: extremely rare in children; most prevalent in 5th/6th decade, usually benign (60–70%). May occur anywhere in GI tract—mainly stomach (70%), small bowel (30–35%), and anorectum (7%). Often arises from mesentery/omentum. Tumor usually large when detected (> 5 cm). Malignant variant has 61% metastasis rate (to liver, lung, peritoneum, rarely bone).
Imaging:

- **Projection radiography/FL:** mass effect/displacement
- **US/CT/MRI:** heterogeneous tumor, well circumscribed, with border of variable thickness. Enhances after contrast administration. Central hemorrhage/necrosis, cystic changes. Smaller tumors (< 5 cm) with homogeneous enhancement are usually benign
- **PET/PET-CT:** detects fewer lesions than does CT, more accurate in distinguishing active tumor from necrosis. PET-CT: better anatomic orientation than PET alone

Course: positive response to tyrosine kinase inhibitors—cyst formation, decrease in central density.

Mesenchymal Tumors

General: all types of benign/malignant mesenchymal tumors as well inflammatory pseudotumors may occur in children. Common: teratoma, fibrolipoma, vascular tumor, mesenteric cyst.
Imaging: US/MRI/CT—corresponding manifestations at various sites.

Case Study 8.13

Clinical presentation: 2-year-old boy with increasing abdominal distention and pain

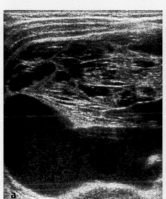 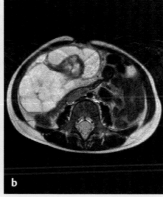

Fig. 8.32a, b

Findings: axial US scan (**a**)—mass with multiple cysts and areas of increased echogenicity consistent with intralesional hemorrhage. Axial T2-weighted MRI (**b**)—same as US, multiple cysts.
Diagnosis: abdominal mesenteric lymphangioma.

Lymphangioma

See also Sect. 8.6.

General: lymphatic malformation, often of huge proportions. Solid and cystic components, often with secondary intralesional hemorrhage. DD: mesenteric cyst, GI duplication/MD, other abdominal cysts (ovarian, choledochal, renal, etc.), fluid-filled bowel segments, encapsulated ascites/chronic confined perforation.

Imaging: US/CT/MRI—septated and fluid-filled cavities, not confluent ("multicystic"), may appear heterogeneous due to intralesional hemorrhage, with fluid-level and sedimentation effects. Scant vascularity—only in septa (which may show minimal enhancement; Case Study 8.13, **Fig. 8.32**). Regional lymph nodes, possible solid components.

! Caution: mesenchymal–angiomatous mixed tumor.

Bibliography

1 Gorincour G, Kokta V, Rypens F, Garel L, Powell J, Dubois J. Imaging characteristics of two subtypes of congenital hemangiomas: rapidly involuting congenital hemangiomas and non-involuting congenital hemangiomas. Pediatr Radiol 2005; 35(12): 1178–1185

2 Jha P, Chawla SC, Tavri S, Patel C, Gooding C, Daldrup-Link H. Pediatric liver tumors—a pictorial review. Eur Radiol 2009; 19(1): 209–219

3 O'Sullivan PJ, Harris AC, Ho SG, Munk PL. The imaging features of gastrointestinal stromal tumours. Eur J Radiol 2006; 60(3): 431–438

4 Peddu P, Huang D, Kane PA, Karani JB, Knisely AS. Vanishing liver tumours. Clin Radiol 2008; 63(3): 329–339

5 Roebuck D. Focal liver lesion in children. Pediatr Radiol 2008; 38(Suppl 3): S518–S522

6 Roebuck DJ, Sebire NJ, Pariente D. Assessment of extrahepatic abdominal extension in primary malignant liver tumours of childhood. Pediatr Radiol 2007; 37(11): 1096–1100

7 Slovis T. Caffey's Pediatric Diagnostic Imaging. 11th ed. Vol II, Sect. VI—The Abdomen, Pelvis and Retroperitoneum. Philadelphia: Mosby/Elsevier; 2008: 1929–1945, 1977–1981, 1992–1996, 2154–2157, 2205–2213

8 Steigen SE, Eide TJ. Gastrointestinal stromal tumors (GISTs): a review. APMIS 2009; 117(2): 73–86

9 Stringer D, Babyn P. Pediatric Gastrointestinal Imaging and Intervention. Hamilton, Ontario: B.C. Decker; 2000: Ch 8, 290–293; Ch 12, 643–659

8

8.6 Important Tumors of Muscle, Bone, and Soft-Tissue

Thekla von Kalle

Bone Tumors

Benign Bone Tumors

Osteoid Osteoma (Osteoblastoma)

Presentation, DD: benign osteoblastic lesion with central nidus. Most prevalent in second decade. Predominantly cortical—in long tubular bones (proximal femur), vertebral appendages. Typical nocturnal pain—responds well to inhibitors of prostaglandin synthesis. **Osteoblastoma:** nidus > 1.5 cm, perifocal sclerosis/pain often less than with osteoid osteoma. DD: Brodie abscess, arthritis, stress fracture, spondylolysis (when in lower lumbar spine).

Imaging:

- **Radiographs:** sclerotic zone with round or oval, lucent central nidus

- **MRI/CT/scintigraphy:** if radiographs equivocal. Advantage of CT = more experience with minimally invasive therapies (e.g., percutaneous radiofrequency ablation/thermocoagulation). MRI: often shows pronounced perifocal edema → caution: do not mistake for malignant tumor. In case of intra-articular involvement: effusion and synovitis

> When nidus in bone marrow or close to joint—sclerosis often absent (**Fig. 8.33**) → difficult to diagnose by radiography and CT. Highly vascularized nidus can be detected by triple-phase scintigraphy/dynamic ce-MRI/dynamic ce-CT.

MRI was long considered unsuitable. But high-resolution sequences, fat saturation, and dynamic contrast-enhanced protocols can accurately diagnose

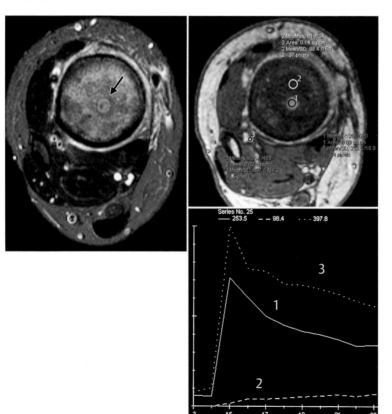

Fig. 8.33 School-aged child with pain in distal lower leg, worse at night. MRI: axial STIR sequence (left) shows extensive edema in bone marrow and periosteum with round lesion at center (arrow). No perifocal sclerosis on radiographs. Dynamic contrast enhancement study (right) with a series of rapid T1-weighted 3D GRE sequences = enhancement in central lesion (curve 1) parallel to signal intensity in vessel (curve 3). Intramedullary edema shows minor enhancement (curve 2). Interpretation: nidus of osteoid osteoma in bone marrow of distal tibia.

or exclude osteoid osteoma without radiation exposure, even in difficult cases (**Fig. 8.33**).

Chondroblastoma

Presentation, DD: frequently painful benign tumor of cartilaginous origin. Most common in second decade. Proximal epiphysis of humerus and knee region. Up to 50% extend beyond growth plate to metaphysis, usually do not expand bone. Periosteal reaction in adjacent metaphysis may occur. Benign dissemination to lung has been described. DD: rare lesions including intraosseous ganglion, osteomyelitis, eosinophilic granuloma, chondroma, low-grade chondrosarcoma, osteosarcoma. Giant cell tumor always metaphyseal in patients with open growth plates.

> Epiphyseal tumor in a child with open growth plates = almost always chondroblastoma.

Imaging:
- **Radiographs:** round or lobulated epiphyseal lucency with sharp outlines and fine sclerotic rim
- **CT:** depicts central calcifications best
- **MRI:** T1-weighted—variable contrast enhancement; T2-weighted—inhomogeneous, hypo- to hyperintense. Typical perifocal edema = distinguishes chondroblastoma from other chondroid tumors. Fluid levels rare. Rarely coexists with secondary aneurysmal bone cyst (ABC). Important for preoperative planning: relationship to growth plate, subchondral cortical bone, and articular cartilage

Giant Cell Tumor

Presentation, DD: painful, aggressive tumor with rich blood supply. Only 20% in patients < 20 years of age. Typical location in epiphyses of knee region. In patients with open growth plates, very rare and always metaphyseal. Rare pulmonary metastases. In adolescents, important DD to osteosarcoma, (solid) ABC, osteomyelitis. Diagnosis always established histologically.
Imaging:
- **Radiographs:** usually show well-circumscribed geographic osteolytic area—rarely with sclerotic margins
- **MRI:** detects extent beyond bone. T1- and T2-weighted sequences = low to moderate signal

intensity, marked contrast-enhancement. Occasionally, cystic components and fluid levels.

Malignant Bone Tumors

Osteosarcoma (Osteogenic Sarcoma)

Presentation, DD: most common malignant osteogenic tumor. Peak incidence: 15 to 25 years of age. Occurs mainly in metaphyses of long tubular bones (~ 50% around the knee), very rare in axial skeleton. Metastasizes mainly to bone and lung. Skip lesions = rare satellite tumors in same/adjacent bone, not contiguous with primary tumor. Most important DD: Ewing sarcoma, ABC, osteomyelitis/osteitis, lymphoma, myositis ossificans, giant cell tumor. Stress fracture and osteoid osteoma can be differentiated by absence of soft tissue component.

> Diagnosis is always established histologically.

Imaging: examination and biopsy at specialized centers according to guidelines of study groups, EURAMOS (European and American Osteosarcoma Study Group), COSS (Cooperative Osteosarcoma Study Group), EOI (European Osteosarcoma Intergroup), SSG (Scandinavian Sarcoma Group), ISG (Italian Sarcoma Group): links and contacts at www.ctu.mrc.ac.uk/euramos/default.asp, coss.olgahospital-stuttgart.de; COG (North American Children's Oncology Group, www.childrensoncologygroup.org).

Before biopsy, primary tumor and affected bone should be completely depicted by radiography and by MRI (or CT) before and after administration of contrast material (**Table 8.6**).
- **Radiographs:** typically mixed pattern of sclerosis and aggressive osteolysis, interrupted periosteal reaction (Codman triangle, spicules; **Fig. 8.34**). Occasional lamellar periosteal reaction (small-cell osteosarcoma), predominance of osteolysis (telangiectatic osteosarcoma)
- **MRI:** best depicts soft tissue mass, intramedullary extent, peritumoral edema, relation to neighboring joint, epiphyseal plate, muscles, vessels, nerves (**Fig. 8.34**). Often only small decrease in volume of ossified tumor matrix after neoadjuvant chemotherapy → monitor response by MRI: enlargement of necrotic areas, reduction of contrast enhancement. Dynamic contrast-enhanced study (**Fig. 8.33**) essential.

8

Table 8.6 Diagnosis of bone tumors by MRI (adapted from COSS and EWING study group recommendations). STIR sequence can be replaced by fs T2-weighted SE. Good image quality and high spatial resolution are essential. Sequence parameters should be adjusted in patients with metal implants (SE and subtraction, no fs)

Diagnostic goal	Purpose	MRI protocol
Complete, detailed visualization of primary tumor before biopsy	Volumetry, most favorable biopsy site, (avoid necrotic tumor areas)	STIR axial, cor (sag) 4–6 mm; 3D T1w GRE dynamic ce study; subtraction analysis if required; consider DWI
Delineation of tumor and perifocal edema	To plan surgical resection	STIR; postcontrast T1w SE with fs cor, sag; pixel ≤ 1 mm, slice thickness 2–3 mm
Delineation of adjacent muscles, joints, nerves, epiphyseal plates, vessels	To plan surgical resection	PDw axial; T1w SE with fs postcontrast axial, cor (sag); pixel ≤ 1 mm, slice thickness 2–3 mm
Complete visualization of affected bone and adjacent joints (whole limb and opposite site, for length determination)	Exclude skip lesions; to plan prosthetic implants	STIR and T1w SE before contrast, cor or sag, with large field of view
Osteosarcoma: response to treatment	Changes in tumor structure, necrosis, decrease in contrast-enhancement	3D dynamic ce study, subtraction analysis if required; consider DWI
Ewing sarcoma: response to treatment	Decrease in tumor volume	T1w SE with fs after contrast in at least 2 planes (alternative: 3D GRE with fs)
Follow-up	Exclude local recurrence or distinguish from postoperative changes	STIR axial, cor (sag); T1w SE pre-contrast and with fs post-contrast, axial, cor (sag), pixel ≤ 1 mm, slice thickness 2–4 mm; dynamic ce series

Key: fs, fat saturation; cor, coronal; sag, sagittal; ce, contrast enancement; DWI, diffusion-weighted imaging; T1w, T1-weighted; PDw, proton-density weighted.

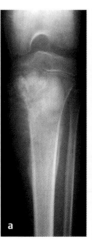
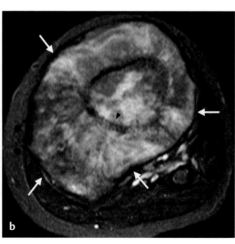

Fig. 8.34a, b Ten-year-old boy with left knee pain and swelling of proximal lower leg. AP radiograph (**a**) = osseous process in proximal tibial metaphysis. Mixed sclerosis and osteolysis. Lateral lamellar periosteal reaction, medial spicules and Codman triangle. MRI (**b**) = axial STIR sequence (6 mm): Hyperintense bone tumor growing through Volkmann canals (arrowhead). Large subperiosteal soft-tissue tumor (arrows). Osteosarcoma of proximal left tibia (histologically confirmed).

- **Additional imaging:** detection of metastases—pulmonary CT, bone scintigraphy, radiographs/MRI/CT. Roles of diffusion imaging to assess tumor response as well as PET-CT and whole-body MRI are being evaluated

Ewing Sarcoma (PNET)

Presentation, DD: second-most common primary malignant bone tumor in children and adolescents (median age 15 years). Predominantly affects diaphysis/metaphysis of long bones (25% in femur) and axial skeleton (**Fig. 8.35**). Main sites of metastases: lung, skeleton. Skip lesions. DD: aggressive forms of osteomyelitis, eosinophilic granuloma, osteosarcoma.

> Diagnosis should always be established histologically.

Imaging: examination and biopsy at specialized centers according to guidelines of the joint therapy protocol EWING 2008: GPOH (Gesellschaft für Pädiatrische Onkologie und Hämatologie, www.kinderkrebsinfo.de), CCLG (Children's Cancer and Leukaemia Group, www.cclg.org.uk), COG (c.f. osteosarcoma), SFCE (Société Française de Lutte contre les Cancers et Leucémies de l'Enfant et de l'Adolescent, www.sfce.org), EORTC (European Organisation for Research and Treatment of Cancer, www.eortc.be), SAKK (Swiss Group for Clinical Cancer Research, www.sakk.ch), SSG (cf. osteosarcoma).

Before biopsy, tumor and affected bone should be completely depicted by radiography and by MRI (or CT) before and after administration of contrast material (**Table 8.6**).

- **Radiographs:** whole primary tumor and affected bone—permeative/moth-eaten osteolysis, interrupted lamellar periosteal reaction, occasional spicules/Codman triangle. Frequent osteosclerotic components if in pelvis
- **MRI:** same as osteosarcoma. Spinal involvement—specify affected segment(s)!
  Volumetry important for prognosis and radiologic assessment of tumor response to chemotherapy (measurement of largest tumor dimensions in three perpendicular planes)

> In case of complex tumor shape, volume estimation is simplified by comparative volumetry based on contrast-enhanced 3D sequences.

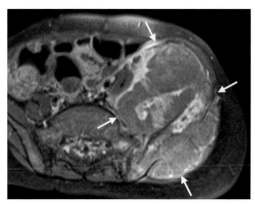

Fig. 8.35 Three-year-old boy limping due to a painful left hip. US (to exclude transient synovitis of hip) showed expansion of iliopsoas muscle. Axial contrast-enhanced T1-weighted TSE sequence with fat saturation (3 mm) shows large soft-tissue mass (arrows) arising from left iliac wing. Ewing sarcoma (histologically confirmed).

- **Metastases:** pulmonary CT, bone scintigraphy, radiographs, or MRI/CT. Role of PET-CT and whole-body MRI being evaluated

Metastases

Presentation, DD: most common origin of skeletal metastases in children: neuroblastoma; in adolescents: osteosarcoma, Ewing sarcoma. DD: multifocal bone involvement by LCH, CRMO. Primary lymphoma of bone. Less common: solitary bone lesions in leukemia ("chloromas"). Differentiation by biopsy and histology.
Imaging: same as for primary bone tumors.

Soft Tissue Tumors

Benign Soft Tissue Tumors

Hemangioma

Presentation, DD: benign neoplasm, most common soft tissue tumor in children.

Congenital hemangiomas—often regress spontaneously in first weeks of life (RICH = rapidly involuting congenital hemangiomas). Some remain at the same size (NICH = noninvoluting congenital hemangiomas).

Infantile hemangiomas typically proliferate during first months of life, then undergo gradual spon-

8

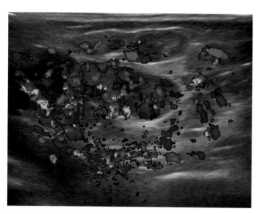

Fig. 8.36 Preauricular swelling in a 2-month-old infant. US with 12-MHz linear probe and CDS at sensitive settings (low flow velocity and wall filter, high gain) demonstrates mass in right parotid gland with hyperechoic and hypoechoic components. With less probe compression, numerous flow signals appear even in superficial areas. Infantile hemangioma of parotid gland.

taneous regression, often with scar formation. May occur in all body regions, most commonly in head and neck region (e.g., parotid gland, **Fig. 8.36**). Large/multiple cutaneous hemangiomas (hemangiomatosis) may be associated with hepatic hemangiomas/hemangioendotheliomas (see Sect. 8.5). DD rare in infancy: infantile fibrosarcoma, myofibromatosis, RMS. Histology needed only in case of atypical appearance. Beyond early childhood (> 2 years of age) requires thorough workup that may have to include histology.

Imaging:
- **US** with high-quality (color) Doppler scan (CDS) = high diagnostic specificity (98%) for infantile hemangiomas: well-circumscribed mass of moderate to high echogenicity with numerous arteries and veins. Document all margins of lesion (e.g., do not miss intraorbital extension). Spectral pattern and calibers of feeding arteries = hemodynamic information, useful for follow-up during treatment—always try to do spectral analysis.

> Superficial low-flow hemangiomas may be compressed by US probe (**Fig. 8.36**) and elude diagnosis → use ample gel.

- **MRI:** if US findings not typical or do not define full extent. High T2-weighted signal intensity (STIR), typical flow voids. **Dynamic contrast-en-**

hanced study = typical vascular signal intensity curve, aids in differentiation from other tumors

Vascular Malformations

Presentation, DD: malformations, no neoplasms (unlike hemangioma). May occur in all body regions. Differentiate simple capillary, arterial, and venous malformations from combined forms. Lesions may enlarge with body growth or by increased vascular dilatation. Require differentiation from hemangioma due to different treatment options.

Imaging:
- **US:** abnormal blood vessels without soft-tissue mass. Phleboliths = evidence for venous malformation (slow blood flow). Doppler can detect arteriovenous shunt by typical waveform (= pulsatile flow and high diastolic velocity, also in veins). Important to define feeding and draining vessels (before planned intervention)
- **MRI:** for further investigation; should preferably include dynamic contrast-enhanced series or MRA. Indications same as for hemangioma. Consider coexisting malformations (e.g., Klippel–Trenaunay syndrome, Proteus syndrome), which can be accurately identified by MRI
- **Conventional angiography**: in selected cases, especially for embolization

Lymphangioma

Presentation, DD: benign cystic soft-tissue tumors in children. May affect all body regions, most common in head and neck. Variable extent; may grow very large even in utero (50% congenital). Frequent local growth and extension along layers of connective tissue between organs/in muscles. Spontaneous regression may occur. Acute enlargement is usually due to spontaneous intralesional hemorrhage. May coexist with hemangioma.

Imaging:
- **US:** typical contiguous large cysts with thin septa (**macrocystic lymphangioma**). Fluid level after intralesional hemorrhage (consider scan orientation!). **Microcystic lymphangioma**—hyperechoic, may be difficult to diagnose in case of very small cysts. Mixed forms occur
- **MRI:** when US cannot depict whole lesion due to complex extension (e.g., from neck into mediastinum). Used preoperatively to delineate vital structures (e.g., trachea, brachial plexus). More sensitive than US for detecting fluid levels

Lipoma

Presentation, DD: common subcutaneous soft-tissue tumor in children.

Superficial lipomas—subcutaneous, slow-growing, circumscribed mass with soft or tense consistency. **Deep lipomas**—less common, usually larger, margins may be infiltrating and ill-defined. DD—other rare lipomatous tumors (see WHO Classification http://www.iarc.fr/en/publications/pdfs-online/pat-gen/index.php). Fibrous hamartoma of infancy (shoulder girdle, most common in male infants) may contain large fat components. Liposarcoma—very rare in children.

Imaging: US: high-resolution linear probe—homogeneous structure and echogenicity with thin septa; typically resembles normal subcutaneous adipose tissue. Larger lipomas are often more heterogeneous, calcifications rare. In case of non-adipose components and thick nodular septa, DD includes lipoblastoma (age < 3 years) or, very rarely, well-differentiated liposarcoma (age > 10 years) → MRI and histologic confirmation indicated.

> Compression and palpation with US probe aid delineation of subcutaneous lipoma.

Subcutaneous Granuloma Anulare

Presentation, DD: benign inflammatory process of subcutaneous tissue. Painless subcutaneous nodules, usually pretibial. Patients typically < 5 years old. Usually diagnosed clinically—DD includes hematoma, FB granuloma.

Imaging:
- **US:** thickened hypoechoic septa/lymphatic vessels in subcutaneous tissue = focal edema. Changes do not spread to other tissue layers.
- **MRI:** only in atypical cases—focal subcutaneous edema and contrast-enhancement

Fibromatosis Colli

Presentation, DD: benign proliferation of fibroblasts in lower third of sternocleidomastoid muscle. Incidence = 0.4% of all live births. Age = 2 weeks to 2 months. Classified among benign juvenile fibromatoses. Association with abnormal intrauterine position. Treatment = physical therapy. Diagnosed clinically.

Imaging: US only in clinically equivocal cases. High-resolution linear probe shows spindle-shaped hy-

perechoic muscle expansion and increased vascularity.

Note: Typical presentation not an indication for MRI, never for CT!

Foreign Body Granuloma

Presentation, DD: posttraumatic, at any age, usually affecting hands or feet. Symptoms are due to swelling, joint effusion.

Imaging:
- **US:** thorough examination with high-resolution linear probe—most soft tissue FBs can be located; usually hyperechoic with associated acoustic shadowing/scattering. History and surrounding tissue abnormalities (granuloma, abscess, fistula, hematoma) suggest correct diagnosis
- **Radiographs:** useful for radiopaque material

> MRI rarely necessary—acquire with sufficiently high resolution (slice thickness < half of anticipated FB size); multiaxial, high-resolution 3D sequence may be required.

Hematoma

Presentation, DD: causative trauma not always remembered.

Imaging:
- **US:** findings depend on extent and age of hemorrhage. Size decreases over time (differentiate it from neoplasm)

> Hematomas change their echogenicity and internal echo pattern within days (shortly after trauma) to weeks (later course). May calcify.

- **MRI:** in doubtful cases—can detect methemoglobin (high T1 signal intensity) and hemosiderin (low signal intensity in T2 GRE)

> Organizing hematomas may show marked contrast-enhancement. In case of nodular enhancement, consider intratumoral hemorrhage.

Myositis Ossificans Traumatica

Presentation, DD: benign response to trauma, may be mistaken for malignancy. Painful soft tissue mass in muscle/tendon attachment. In adolescents/young adults more frequently than in children. Trauma not always remembered = thorough

8

history needed. May be difficult to distinguish from malignant tumor by imaging alone.

> True bone neoplasm in injury, may be mistaken for osteosarcoma even histologically → use biopsy with caution. Reference pathology may be required.

DD: exostosis, paraosseous osteosarcoma, nontraumatic myositis ossificans, progressive ossifying fibrodysplasia.

Imaging:

- **US:** like hematoma; in addition, calcifications with acoustic shadows
- **Radiography** (or CT): demonstrates typical calcification and/or ossification
- **MRI:** if radiographic and US findings equivocal; shows hemosiderin deposition and calcification (T1 +T2 GRE); however, differentiation not possible without radiograph!

> Affected area may show significant edema and marked contrast-enhancement.

Malignant Soft Tissue Tumors

Rhabdomyosarcoma

Presentation, DD: most common soft tissue sarcoma in children.

Embryonal RMS (55–70% of all RMS—infants, preschool and school-age children), most common in head and neck region (46%; e.g., orbit, pterygo-

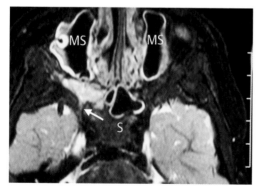

Fig. 8.37 Status post adenectomy in a 6-year-old boy. Surgical specimen contained parts of malignant tumor. MRI: axial STIR image (3 mm) at level of maxillary sinuses and sphenoid bone (S). Hyperintense tumor posterior to right maxillary sinus has invaded skull base via foramen rotundum (arrow). Finding confirmed by contrast-enhanced fat-saturated T1-weighted MRI (not shown). RMS of right pterygopalatine fossa (histologically confirmed).

palatine fossa) with invasion of skull base foramina (**Fig. 8.37**) and urogenital region (38%; e.g., bladder, prostate, vagina—see Chapter 5).

Alveolar RMS (up to 45% of all RMS, school-age children and adolescents) usually occurs in limb muscles, less favorable prognosis.

Prognosis depends on histology, size, location, extension. DD: other soft tissue sarcomas (e.g., synovial sarcoma) less common in children. See WHO Classification (http://www.iarc.fr/en/publications/pdfs-online/pat-gen/index.php).

> Diagnosis relies on histology after open or image-guided biopsy (MRI/US/CT).

Imaging: primary diagnosis and treatment/monitoring for recurrence at specialized centers by experienced pediatric radiologists according to guidelines of study groups: EPSSG (European Pediatric Soft-Tissue Sarcoma Study Group: http:/epssg.cineca.org), CWS (Cooperative Weichteilsarkom Studiengruppe cws.olgahospital-stuttgart.de), COG STS (Children's Oncology Group, Soft Tissue Sarcoma Committee, USA, http://www.cancer.gov/cancertopics/types/childrhabdomyosarcoma).

- **US:** nonspecific; can detect and describe tumor, sometimes detects hypervascularity (CDS)
- **MRI:** modality of choice—demonstrates primary tumor (alternative: CT) as circumscribed or invasive complex mass. Low T1-weighted signal intensity, high T2-weighted signal. Enhances markedly after Gd, except for necrotic areas. Recommended = high-resolution sequences (voxel ≤ 1 × 1 × 4 mm) before (T2 with fat saturation, STIR) and after administration of contrast material (T1 with frequency-selective fat saturation or subtraction analysis) in at least two orientations. Dynamic contrast-enhanced study and DWI help to distinguish tumor from edema/necrosis. 3D sequences facilitate volumetry of tumors with complex shape

> Essential for staging and treatment decisions = tumor size (≤ 5 cm/> 5 cm), tumor volume over time, precise description of location (e.g., parameningeal, nonparameningeal), extent, invasiveness, and lymph node involvement.

- **Additional imaging:** pulmonary CT, bone scintigraphy, abdominal US, lymph node US. Role of PET-CT and whole-body MRI—still being evaluated

Case Study 8.14

Clinical presentation: 3-year-old boy refused to bear weight on his left leg. US and MRI prompted referral for suspected malignancy. No trauma observed.
Imaging options: US, radiography, MRI, CT.

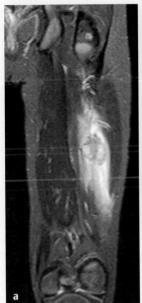
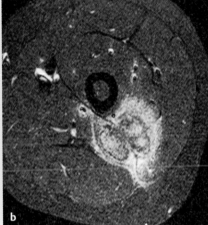
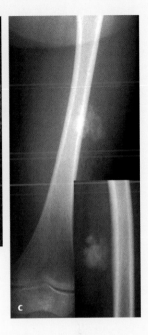

Fig. 8.38a–c
Available images and findings: US—inhomogeneous, poorly circumscribed intramuscular area with central acoustic shadow. MRI—coronal STIR (**a**) shows 3-mm soft-tissue lesion with inhomogeneous hypointense center crossing muscle border, extensive perifocal edema. Fat-saturated T1-weighted image after Gd (**b**) shows marked contrast-enhancement. AP and lateral radiograph (**c**) show soft tissue calcification/ossification not in contact with bone.
Further course: spontaneous regression.
Diagnosis: myositis ossificans.
DD: exostosis, nontraumatic myositis ossificans. Osteosarcoma in adolescence (extremely rare in young children).
Radiologic therapy: none.
With clear-cut history, US and radiographs were sufficient to make diagnosis. Without trauma history, always check and document regression of findings (e.g., with radiographs and US). If MRI is evaluated together with radiographs, radiation exposure by CT can be avoided.

8

Infantile/Congenital Fibrosarcoma

Presentation, DD: 12% of all malignant soft tissue tumors in infants; favorable prognosis!

Congenital (up to 80%), rare after 2 years of age. Occurrence: limbs 50%, trunk 19%, head and neck 16%. Tumor may grow rapidly and infiltrate multiple tissue layers. Spontaneous regression rare. Rarely metastasizes. DD: hemangioma, myofibroma, rarely malignant nerve sheath tumor.

Imaging:
- **US:** shows often tortuous tumor vessels with rapid blood flow
- **MRI:** detailed examination based on study group guidelines (cf. RMS) necessary to ensure complete resection. High rate of local recurrence

Bibliography

1 Bianchi S, Martinoli C. Ultrasound of the Musculoskeletal System. Berlin, Heidelberg: Springer; 2007

2 Dubois J, Garel L. Imaging and therapeutic approach of hemangiomas and vascular malformations in the pediatric age group. Pediatr Radiol 1999; 29(12): 879–893

3 Fletcher CDM, Unni KK, Mertens F, eds. World Health Organization, Classification of Tumours. Pathology and Genetics of Tumours of Soft Tissue and Bone. Lyon: IARC Press; 2002. Website: http://www.iarc.fr/en/publications/pdfs-online/pat-gen/index.php; status: 30 Nov 2009

4 Freyschmidt J, Ostertag H, Jundt G. Knochentumoren. 2nd ed. Berlin, Heidelberg: Springer; 2003

5 Kan JH, Kleinman PK. Pediatric and Adolescent Musculoskeletal MRI. A Case-Based Approach. New York: Springer; 2007

6 Kransdorf MJ, Murphey MD. Imaging of Soft Tissue Tumors. 2nd ed. Philadelphia: Lippincott Williams & Wilkins; 2006

7 Laor T. MR imaging of soft tissue tumors and tumorlike lesions. Pediatr Radiol 2004; 34(1): 24–37

8 Oka K, Yakushiji T, Sato H, Hirai T, Yamashita Y, Mizuta H. The value of diffusion-weighted imaging for monitoring the chemotherapeutic response of osteosarcoma: a comparison between average apparent diffusion coefficient and minimum apparent diffusion coefficient. Skeletal Radiol 2010; 39(2): 141–146

9 von Kalle T, Langendörfer M, Fernandez FF, Winkler P. Combined dynamic contrast-enhancement and serial 3D-subtraction analysis in magnetic resonance imaging of osteoid osteomas. Eur Radiol 2009; 19(10): 2508–2517

10 Zampa V, Bargellini I, Ortori S, Faggioni L, Cioni R, Bartolozzi C. Osteoid osteoma in atypical locations: the added value of dynamic gadolinium-enhanced MR imaging. Eur J Radiol 2009; 71(3): 527–535

8.7 Systemic Oncologic Diseases

Doris Zebedin, Erich Sorantin

Langerhans Cell Histiocytosis

Definition: tumorlike proliferation of dendritic cells having phenotypic characteristics of epidermal Langerhans cells. Etiology unknown. Peak incidence = first decade of life. Male preponderance— m : f = 4 : 3.

Clinical manifestations:

- Monosystemic LCH: eosinophilic granuloma (70%)
- Multisystemic LCH: acute disseminated fulminated form = Letterer–Siwe disease, chronic disseminated form = Hand–Schüller–Christian disease

Imaging: recommended for more complete workup —bone scintigraphy, radiographic skeletal survey or spot films of positive scans in scintigraphy, chest radiographs, thin-section chest CT (**Fig. 8.39**), MRI of brain/sella turcica (or whole-body MRI). Typical radiological findings:

- Skeletal: punched-out osteolytic medullary lesions in calvarium, no sclerotic margin, with soft tissue component (DD: epidermoid). Only healed lesions have sclerotic margin (Case Study 8.15, **Fig. 8.40**). Endosteal scalloping in meta- and diaphysis of long bones. Vertebra plana (Calvé disease) in spine
- Infiltration of neurohypophysis and osteolytic lesion of sphenoid bone
- Infiltration of liver/spleen: diffuse, granulomatous, with or without organ enlargement
- Lung: centrilobular nodules 1 to 60 mm in size with indistinct margins; uniform small and large subpleural cysts with bizarre shapes; interstitial fibrosis

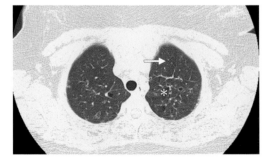

Fig. 8.39 Thin-section chest CT. Langerhans cell histiocytosis with pulmonary involvement—cysts, centrilobular nodules.

Case Study 8.15

Clinical history: suspicion of head injury (arrows) on lateral skull radiograph.

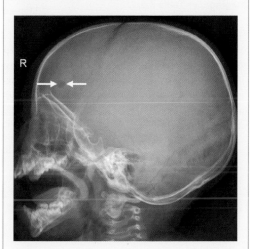

Fig. 8.40

Findings: 5-mm osteolytic lesion in frontal region of calvarium with sclerotic margin.
Diagnosis: healing eosinophilic granuloma (DD: epidermoid).
Further imaging: US—with eosinophilic granuloma, inner table not definable at affected site; if present → eosinophilic granuloma very unlikely. If findings equivocal: MRI. Eosinophilic granuloma → complete destruction of calvarium, contrast enhancement of lesion and adjacent meninges.
Treatment: corticosteroids and cytostatic agents for multisystem involvement.

Typical sparing of costophrenic angles—DD: idiopathic pulmonary fibrosis. Diagnosis is always established by biopsy. LCH = known imaging chameleon—frequently associated with unexpected findings and very diverse manifestations.

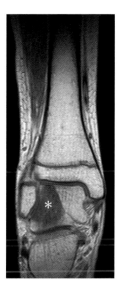

Fig. 8.41 Chloroma of talus. Coronal T1-weighted MRI of ankle joint shows absence of fat marrow signal in lateral half of talar dome (*). *Histology*: recurrence of acute myeloid lymphoma.

Childhood Leukemias

Definition: malignant clonal neoplasia with abnormal differentiation of hematopoietic cells (lymphatic/myeloid) in bone marrow. Median age for acute lymphoblastic leukemia (ALL) = 4.7 years. Prognosis for ALL = 80% survival rate.

Classification:

- Acute leukemias: immature cells; most common form = ALL
- Chronic leukemias: mature cells (chronic lymphoblastic leukemia, chronic myeloid leukemia)
- Special form: chloroma = extramedullary tumorlike proliferation of myeloid precursor cells (**Fig. 8.41**); initial manifestation/recurrence of acute myeloid leukemia (AML) (see also Sect. 8.6)

Imaging:

- **Skeletal radiography:** metaphyseal lucent bands, diffuse osteoporosis, focal lytic lesions
- **Chest radiography and CT:** focal homogenous opacities or diffuse peribronchial and perivascular lung infiltrates (HRCT), inflammatory/hemorrhagic infiltrates, hilar and mediastinal lymph node enlargement
- **US**—mediastinum (thymus), abdomen, lymph nodes: moderate hepato-splenomegaly. Bilateral renal enlargement, urate nephropathy (medullary deposits/stone). Bilateral, asymmetric lymphadenopathy, have atypical morphology,

8

may form conglomerate mass. Frequent infiltration of testis/ovary

> Infiltration of testis/ovary may result in torsion at atypical age. Also sanctuary for residual tumor in younger age = possible and common site of recurrence

- **CT/MRI:** chest and abdomen (also for staging, see findings above) and neurocranium (leukemic meningeosis = specific complication of ALL)

Treatment: combination chemotherapy, allogeneic hematopoietic stem cell transplantation.

Malignant Lymphomas in Children

Definition: proliferation of abnormal lymphocytes in lymphatic and other organs (bone marrow). Age: Hodgkin lymphoma = second to third decade; NHL = first to second decade.

Classification and staging: Ann Arbor Staging Classification for Hodgkin lymphoma (**Table 8.7**) and **St. Jude Children's Research Hospital Staging Classification** for NHL (**Table 8.8**).
Imaging: See **Table 8.9**.

All imaging studies show extranodal lymphomatous infiltration of parenchymal organs, bowel loops, and intranodal infiltration with enlarged lymph nodes in affected regions. Lesions often show little contrast enhancement; sometimes difficult to identify specific entities and make DD. Organ involvement = diffuse or nodular, with or without organ enlargement.

> Determine smallest lymph node diameter (axial image). Nodal diameters region-specific (e.g., > 10 mm abnormal in neck, > 15 mm at mandibular angle). Diagnosis is always histological → excision of representative lymph node/biopsy of affected tissue.

Table 8.7 Ann Arbor Staging Classification for Hodgkin lymphoma

Stage	Findings
I	Involvement of single lymph node region (I) or lymphoid structure (e.g., spleen, thymus, Waldeyer ring) or localized involvement of single extralymphatic organ or site (IE)
II	Involvement of two or more lymph node regions on same side of diaphragm (II) or localized contiguous involvement of single extranodal organ or site and lymph node region on same side of diaphragm (IIE); number of anatomic sites should be indicated by subscript (e.g., II$_2$)
III	Involvement of lymph node regions on both sides of diaphragm (III), plus localized involvement of extranodal organ site (IIIE) or simultaneous involvement of spleen (IIIS) or simultaneous involvement of both (IIIE + S)
IV	Diffuse or disseminated (involvement of one or more extranodal organ sites or tissues with or without associated lymph node involvement

Table 8.8 St Jude Children's Research Hospital Staging Classification for non-Hodgkin lymphoma

Stage	Findings
I	Single nodal or extranodal tumor without local spread outside abdomen and mediastinum
II	Single tumor with regional node involvement, two or multiple nodal and/or extranodal sites of involvement on same side of diaphragm or primary GI-tract tumor (resected) with or without regional node involvement
III	Tumors or nodal areas of involvement on both sides of diaphragm - Any primary intrathoracic tumors - All extensive intraabdominal disease - Paraspinal or epidural tumors
IV	Bone marrow disease or CNS disease regardless of other sites of involvement

Table 8.9 Diagnostic steps in imaging evaluation of children with lymphoma

Imaging Study	Indication
US study of neck, abdomen, pelvis, and inguinal region	Evaluation of superficial and abdominal lymph nodes or parenchymatous organs, bowel loops, and testes
Chest radiography	Preliminary evaluation of mediastinum and lungs
CT of neck	Evaluation of Waldeyer ring with cervical lymph node involvement
Chest CT	Detailed evaluation of mediastinum, lungs, pericardium, pleura, and chest wall
CT of abdomen and pelvis	Evaluation of parenchymatous organs, lymph nodes, and mesentery, peritoneum, and pelvic organs
MRI of CNS	Indicated only in cases of suspected CNS disease
Whole body MRI	Being evaluated
^{99m}Tc bone scan	Indicated for bone assessment only in children with bone pain and elevated alkaline phosphatase levels
^{67}Ga scan	Useful as whole-body screening modality
FDG PET and PET-CT	Role in children still to be defined; possibly useful in follow-up

DD: lymph node metastasis—conglomerate nodal mass, rarely with necrosis; more often shows homogeneous signal at MRI. DD includes any other systemic malignant/inflammatory disease with multiorgan involvement.

Bibliography

1 Brisse H, Pacquement H, Burdairon E, Plancher C, Neuenschwander S. Outcome of residual mediastinal masses of thoracic lymphomas in children: impact on management and radiological follow-up strategy. Pediatr Radiol 1998; 28(6): 444–450

2 Carrol BA. Lymphoma. In: Goldberg BB, ed. Ultrasound in Cancer. Clinics in Diagnostic Ultrasound. Vol 6. New York: Churchill Livingstone;1981: 52–67

3 Dähnert W. Radiology Review Manual. Philadelphia: Lippincott Williams & Wilkins; 2003: 509–510, 491–493, 923–924

4 Bohndorf. K, Imhof H, Pope TL. Musculoskeletal Imaging: a Concise Multimodality Approach. Stuttgart: Thieme; 2001: 208–210

5 Stull MA, Kransdorf MJ, Devaney KO; Musculosceletal Imaging. Langerhans cell histiocytosis of bone. Radiographics 1992; 12(4): 801–823

6 Guermazi A. Radiological Imaging in Hematological Malignancies (Medical Radiology). Berlin: Springer; 2004: 351–364

7 Schmidt S, Eich G, Geoffray A, et al. Extraosseous langerhans cell histiocytosis in children. Radiographics 2008; 28(3): 707–726; quiz 910–911

8 Toma P, Granata C, Rossi A, Garaventa A. Multimodality imaging of Hodgkin disease and non-Hodgkin lymphomas in children. Radiographics 2007; 27(5): 1335–1354

8

9 Syndromes, Metabolic Disorders, and Other Characteristic Features in Children

Heimo Nemec

9.1 Introduction

Radiological research into known syndromes associated with skeletal anomalies began shortly after implementation of radiology in human medicine → imaging quickly became indispensable tool for diagnosing syndromic conditions.

Recent years = paradigm shift—growing importance of prepubescent/fetal/family examinations and human genetics = early detection of most syndromic changes = scheduled delivery. Even so, radiology still critical tool for diagnosis of suspected syndromes.

Imaging modalities:

- **Radiography:** essential for diagnosing syndromes—provides thorough, targeted examination of affected skeletal regions in suspected syndromic diseases; sometimes used for complete skeletal survey (see also Sections 7.1, 7.2)
- **US:** rapidly available noninvasive test, excellent for detection and follow-up of organic changes in metabolic disorders
- **MRI:** nonionizing modality for diagnosing cerebral changes in children with syndromes and metabolic disorders

> This chapter is intended to illustrate essential imaging techniques and findings for common or important entities, rather than cover all relevant aspects.

9.2 Hormone Deficiencies and Growth Disorders

Pediatric growth problems are often indicators of metabolic disorders—several factors should be considered to avoid misinterpretations (**Table 9.1**). Compare with normal population/percentile curves broken down by gender and ethnicity.

Table 9.1 Nonnutritional factors that affect body growth in children

Factors that affect predicted body height
Gender
Height of parents
Ethnicity origin
Geographical region

Constitutional Growth Delay

Slow pediatric growth rate with delayed but normal puberty and normal adult height (as predicted from paternal and maternal height). Parents often found to have similar history. Constitutional growth delay (CGD) = normal variant of growth.

Diagnosis based on "skeletal age" of left hand = comparing radiographs with standard atlas—Greulich and Pyle (1959), Maresh (1955), Tanner et al. (1975), or Cole et al. (1988) (see also Sect. 7.1).

Tall Stature

Definition: body height > 75th percentile (relative to healthy children of equal age).

Table 9.2 Changes associated with Marfan syndrome

Cardiac valve defects
Aortic dissection
Retinal detachment
Glaucoma
Tall stature
Increased incidence of pneumothorax

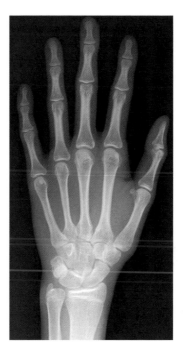

Marfan Syndrome

Etiology: mutation in fibrillin gene (long arm of chromosome 15). Autosomal dominant inheritance; incidence = 1 : 5,000 worldwide.

Clinical features: connective tissue weakness and associated changes: tall stature and long limbs, hypermobile joints, increased risk of aortic dissection (**Table 9.2**).

Imaging: radiography—long fingers (arachnodactyly, **Fig. 9.1**), carpal angle > 140° (angle formed by line tangent to proximal surfaces of scaphoid and lunate and line tangent to proximal margins of triquetrum and lunate). Pectus excavatum/carinatum (**Fig. 9.2**). Dislocations of hip and sternoclavicular joints.

Fig. 9.1 Marfan syndrome. Radiograph of hand shows elongated phalangeal bones (arachnodactyly) in adolescent male with Marfan syndrome.

Wiedemann–Beckwith Syndrome

Etiology: exomphalos–macroglossiagigantism (EMG) syndrome. Change in chromosome 11 (Igf2 gene). Autosomal dominant inheritance.

Clinical features: macroglossia, birth weight/length usually ↑. Nonuniform growth, sometimes with hemihypertrophy. Craniofacial dysmorphia—possible microcephaly, frequent midfacial hypoplasia. Increased incidence of omphalocele/umbilical hernia. Increased cancer risk (Wilms tumor, hepatoblastoma).

Imaging: US, radiography.

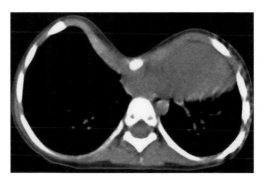

Fig. 9.2 Funnel chest. Unenhanced axial CT scan shows funnel-chest depression of sternum displacing heart toward left side. Scan taken before implantation of Nuss bar. Note: low-dose scan (i.e., 80 kV, 63 mAs) adequate for this indication.

- Visceromegaly, especially nephro-/hepatomegaly, hemihypertrophy, renal parenchymal cysts and cystic adrenal changes (**Fig. 9.3**)
- Possible accelerated bone growth, midfacial hypoplasia. Mental development ranges from normal intelligence to severe retardation

9

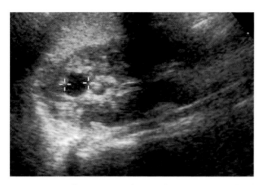

Fig. 9.3 Syndromic simple renal cyst. Longitudinal US scan of left flank shows simple renal parenchymal cyst 8.5 mm in diameter with posterior acoustic enhancement in upper third of left kidney—nonspecific finding that may occur in various syndromes or trisomy, for example.

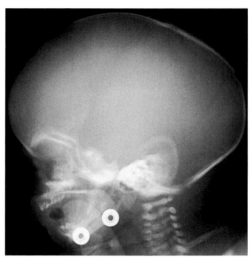

Fig. 9.4 Dolichocephaly. Lateral skull radiograph in Sotos syndrome shows elongated head shape with prominent occiput (dolichocephaly).

Sotos Syndrome

Etiology: congenital somatomegaly caused by mutation on NSD1 gene (chromosome 5). Autosomal dominant inheritance.

Clinical features: all physical growth parameters (height, weight, body circumference) > 97th percentile. Acromegaly (affecting phalanges more than metacarpals) = large hands and feet. Head = increased growth, prominent forehead. Poor motor coordination, delayed intellectual development (mental retardation). As in Wiedemann–Beckwith syndrome, cancer risk increased (Wilms tumor, hepatocellular carcinoma, small-cell lung cancer, etc.).

Imaging: US, radiography. Large, elongated head (dolichocephaly, **Fig. 9.4**). Hypertelorism (nonspecific). Large hands with long phalanges.

> At US, give particular attention to possible tumors of liver and kidneys.

Short Stature

Definition: body height less than third percentile (relative to healthy children of equal age). May present as abrupt cessation of initially normal growth. Prenatal causes include maternal drug use (alcohol, nicotine, opiates) and maternal infections

Table 9.3 Possible causes of short stature

Prenatal causes	
Toxic exposure	Fetal alcohol syndrome
	Toxoplasmosis
	Rubella
Syndromes	Seckel syndrome
	Microcephalic osteodysplastic dwarfism (**Fig. 9.5**)
	Achondroplasias
	Trisomy 21
Postnatal causes	
Deficiency states	Vitamin deficiency
	Malnutrition
	Celiac disease
Chronic diseases	Anemias
	Congenital heart disease
	Adrenal insufficiency
Metabolic diseases	Diabetes
	Glycogen storage disease
Endocrine diseases	Somatotropin deficiency
Hypothyroidism	

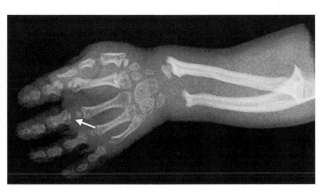

Fig. 9.5   Microcephalic osteodys-plastic primordial dwarfism type 2 (MOPD II). Radiograph of hand and forearm shows shortening and thickening of metacarpals and phalanges plus shortening and deformity of forearm bones. Cortical bone density greatly increased at some sites, especially in forearm. Osteopenia of hand bones. Proximal phalanges have fine cone-shaped epiphyses (arrow).

during pregnancy. Other causes: deficiency states, chronic diseases, syndromes, metabolic defects, radiation, chemotherapy, etc. (**Table 9.3**).

Imaging: radiography—skeletal segments shortened, often deformed (especially the limbs). Disproportionate bone lengths (**Fig. 9.5**). Osteopenic bone matrix in deficiency diseases.

9.3   Adrenal Involvement in Hormonal Disorders

General: adrenal glands can be clearly defined with US, especially in small children (**Fig. 9.6**). Adrenal hormones (corticosteroids, mineralocorticoids, sex hormones) are synthesized from cholesterol (**Fig. 9.7**). Tumors/hemorrhage may cause adrenal dysfunction with abnormalities of hormone synthesis. Dysfunction may be primary or secondary.

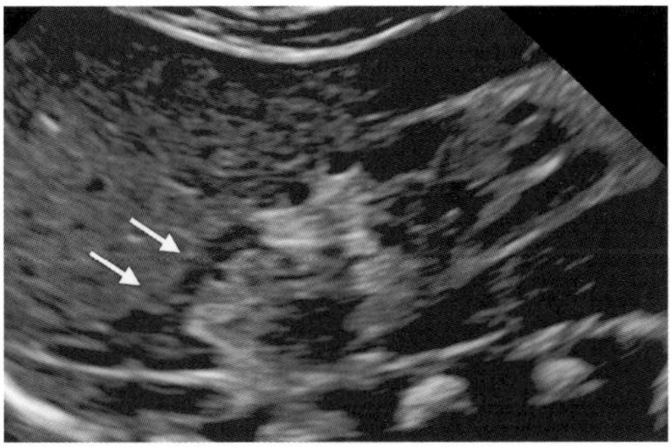

Adrenal Hypofunction, Adrenal Insufficiency

Primary (= functional disorder in adrenal gland itself) and secondary (= caused by disease of pituitary anterior lobe) (**Table 9.4**).

Addison Disease

Definition: adrenal hypoplasia, adrenocortical destruction due to chronic process.
Etiology:
- Autoimmune adrenalitis
- Metabolic diseases and syndromes (Zellweger syndrome, adrenoleukodystrophy, etc.)
- Amyloidosis, metastases, hemorrhage, infectious diseases, Waterhouse–Friedrichsen syndrome

Fig. 9.6   Normal adrenal gland. Longitudinal US scan of right flank with high-resolution curved-array probe. Transhepatic scan shows typical Y-shaped configuration of normal neonatal adrenal gland (arrows).

Table 9.4   Classification of adrenal insufficiency

Primary adrenal insufficiency	Addison disease
	Congenital adrenal hypoplasia
	Familial corticosteroid insufficiency
	Mineralocorticoid deficiency
Secondary adrenal insufficiency	Adrenocorticotropin deficiency
	Panhypopituitarism

9

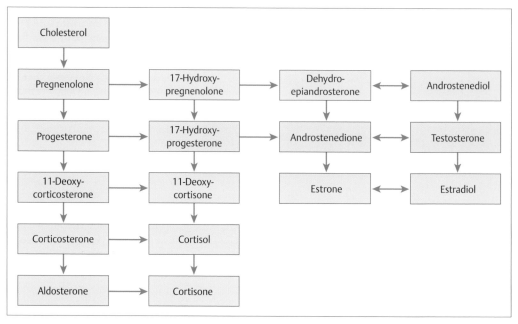

Fig. 9.7 Steroid biosynthesis in adrenal cortex.

Autoimmune Adrenalitis

Infiltration of adrenal gland by lymphocytes—accounts for 70 to 80% of all Addison disease cases. Possible involvement of other organs in polyendocrine syndromes (e.g., autoimmune thyroiditis, diabetes mellitus, etc.).

Clinical features: general weakness, rapid fatigability, loss of appetite, vomiting (may lead to anorexic appearance), salt craving, hyperpigmented skin; abdominal pain common.

Imaging: adrenal calcifications, hypertrophic kidneys, small adrenal glands

Adrenoleukodystrophy

X-linked recessive. Addison disease associated with rapid demyelination of white matter due to deficient breakdown of long-chain fatty acids (deposited mainly in adrenal cortex and cerebral white matter)—see also Sect. 4.1.

Clinical features: adrenal changes typical of Addison disease. Symmetrical areas of demyelination in cerebral white matter, starting in occipital lobes (**Fig. 9.8**).

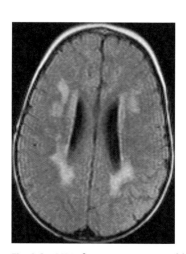

Fig. 9.8 MRI of neurocranium in Addison disease. Axial MRI of cerebrum (FLAIR sequence) shows symmetrical periventricular white matter lesions in 18-month-old girl with Addison disease.

Adrenogenital Syndrome

Adrenogenital syndrome (AGS) refers to group of metabolic diseases characterized by abnormal adrenal hormone production. Sex hormones are not affected → virilization in girls, premature puberty in boys. Abnormal salt levels in blood due to decreased aldosterone production. Autosomal recessive disorder marked by deficiency of 21-hydroxylase enzyme.

Clinical features: three types of AGS:

1. AGS without salt loss: in girls = clitoral hypertrophy, early pubic and axillary hair growth, male pubic hair pattern (hirsutism); in boys = penis usually enlarged; body growth is initially rapid, then ceases due to premature closure of epiphyseal plates
2. AGS with salt loss: insufficient aldosterone production → salt loss, neonatal onset of hyponatremia and hyperkalemia, metabolic acidosis; other features same as in type 1
3. Late-onset AGS: manifestations appear later, with premature pubic hair growth. Males infertile, menstrual abnormalities in females. Body growth is usually decreased

Imaging: US and radiography (plus MRI if necessary). Findings nonspecific: premature closure of growth plates, premature calcification of cartilaginous rib attachments; small uterus (**Fig. 9.9**). Increased pneumatization of mastoid and paranasal sinuses.

Adrenal Hyperfunction

Definition: conditions marked by excessive production of corticosteroids or mineralocorticoids.

Corticosteroid Excess

General: Cushing disease: collective term for all diseases based on adrenocortical hyperfunction = increased corticosteroid production. Cause may be pituitary microadenoma or iatrogenic (exogenous corticosteroid excess = most frequent cause). Tumor-related adrenal hyperfunction rare in children.

Clinical features: truncal obesity, marked weight gain accompanied by decreased muscle mass, polydipsia, polyuria, short stature.

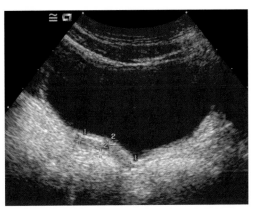

Fig. 9.9 Adrenogenital syndrome (AGS)—congenital adrenal hyperplasia. Midsagittal lower abdominal US scan shows somewhat small uterus (++) behind fluid-filled bladder of 9-year-old girl with known AGS. Note: uterus (and ovaries) may usually remain small for some time before puberty.

Imaging:

- **Radiography:** osteoporosis, increased susceptibility to fractures with excess callus formation; cystic skeletal changes
- **MRI/CT/US:** pituitary adenoma (microadenoma may not be visible even on MRI!). Adrenal tumor (US, MRI, rarely CT); (symmetrical) adrenal hyperplasia

Mineralocorticoid Excess

Three types: primary and secondary hyperaldosteronism, pseudoaldosteronism.

Primary Hyperaldosteronism

Rare in children, characterized by increased aldosterone production.

Causes: autonomous aldosterone synthesis (Conn syndrome), unilateral adrenocortical adenoma, autonomous bilateral adrenal hypertrophy, adrenocortical carcinoma.

Clinical features: arterial hypertension; polydipsia, muscle weakness.

Imaging: US, MRI/CT—adenoma/carcinoma of adrenal cortex. Sequelae of hypertension (compensated cardiac hypertrophy, etc.).

9

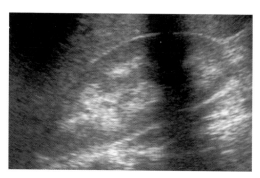

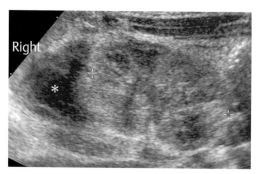

Fig. 9.10   Pseudohyperaldosteronism in 12-year-old girl. Longitudinal US scan through right flank shows increased echogenicity of renal papillae and variably increased echogenicity of medullary pyramids consistent with secondary nephrocalcinosis (grade I–II) in child with known pseudohyperaldosteronism.

Fig. 9.11   Neonatal adrenal hemorrhage. Posteroanterior longitudinal US scan in 1-week-old newborn shows "pseudocystic septated" mass on upper renal pole with typical adrenal shape and no other definable adrenal gland structures. Findings consistent with adrenal hemorrhage (*) undergoing resolution and absorption. Kidney is shown (++).

Secondary Hyperaldosteronism

Associated with increased renin production (Wilms tumor, renovascular malformation, etc.).
Clinical features: arterial hypertension due to elevated serum renin level.
Imaging: nonspecific.

Pseudohyperaldosteronism

Distinguished by fall in aldosterone and renin levels. May result from mutations (enzyme defect) or excessive licorice consumption (inhibits 11β-hydroxysteroid dehydrogenase).
Clinical features: similar to other forms of mineralocorticoid excess.
Imaging: nonspecific; nephrocalcinosis at US (**Fig. 9.10**).

Neonatal Adrenal Hemorrhage

General: usually unilateral, often on right side. May be caused by obstetric trauma, perinatal asphyxia, meningococcal sepsis, systemic diseases; rarely associated with renal vein thrombosis.
Clinical features: possible palpable swelling in flank, rarely hormonal changes (when bilateral).
Imaging:

- **US:** initially shows inhomogeneous, echogenic suprarenal mass (= adrenal gland), which later becomes more hypoechoic, sometimes cystic and septated (**Fig. 9.11**). Size diminishes over time (distinguishing feature from malignant tumor). May no longer be visible by 2 to 6 weeks, depending on initial extent. Residual calcifications may form (Case Study 9.1, **Fig. 9.45a–c**)
- **Abdominal radiograph:** may detect calcification as incidental finding in late phase
- **CT/MRI:** used very rarely in selected cases for DD

DD: (hemorrhagic) neuroblastoma (adrenal tumor), tumors (e.g., segmental cystic nephroma, segmental MCD, Wilms tumor, etc.) of upper renal pole, changes in upper moiety of duplex kidney.

9.4   Abnormalities of Thyroid Gland and Thyroid Metabolism

General: often already present in newborns. Imaging modality of choice = US, can evaluate size, structure, and perfusion of thyroid gland. Size determination = volumetry of single lobe (formula for ellipse: length × width × height × 0.523). Both sides added together, compared with tables of normal values (**Table 9.5**). Prerequisite for this formula = normal gland shape.

Table 9.5 Volume of thyroid gland in children. Reference values for thyroid volume as function of body weight (mean value ±2 standard deviations) (after Hofmann et al. 2005, p. 698)

Body weight	Volume of thyroid gland (mL)		
(kg)	Mean value (m)	m − 2 SD	m + 2 SD
0–5	0.9	0.5	1.8
>5–10	1.4	0.9	2.4
>10–20	2.6	1.4	4.9
>20–30	4.4	2.2	8.8
>30–40	6.3	3.5	11.6
>40–50	10.5	5.3	21.0
>50	10.4	5.3	21.0

Hyperthyroidism

Increased production of thyroid hormones. Rare in children, usually form of Graves disease.

Graves Disease

Definition: antibodies bind to thyroid-stimulating hormone (TSH) receptors → thyroid gland increases thyroid hormone synthesis. Five times more common in females, may be present in newborns (TSH autoantibodies can cross placental barrier). Graves disease (= Morbus Basedow) develops in 1 to 2% children of affected mothers.

Clinical features: goiter, nervousness, irritability, weight loss despite normal appetite, tachycardia, increased sweating, secondary nocturnal enuresis.

Imaging:
- **US:** thyroid gland inhomogeneous, may be nodular with hypoechoic structures (**Figs. 9.12** and **9.13**). With inflammation: enlarged gland with increased vascularity or hyperemia ("thyroid inferno"; Case Study 9.2, **Fig. 9.46a, b**)
- **Scintigraphy:** increased iodine uptake

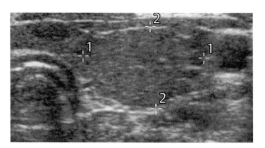

Fig. 9.12   Thyroid nodule in hyperthyroidism. Transverse thyroid US scan with linear probe shows echogenic, relatively homogeneous, well-circumscribed nodule with thyroidlike echo pattern (++) in the thyroid lobe of 8-year-old girl with hyperthyroidism (TSH < 0.01 mU/L).

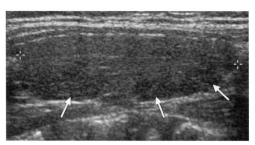

Fig. 9.13   Thyroid changes in Graves disease. Longitudinal US scan with linear probe shows small zones of decreased echogenicity (arrows) in somewhat inhomogeneous thyroid gland that is slightly large for age. Note: sometimes difficult to distinguish parathyroids from nodular changes!

9

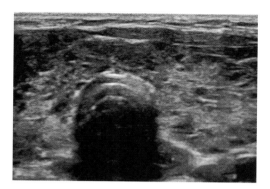

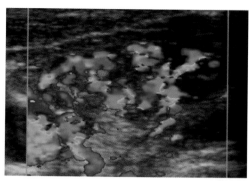

Fig. 9.14 US appearance of Hashimoto thyroiditis. Transverse US scan with linear probe displays small, inhomogeneous left thyroid lobe with focal hypoechoic changes in 10-year-old boy with Hashimoto thyroiditis.

Fig. 9.15 CDS of the thyroid gland in Hashimoto thyroiditis. Transverse US scan with linear probe. Color Doppler sonogram of right thyroid lobe of patient in **Fig. 9.14** shows marked hypervascularity of gland during acute exacerbation of Hashimoto thyroiditis.

Table 9.6 Possible causes of goiter

Dietary iodine deficiency
Hormone resistance
Autoimmune thyropathy (Hashimoto thyroiditis)
Tumors
Cyst formation
Thyroid autonomy
Inflammation

Table 9.7 WHO classification of goiter

Stage	Findings
0	No goiter
1	Thyroid gland visible only when the neck is fully extended
2	Thyroid gland visible in a normal head position
3	Marked thyroid gland enlargement visible at a distance

Hashimoto Thyroiditis

Definition: autoimmune thyroid inflammation with lymphocytic infiltration of gland, usually congenital, often goes undetected for years. Marked initially by enlargement of the thyroid gland (hypertrophic type), eventually giving way to thyroid atrophy (atrophic type). Often coexists with diabetes mellitus, Down syndrome.

Clinical features: painless swelling of thyroid gland, possible signs of hyperfunction (nervousness, sweating, sleep disturbances) or hypofunction (lethargy, weight gain, muscle weakness).

Imaging:

- **US:** enlarged thyroid gland with inhomogeneous structure that includes focal hypoechoic changes (**Fig. 9.14**). Advanced cases show nodular transformation with hyperechoic gland. In chronic cases gland small and difficult to distin-

guish from surrounding cervical soft tissues. Perfusion may be markedly increased in acute stage (**Fig. 9.15**)

- **Scintigraphy:** decreased uptake

Goiter

Definition: enlarged thyroid gland that may include nodular components. Variety of possible causes (**Table 9.6**). Classified by hormonal status as euthyroid, hyperthyroid, or hypothyroid. WHO criteria for staging (**Table 9.7**).

Clinical features: palpable/visible swelling at base of neck. Globus sensation due to tracheal displacement by large nodular goiter. Other clinical signs depend on hormonal change.

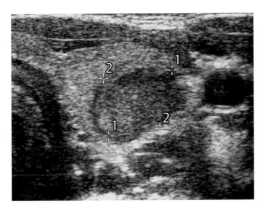

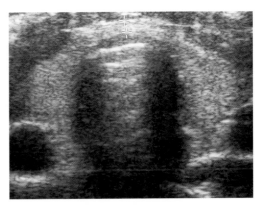

Fig. 9.16 US appearance of goiter. Transverse US scan with linear probe shows large, hypoechoic nodular goiter bounded by relatively well-defined pseudocapsule (++) in thyroid left lobe.

Fig. 9.17 Congenital hypothyroidism. Transverse US scan with linear probe shows small thyroid gland with somewhat coarse texture in 8-year-old girl with congenital hypothyroidism. Thyroid isthmus (++) measures only 1.5 mm in thickness.

Imaging: US—thyroid enlargement (thyroid lobes overlap cervical vessels), possible nodular changes (**Fig. 9.16**). Inflammation or marked hyperfunction → hypervascularity.

Hypothyroidism

Definition: congenital/acquired hypofunction of thyroid gland—detected by neonatal screening. Incidence = 1 : 4,000, female-to-male ratio = 2 : 1.

Three types:

- Primary hypothyroidism: thyroid gland itself diseased, causing impaired thyroid hormone production
- Secondary hypothyroidism: result of pituitary disease; TSH production absent or diminished
- Tertiary hypothyroidism: originates in hypothalamus; TRH production impaired

Clinical features: signs and symptoms depend on type.

- Congenital hypothyroidism: prolonged neonatal jaundice, decreased muscle tone, sleepiness, constipation, hypothermia, bradycardia, umbilical hernia, retardation
- Acquired hypothyroidism: goiter, fatigue, menstrual irregularities, short stature, delayed bone age

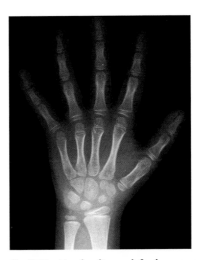

Fig. 9.18 Hand radiograph for bone age assessment. Same patient as in **Fig. 9.17**. Her bone age (based on radiograph of left hand) corresponds to that of 6½-year-old girl. Carpal bones too small, epiphyseal plates too wide = insufficient closure for age = growth retardation.

Imaging:

- **US:** thyroid gland hypotrophic to atrophic with decreased echogenicity and vascularity (**Fig. 9.17**). Radiographic delay of bone growth (**Fig. 9.18**)
- **Scintigraphy:** decreased uptake

9

Congenital Primary Hypothyroidism

Most common pediatric form of hypothyroidism. Prevalence 1 : 4,000; girls affected twice as often as boys. Usually marked by hypoplasia/aplasia of thyroid gland. Other causes: receptor disorders, abnormal hormone production due to enzyme defects.

Acquired Primary Hypothyroidism

Usually occurs in Hashimoto thyroiditis (advanced to main cause by iodine prophylaxis), iodine deficiency, after chemotherapy or radiation.

Acquired Secondary and Tertiary Hypothyroidism

Most often caused by cerebral tumor surgery or radiation to brain.

9.5   Typical Bony Changes in Syndromic Disorders

Some syndromes are associated with marked and impressive skeletal changes, others with only subtle changes. Detecting these changes = important task of radiology—interpreting within context of clinical and physiognomonic changes supplies important evidence for detection and diagnosis of syndromes.

Sagittal Cleft (Butterfly Vertebra)

Congenital cleft vertebra composed of two lateral hemivertebrae (**Fig. 9.19**). Suggestive of:

- VACTER(L) association (see Sect. 2.5 and 7.2)
- Alagille syndrome (vertebral body changes, liver anomaly—arteriohepatic dysplasia, pulmonic stenosis, ocular malformation; autosomal dominant)

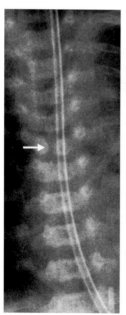 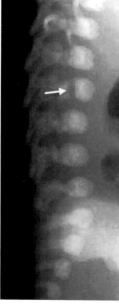

Fig. 9.19   Vertebral body cleft (VACTERL association). Detail from AP chest radiograph reveals sagittal clefts in T6 and T7 vertebrae. Gastric tube.

Fig. 9.20   Vertebral body changes in trisomy. Lateral spinal radiograph shows frontal lumbar cleft (arrow) in newborn with known trisomy 13. Note also ovoid shape of vertebral body.

Fig. 9.19   **Fig. 9.20**

Frontal Cleft

Coronal cleft in vertebral bodies (**Fig. 9.20**).
- Trisomy 13: autosomal dominant inheritance; characterized by spondylometaepiphyseal dysplasia, disproportionate short stature, progressive dysplasia of axial and limb bones, flat facial contour, marked articular cartilage changes—histologic "Swiss cheese" pattern
- Other associated conditions: Kniest syndrome, Larsen syndrome, mucolipidosis II

Lateral or Posterior Hemivertebra

Absence of vertebral ossification center (**Fig. 9.21**). Found in VACTERL and Klippel–Feil syndrome.

Klippel–Feil Syndrome

Rare, autosomal recessive.
Clinical features: short neck, decreased ROM at occipitocervical junction. Severe auricular changes and hearing loss.
Radiologic manifestations: cervical block vertebrae, hemivertebrae, renal agenesis.

Congenital Block Vertebrae

Congenital fusion of ossification centers. Found in Klippel–Feil syndrome and trisomy 18.

Trisomy 18 (Edwards Syndrome)

General: three copies of chromosome 18. Incidence = 3 : 10,000. Girls predominate. Risk increases with maternal age. Several types—most common forms = free trisomy 18 (extra chromosome present in all cells) and mosaic trisomy 18 (extra chromosome present in some but not all cells).
Clinical features: symptoms vary in severity, always occur in combination.
Imaging:
- **Prenatal:** US and amniotic fluid examination = polyhydramnios, polydactyly, flexion contractures of fingers, cardiac anomalies (ventricular septal defects, atrioventricular canal), dolichocephaly, small mouth, increased incidence of omphalocele
- **Postnatal:** various modalities; signs usually combined, variable severity/expression = choroid plexus cysts, polydactyly, contractures, urogenital anomalies, vertebral blocking (**Fig. 9.22**)

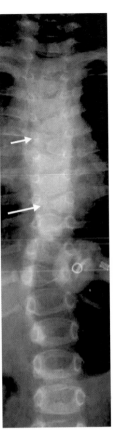

Fig. 9.21 Multiple neonatal syndromic vertebral body changes. AP radiograph of spine shows multiple, varied vertebral body deformities with hemivertebra (short arrow) and butterfly vertebra (long arrow) in child with VACTERL. Percutaneous endoscopic gastrostomy tube in left paramedian upper abdomen (o).

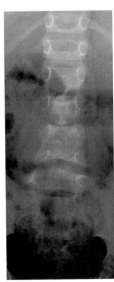

Fig. 9.22 Vertebral blocking. AP spot radiograph of spine demonstrates fusion of L3 and L4 vertebrae (boy with trisomy 18).

9

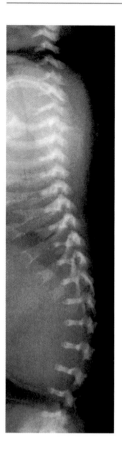

Fig. 9.23   Platyspondyly. Full-length lateral radiograph of spine shows flat vertebral bodies and short bifid ribs in neonate with type 1 thanatophoric dysplasia. Child died shortly after from respiratory failure.

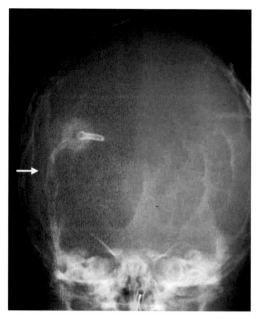

Fig. 9.24   Skull radiograph in Arnold–Chiari malformation with hydrocephalus. AP skull film shows distinct regional bone defects, some filled with fibrous tissue, consistent with lacunar skull in Arnold–Chiari malformation and internal hydrocephalus. Ventriculoperitoneal shunt (arrow), gastric tube.

Platyspondyly

Congenital reduction of vertebral body height (**Fig. 9.23**). Found in thanatophoric dwarfism (see Sect. 9.6).

Skull

Often bears changes pathognomonic for certain syndromes. Examples follow.

Lacunar Skull (Lückenschädel)

Defects in inner table of skull, usually with intact outer table (**Fig. 9.24**), often associated with increased intracranial pressure and spina bifida. Found in Arnold–Chiari malformations (**Fig. 9.25**) and MMC (see Sect. 4.1).

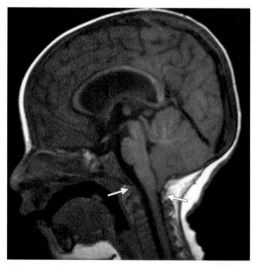

Fig. 9.25   Chiari I malformation in a 1-year-old boy. Midsagittal T1-weighted MRI shows cerebellar tonsillar herniation into foramen magnum (arrow).

Cloverleaf Skull

Premature fusion of coronal, lambdoid, and squamous sutures—give skull a cloverleaf shape (see also Sect. 4.1). Usually associated with increased intracranial pressure and other cranial abnormalities. Found in Apert syndrome (see Sect. 9.4) and Crouzon syndrome.

Craniofacial Dysostosis (Crouzon Syndrome)

Rare, autosomal dominant condition marked by premature fusion of coronal suture (**Fig. 9.26**) and premature ossification of other sutures. Midfacial hypoplasia.
Clinical features: divergent strabismus, exophthalmos, mild mental retardation. Often associated with obstructive airway disease and cor pulmonale.
Imaging: radiography, US, MRI, possibly 3D CT—brachycephaly, premature synostosis, internal hydrocephalus, aural atresia.

> Many types of craniosynostosis occur in syndromes—but can be interpreted as syndromic only on basis of other clinical and radiologic findings.

Limbs

Subject to many possible malformations—some typical examples listed along with possible associated syndromes. See also Sections 7.1 and 7.2. Examples below illustrate only small fraction of possible limb anomalies.

> Many syndromes associated with osseous changes display bony malformations typical of particular syndrome. But every skeletal malformation does not necessarily indicate a syndrome.

Polydactyly

See **Fig. 9.27**.

Presence of sixth digit (hexadactyly) most common. Autosomal dominant inheritance. Treatment consists of surgical removal for cosmetic and functional indications.

Possible association with Edwards syndrome (trisomy 18), Ellis–van Creveld syndrome, short rib-polydactyly syndrome, etc.

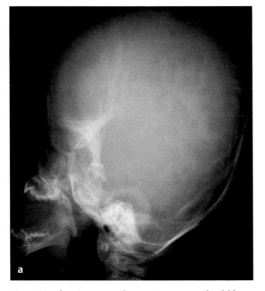
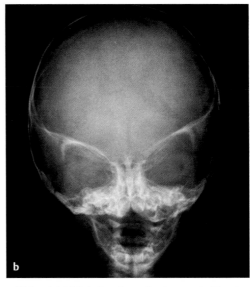

Fig. 9.26a, b   Apert syndrome in a 4-month-old boy. Lateral (**a**) and AP (**b**) skull radiographs show typical brachycephaly with short head, steep flat forehead, and atrophic auditory canal. Cranial sutures already fused.

9

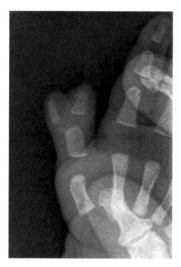
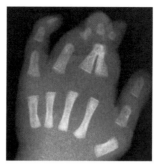
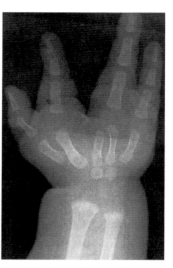

Fig. 9.27 Polydactyly. Spot radiograph shows polydactyly of right thumb in otherwise healthy neonate.

Fig. 9.28 Symphalangism. Radiograph of right hand shows fusion of proximal phalanges of second through fourth rays in Apert syndrome.

Fig. 9.29 Adactyly in Kniest syndrome. Radiograph of right hand in 6-month-old boy shows absence of third ray with third metacarpal abutting the fourth. (With kind permission from Ebel et al. 1995, p. 334.)

Arachnodactyly

Abnormally long, slender "spiderlike" fingers. A feature of Marfan syndrome (see Sect. 9.2).

Syndactyly

Two or more fingers or toes fused together/fail to separate. Feature of Apert syndrome, also trisomy 13 and 18.

Symphalangism

Fusion of phalangeal bones (**Fig. 9.28**). Detection often delayed. Found in Apert syndrome, diastrophic dwarfism, or as anomaly with brachydactyly.

Adactyly

Congenital absence of one or more fingers, often with intact metacarpals (**Fig. 9.29**). Found in **Kniest syndrome** (among others) = rare type II collagen disease with autosomal dominant inheritance. Features include adactyly, disproportionate short stature, dysplasia of axial and limb bones, cleft palate, and osteoporosis.

Lower Limb

Lower limb anomalies common in syndromes. Typical changes: thickened long bones with prominent epiphyses and elongated fibula (relative to tibia; **Fig. 9.30**). Example: achondroplasia (see Sect. 9.6).

- **Clubfoot** (pes equinovarus): typical malformation (**Fig. 9.31**), found in several syndromes (**Table 9.8**). Also associated with oligohydramnios, unfavorable fetal position, and amniotic band syndrome

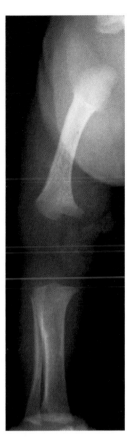

Fig. 9.30 Syndromic changes in the lower limb. A 3-day-old male infant with short, stout lower limb. Fibula appears elongated relative to tibia.

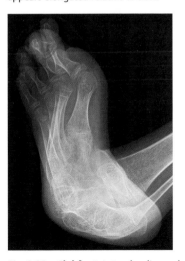

Fig. 9.31 Clubfoot. Lateral radiograph shows clubbing of foot in 17-year-old mentally retarded male.

Table 9.8 Examples of syndromes associated with clubfoot

Homocystinuria
Caudal regression syndrome
Larsen syndrome
Zellweger syndrome
Noonan syndrome
Arthrogryposis

Pelvis

Syndromes commonly associated with pelvic anomalies—especially malformations of iliac wings. Pelvic deformity may also develop secondarily in other diseases (due to inactivity) such as spastic diplegia, MMC, etc.

Caudal Regression Syndrome

In spina bifida, tethered cord, sacral lipoma, lumbosacral dysgenesis, anal atresia (see also Sect. 4.1). Frequent concomitant involvement of lower limbs (e.g., clubfeet). Pelvic skeleton grossly deformed and narrow (**Fig. 9.32**). Consequent scoliosis → marked thoracic asymmetry (**Fig. 9.33**).

Some congenital syndromes also associated with changes in pelvic skeleton (often typical of specific underlying disease) as illustrated in **Fig. 9.34**.

9

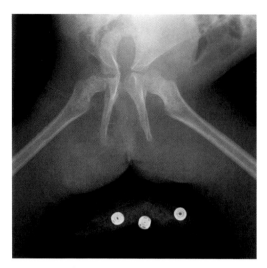

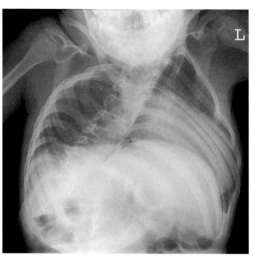

Fig. 9.32 Pelvis in caudal regression syndrome. AP radiograph of pelvis and upper legs shows dysplastic pelvis with fused iliac wings and absence of sacrum in caudal regression syndrome. Hip problems include hypoplastic acetabula and abnormally rotated and partially flattened femoral heads.

Fig. 9.33 Thoracic asymmetry. Chest radiograph in caudal regression syndrome shows massive thoracic asymmetry with right convex scoliosis. Cardiac silhouette displaced to left and compensated. Small, central hypoventilated areas visible in left lung.

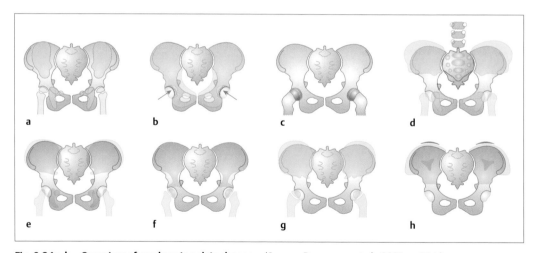

Fig. 9.34a–h Overview of syndromic pelvic changes. (Source: Brossmann et al., 2001, p. 334.)

a Cleidocranial dysplasia.
b Osteogenesis imperfecta.
c Hypothyroidism.
d Achondroplasia.
e Mucopolysaccharidosis type 4 (Morquio syndrome).

f Dysostosis multiplex (mucopolysaccharidosis type I and other mucopolysaccharidoses and mucolipidoses).
g Chondroectodermal dysplasia (Ellis–van Creveld syndrome).
h Osteoonychodysostosis (nail–patella syndrome).

9.6 Examples of Syndromic Conditions with Skeletal Involvement

Many syndromes are diagnosed very early with prenatal US → pregnancy termination or awareness of problems at delivery. Examples of commonly occurring syndromes presented below.

Osteogenesis Imperfecta

General: autosomal dominant, usually point mutation in collagen gene. Incidence = 4 : 100,000 to 10 : 100,000 of live births.
Clinical features: brittle bones with multiple disseminated fractures after minimal trauma → skeletal deformity and frequent growth retardation.
Imaging: radiography—multiple fractures, increasing deformity (**Fig. 9.35**).
Treatment: early institution of physical therapy (to strengthen muscles). Biphosphonate therapy. Recent option: stabilizing telescopic rods inserted into long bones.

Achondroplasia

General: generalized skeletal disease. Incidence (in United States) = 0.3 : 10,000 to 0.6 : 10,000.
Clinical features: disproportionate short stature with proximal limb shortening. Adult height usually < 130 cm. Large skull. Intelligence usually normal. Frequent spinal stenosis and thoracic kyphosis.
Imaging: radiography, US/MRI—large head with frontal bossing (**Fig. 9.36a**). Small foramen magnum. Interpedicular distance in lumbar spine decreases from above downward. Short, broad limbs. Rounded appearance of iliac wings (**Fig. 9.36b**). Internal hydrocephalus (rare complication).
Treatment: increasing use of surgical limb lengthening; decompression of narrow spinal canal (only in patients with neurologic symptoms).

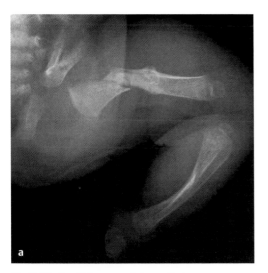

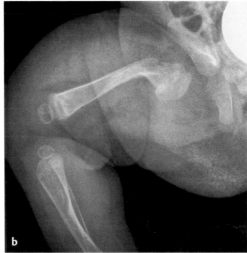

Fig. 9.35a, b Osteogenesis imperfecta.

a Radiograph of left hip and femur in 1-day-old girl shows recent and old fractures of left femur and decreased bone matrix density in osteogenesis imperfecta.

b Radiograph of right leg 12 days later shows new fracture of right femur. Note: Field of view includes portions of lower leg and pelvis due to difficult handling and high fracture risk.

9

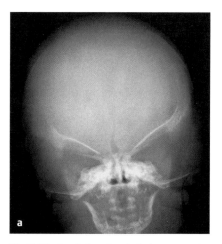

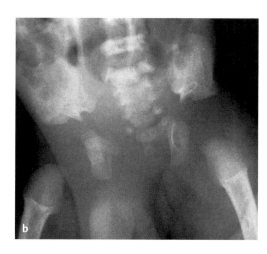

Fig. 9.36a, b   Achondroplasia in a neonate.

a AP skull radiograph shows frontal bossing with "harlequin" appearance of both orbits. Hypoplastic mandible.

b AP pelvic radiograph (without gonadal shielding) shows rounded iliac wings with trident configuration. Thickened ends of femurs. Sagittal cleft visible in sacrum.

Thanatophoric Dwarfism

General: rare malformation based on mutation in type II collagen structural protein gene. Affected children rarely survive first months of life. Incidence = 0.21 : 10,000 to 0.3 : 10,000.

Clinical features: short trunk and short limbs. Large head, pear-shaped body, and small thorax. Frequently, cleft palate and clubfoot.

Imaging: radiography—narrow thorax due to short, slender ribs. Platyspondyly. Limbs short and stout. Iliac wings small and squared (**Fig. 9.37**).

Treatment: none; constricted thoracic cage leads to death from respiratory failure.

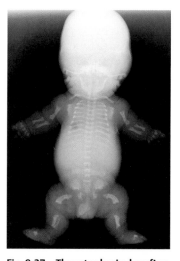

Fig. 9.37   Thanatophoric dwarfism— "postmortem babygram." Thanatophoric dwarfism diagnosed prenatally, neonate died shortly after birth. Findings include very short, slender ribs and marked platyspondyly. Limbs short and stout with "croissant" bowing of femurs. Metacarpals and metatarsals extremely short, and iliac wings squared. Cloverleaf skull.

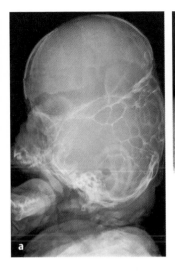

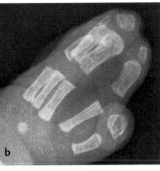

Fig. 9.38a, b Apert syndrome in 6-month-old boy.
a Lateral radiograph shows typical cloverleaf deformity of skull with lacunar, honeycombed occipital bone structure.
b Radiograph of hand shows syndactyly with thickened distal phalanges ("shovel hand").

Apert Syndrome

General: craniofacial malformation. Autosomal dominant inheritance, high rate of new mutations (chromosome 10).

Clinical features: deformed head, extremely high forehead. Other features: hypertelorism, open cleft palate, frequent mental retardation, hearing loss, axillary hypoplasias, syndactyly of hands and feet.

Imaging: radiography, US/MRI/3D CT—brachycephaly (**Fig. 9.38a**), maxillary hypoplasia, hydrocephalus, syndactyly (**Fig. 9.38b**).

Treatment: often treated by cranial surgery, myringostomy, surgical separation of fused digits, repair of cleft palate, psychological support.

Treacher Collins Syndrome (Mandibulofacial Dysostosis)

General: rare, autosomal dominant disorder based on mutation of TCOF1 gene. Incidence = 1 : 50,000 live births (**Fig. 9.39**).

Clinical features: gross deformities include mandibular hypoplasia and frequent microtia with absence of external auditory canal. Cardiac anomalies. Often associated with choanal atresia—note when attempting nasogastric intubation!

Imaging: radiography, CT—hypoplastic mandible, underdeveloped zygoma (**Fig. 9.40a**). Choanal atresia. Middle/inner ear changes with hypoplastic middle ear cavity. Absence of external auditory canals with auricular anomalies (**Fig. 9.40b**).

Treatment: multiple surgical procedures, psychological support.

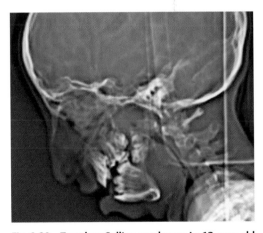

Fig. 9.39 Treacher Collins syndrome in 12-year-old girl. Lateral CT scout view displays typical facial features with shortened mandibular rami and deformed jaws with small maxilla. Skull disproportionate, with prominent nose and neurocranium too large relative to jaw. Zygomatic arches absent.

9

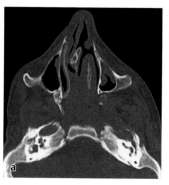
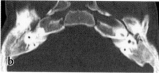

Fig. 9.40a, b   Treacher Collins syndrome.
a Axial CT scan of facial skeleton shows bilateral absence of zygomatic arches, mucosal swelling in both maxillary sinuses, and dystrophy and destruction of nasal septum.
b Axial CT scan through petrous pyramids shows bilateral atresia of external auditory canals. Note absence of auricles and mastoid air cells.

9.7   Metabolic Disorders

This section reviews selected metabolic disorders that may have typical radiologic features. Enzymatic and molecular tests are primary tools for diagnosing metabolic disorders.

Role of imaging: follow-up of organic/cerebral changes. May show evidence of systemic (metabolic) disease in cases with very early/atypical manifestations. Helpful in narrowing DD.

Hunter Syndrome (Mucopolysaccharidosis Type II)

General: lysosomal metabolic disease, X-linked recessive.

Clinical features: large range of clinical findings—from very severe retardation to mild forms without cognitive impairment. Typical "orange peel" skin (clusters of pale cutaneous nodules). Enlarged tongue, fleshy lips. Conductive and sensorineural hearing loss, frequent optic nerve atrophy. Increasing cardiac involvement—may lead to heart failure. Possible progressive mental retardation and pyramidal tract signs, depending on type.

Imaging: radiography, US, MRI—skeletal changes (dysostosis multiplex, barrel-shaped vertebrae). Hepatomegaly with diffuse damage to liver parenchyma—visceromegaly (**Fig. 9.41**). Cerebral atrophy (**Fig. 9.42**).

Treatment: enzyme therapy (Elaprase).

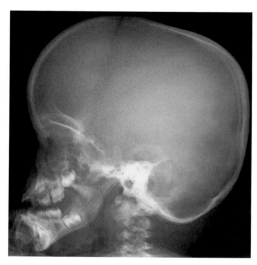

Fig. 9.41   Mucopolysaccharidosis in 2-year-old boy.
Lateral skull radiograph displays frontal bossing in mucopolysaccharidosis type II (Hunter syndrome).

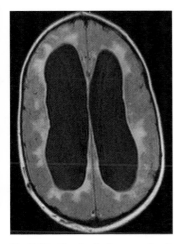

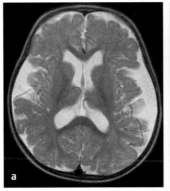

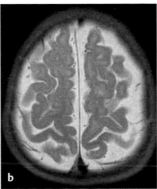

Fig. 9.42 Cerebral changes in 4-year-old boy with mucopolysaccharidosis. Axial MRI of neurocranium (FLAIR sequence) in Hunter syndrome shows marked dilatation of inner CSF spaces, white matter rarefaction, and periventricular demyelination.

Fig. 9.43a, b Glutaric aciduria type 1 in 18-month-old boy. Axial MRI of neurocranium, T2-weighted sequence.
a Dilatation of outer CSF spaces plus typical accentuation of sylvian fissure. Inner CSF spaces enlarged due to lack of age-appropriate myelination.
b CSF spaces markedly enlarged due to external cerebral atrophy.

Glutaric Aciduria Type 1

General: impaired breakdown of amino acids lysine, tryptophan, and hydrolysine. High levels of glutaric acid and 3-hydroglutaric acid detected in all body fluids.

Clinical features: usually undetected until first catabolic crisis. Encephalopathy = severe dystonic-dyskinetic symptoms. Slightly decreased muscle tone, irritability, nervousness. Macrocephaly (early sign).

> Acute encephalopathic crisis may be mistaken for "encephalitis" due to frequency of crises during/after infection.

Imaging:
- **(US), MRI:** detection and follow-up of cerebral changes (deficient myelination, white matter rarefaction) with predominantly frontal atrophy (**Fig. 9.43**)
- **US:** organomegaly, signs of hepatopathy.

Treatment: diet low in lysine/tryptophan. Rapid treatment of metabolic disorders. Early treatment → child goes on to normal development.

Rickets

Vitamin D Rickets

General: rare in Central Europe owing to population-wide vitamin D prophylaxis. Causes = lack of prophylaxis, vegetarian diet, rarely abnormalities of synthesis, renal failure, severe GI malabsorption, prolonged stay in ICU (premature infants/neonatology).

Clinical features: susceptibility to infections and neurologic seizures, tetany.

Imaging: radiography, possibly US—"rachitic rosary" pattern (**Fig. 9.44**). Bilateral genu varum/valgum. Growth plate changes—inadequate/immature development of metaphyseal bone structures, epiphyseal cupping, fraying.

Treatment: vitamin D prophylaxis. Vitamin D supplementation for 3 to 6 weeks.

9

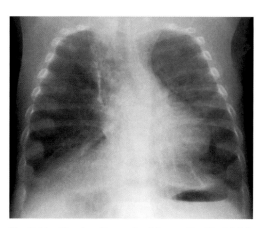

Fig. 9.44 Chest radiograph of 5-month-old girl following prolonged ICU stay after premature delivery. Prominent knobs at costochondral joints of most ribs create "rosary-bead" pattern in iatrogenic rickets associated with prolonged parenteral nutrition.

Hypophosphatemic Rickets

Synonyms: vitamin D-resistant rickets, "phosphate diabetes."

Phosphate deficiency → mineralization ↓, leading to osteoporosis. X-linked dominant.

Clinical features: hyperphosphaturia (familial, neoplasia, Fanconi syndrome), growth disorders, bowlegs.

Imaging: radiography—decreased bone matrix, pseudofractures; rarely, bony narrowing of the spinal canal.

Treatment: administration of elemental phosphorus.

Hyperparathyroidism

Increased parathyroid hormone production by parathyroid glands, decalcification of bones due to increased renal phosphate excretion. Types:

- Primary hyperparathyroidism: parathyroid adenoma
- Secondary hyperparathyroidism: renal failure and decreased $1,25(OH)_2$ vitamin D synthesis
- Tertiary hyperparathyroidism: in response to prolonged secondary hyperparathyroidism—may become autonomous

Clinical features: of primary hyperparathyroidism: hyperphosphaturia, growth abnormalities.

Imaging: radiography, possibly US—as described above (skeletal changes).

Treatment: for primary hyperparathyroidism—removal of parathyroid adenoma, subtotal removal of parathyroid glands.

Bibliography

1 Baraitaser M, Winter RM. Fehlbildungssyndrome. 2nd ed. Bern: Hans Huber; 2001
2 Baujat G, Cormier-Daire V. Sotos syndrome. Orphanet J Rare Dis 2007; 2: 36
3 Brossmann J, Czerny C, Freyschmidt J, eds. Grenzen des Normalen und Anfänge des Pathologischen in der Radiologie des kindlichen und erwachsenen Skeletts. Stuttgart: Thieme; 2001
4 Chaabouni M, Fersi M, Belghith N, et al. Treacher–Collins syndrome: clinical and genetic aspects apropos of 4 cases of which 1 is familial. [Article in French] Tunis Med 2007; 85(10): 885–890
5 Cole AJL, Webb L, Cole TJ. Bone age estimation: a comparison of methods. Br J Radiol 1988; 61(728): 683–686
6 Ebel KD, Willich E, Richter E. Differenzialdiagnostik in der pädiatrischen Radiologie, Vol. 1. Stuttgart: Thieme; 1995
7 Freyschmidt J, Sternberg A, Brossmann J, Wiens J. Koehler/Zimmer's Borderlands of Normal and Early Pathological Findings in Skeletal Radiography. 5th ed. Stuttgart: Thieme; 2003
8 Greulich WM, Pyle SI. Radiographic Atlas of Skeletal Development of the Hand and Wrist. 2nd ed. Stanford, CA: Stanford University Press; 1959
9 Hunter D, Baxter PJ, Adams PH. In: Tar-Ching AW, Cockcroft A, Harrington JM, eds. Hunter's Diseases of Occupations. 9th ed. London: Hodder-Arnold; 1999
10 Leonard NJ. Sacrococcygeal teratoma in two cases of Sotos syndrome. Am J Med Genet 2000; 95: 182–184
11 Maresh MM. Linear growth of long bones of extremities from infancy through adolescence; continuing studies. AMA Am J Dis Child 1955; 89(6): 725–742
12 Munné S, Sandalinas M, Magli C, Gianaroli L, Cohen J, Warburton D. Increased rate of aneuploid embryos in young women with previous aneuploid conceptions. Prenat Diagn 2004; 24(8): 638–643
13 Oestreich AE. Growth of the Pediatric Skeleton. Berlin, Heidelberg: Springer; 2008

Case Study 9.1

History and clinical presentation: neonate with large abdomen after obstetric trauma and perinatal asphyxia. Uneventful pregnancy. Clinically enlarged abdomen, blood pressure problems, palpable mass in right renal bed.
Laboratory findings: (hemorrhagic?) anemia, hyperbilirubinemia.
Suitable imaging modalities: US, possibly plain radiographs; rarely MRI (or CT if unavailable).

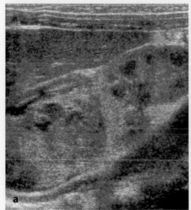
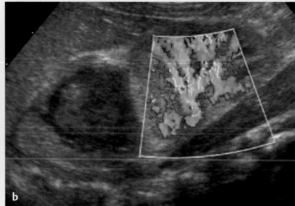

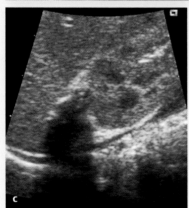

Fig. 9.45a–c

Available images: US including CDS.
Findings: inhomogeneous, well-circumscribed, complex liquid-appearing mass in right adrenal bed (**a**). Mass showed marked complex transformation and enlargement over several days with good vascularity of adjacent right kidney by CDS (**b**). Long-term follow-ups showed eventual calcification with acoustic shadow (**c**).
Diagnosis: adrenal hemorrhage.
DD: neuroblastoma/adrenal gland tumor, complex cystic renal tumor, duplex kidney with disease in upper moiety.
(With kind permission of M. Riccabona, Graz, Austria.)

9

▬▬ **Case Study 9.2** ▬▬

History and clinical presentation: 12-year-old girl with chronic fatigue, pallor, and doughy skin.
Laboratory findings: greatly elevated TSH, low thyroid hormones.
Suitable imaging modalities: US, scintigraphy.

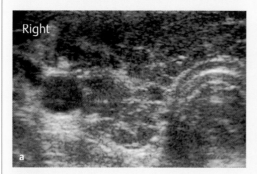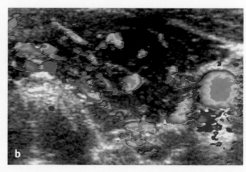

Fig. 9.46a, b

Available images: US with CDS.
Findings: transverse US scan shows (painless) enlargement of thyroid gland—still delineated with inhomogeneous, hypoechoic parenchyma and pseudosepta (**a**). CDS shows increased vascularity (**b**).
Diagnosis: Graves disease (based on images and laboratory findings).
DD: Hashimoto thyroiditis (see **Figs. 9.14** and **9.15**), amyloidosis, goiter. Echogenicity of thyroid parenchyma markedly increased in chronic stage.

14 Santiago J, Muszlak M, Samson C, et al. Malignancy risk and Wiedemann-Beckwith syndrome: what follow-up to provide?. [Article in French] Arch Pediatr 2008; 15 (9): 1498–1502

15 Saudubray JM, Van den Berghe G, Waller JH, eds. Inborn Metabolic Diseases: Diagnosis and Treatment. 5th ed. Berlin: Springer; 2011

16 Siegel MJ,. Pediatric Sonography. 4th ed. Philadelphia: Wolters Kluwer/Lippincott Williams & Wilkins; 2010

17 Slovis TL. Caffey's Pediatric Diagnostic imaging. 11th ed. Philadelphia: Mosby/Elsevier; 2008

18 Sperling MA Pediatric Endocrinology. 3rd ed. Philadelphia: Mosby/Elsevier; 2008

19 Spranger J, Brill P, Poznanski A. Bone Dysplasias. 2nd ed. Munich: Urban & Fischer; 2002

20 Tanner JM, Whitehouse RH, Marshall WA, et al. Assessement of Skeletal Maturity and Prediction of Adult Height (TW2 Method). London: Academic Press; 1975

21 Lachman RS, Taybi H. Taybi and Lachman's Radiology of Syndromes, Metabolic Disorders and Skeletal Dysplasias. 5th ed. Philadelphia: Mosby/Elsevier; 2006

22 Waller DK, Correa A, Vo TM, et al. The population-based prevalence of achondroplasia and thanatophoric dysplasia in selected regions of the U.S. Am J Med Gen et A 2008; 146A(18): 2385–2389

23 Zuppa AA, Sindico P, Savarese I, et al. Neonatal hyperthyroidism: neonatal clinical course of two brothers born to a mother with Graves–Basedow disease, before and after total thyroidectomy. J Pediatr Endocrinol Metab 2007; 20(4): 535–539

Index

Note: Page numbers in italic are references to figures.